Manual
of
Pediatric
Nutrition

JOHN WILEY & SONS, INC.

New York • Chichester • Weinheim • Brisbane • Singapore • Toronto

This book is printed on acid-free paper. ☉

Copyright © 1997 by Twin Cities District Dietetic Association. All rights reserved
Published by John Wiley & Sons, Inc.
Published simultaneously in Canada
Previously published by Chronimed Publishing

No part of this publication may be reproduced, stored in a retrieval system or transmitted in any form or by any means, electronic, mechanical, photocopying, recording, scanning, or otherwise, except as permitted under Sections 107 or 108 of the 1976 United States Copyright Act, without either the prior written permission of the Publisher, or authorization through payment of the appropriate per-copy fee to the Copyright Clearance Center, 222 Rosewood Drive, Danvers, MA 01923, (978) 750-8400, fax (978) 750-4744. Requests to the Publisher for permission should be addressed to the Permissions Department, John Wiley & Sons, Inc., 605 Third Avenue, New York, NY 10158-0012, (212) 850-6011, fax (212) 850-6008, E-Mail: PERMREQ@WILEY.COM.

The information contained in this book is not intended to serve as a replacement for professional medical advice. Any use of the information in this book is at the reader's discretion. The author and the publisher specifically disclaim any and all liability arising directly or indirectly from the use or application of any information contained in this book. A health care professional should be consulted regarding your specific situation.

Library of Congress Cataloging-in-Publication Data:

ISBN 0-471-34917-8

Printed in the United States of America

10   9   8   7   6   5   4   3   2

This revised 3rd edition of the Twin Cities District Dietetic Association (TCDDA) Manual of Pediatric Nutrition is the result of a cooperative effort on the part of the pediatric dietitians from the major children's hospitals, pediatric units, and public health agencies serving children in the Minneapolis/St. Paul metropolitan area. This joint effort was undertaken with the belief that a single manual, written by dietitians with experience and expertise in various areas of pediatrics, would promote continuity in the nutritional care of the pediatric population in the Twin Cities.

The TCDDA Manual of Pediatric Nutrition is similar in format and philosophy to the TCDDA Manual of Clinical Nutrition, yet is devoted to pediatrics, compiling nutrition information from gestation through adolescence. Each section has been reviewed and/or revised and reflects current information and practice. The manual has been produced as a professional resource for dietitians, physicians, dietetic technicians, dietary managers, nurses, other health care professionals, and students or interns.

Although copyrighted, the educational materials are tools to be used for client education in conjunction with physician orders. The loose-leaf format facilitates duplication for this purpose.

The contributors hope that this manual will assist the professional in providing optimal nutritional care for individuals in ambulatory and institutional settings.

Additional Notes

References to the Recommended Dietary Allowances of the National Research Council refer to the Recommended Daily Dietary Allowances which are listed in the appendix of the manual, and published in:

Food and Nutrition Board. Recommended Dietary Allowances, 10th ed, Washington, DC; National Academy of Sciences, National Research Council, 1989.

The Recommended Dietary Allowances are used to evaluate the nutritional adequacy of diets. Calories, calories, Kcal, and kcal, used in this manual all refer to kilocalories.

Acknowledgements

The Committee wishes to thank all of the individuals and organizations who contributed to this project, and for their continued support of the practice of dietetics.

Special thanks to:

Shriners Hospitals for Children/Twin Cities which has generously supported the production of this edition of the manual.

Kathleen Remington, M.A., who provided editorial and technical support.

Authors, Contributors and Diet Manual Committee Members

Susan Marx, M.Ed., R.D. (Co-Chairperson)
Barbara Riniker Daniels, M.S., R.D. (Co-Chairperson)
Karen Travis Moberg, R.D. (Co-Chairperson)

Denise Andersen, M.S., R.D.
Daidre Bakke, R.D.
Lisa Brown, R.D.
Marna Melrose Canterbury, R.D., L.D.
Janie Cooperman, M.S., R.D., C.S.
Mary Colleen Dado, R.D.
JoAnn Daehler-Miller, M.S., R.D.
Heather L. Eskuri, R.D.
Marcia Gahagan Hayes, M.P.H., R.D., L.D.
Eve Gehling, Med, R.D., L.D., C.D.E.
Lori Gross, M.S., R.D., C.N.S.D.
Kimberly Gwynne, R.D., L.D.
Robin B. Herr, R.D., C.D.E.
Dee Jones, R.D., L.D., C.N.S.D.
Jackie Labat, M.S., R.D., L.D., C.D.E.
Janelle Lawler, R.D., L.D.
Melissa Le, R.D.
Dorothy Markowitz, R.D.
Barbara Mertz, R.D.
Cathy Munn, R.D., L.D.
Nancy Roberts, M.S., R.D., C.N.S.D.
Kathleen Schissel, R.D.
Mary Spencer, R.D., L.D., C.D.E.
Jacqueline Vallette Uglow, R.D.
Elizabeth VanOss Tymchuck, M.S., R.D.
Janelle Waslaski, R.D., L.D.
Dixie Willard Wolfe, R.D., C.N.S.D.
Donna Ziemer, M.S., R.D., L.D., C.N.S.D.

Twin Cities District Dietetic Association
MANUAL OF PEDIATRIC NUTRITION

Table of Contents

GENERAL NUTRITION

Nutrition for Life

Food is basic to life. A balanced intake of nutrients is necessary for maintenance and restoration of health. Food consists of different amounts of six basic components: carbohydrate, protein, fat, vitamins, minerals, and water. While no single food contains all of these essential nutrients, eating a variety of foods will help ensure an adequate intake of the different nutrients.

The energy provided by food is measured in calories. An ideal weight can be maintained when calorie intake and expenditure are balanced.

The goal of good nutrition and good health is met by choosing a variety of foods that contain all six basic nutrients in amounts appropriate for each individual's needs. Numerous guidelines have been developed to assist with meeting this goal. The Food Guide Pyramid is the most commonly used. The United States Department of Agriculture (USDA) and the United States Department of Health and Human Services (USDHHS) "Food Guide Pyramid" booklet describes the food pyramid system for choosing a healthy diet. This guide was developed as a device to aid in planning an adequate diet for each day based on the Dietary Guidelines for Americans (USDA and USDHHS, 1990). The Food Guide Pyramid recommends a range of servings needed from each major food group. The exact number of servings needed is determined by an individual's caloric needs, which depends on age, sex, height, weight, provision for growth and activity level. (See pages 33–35 specific guidelines.)

Major Nutrients and Their Sources

Nutrients in food are essential for the normal growth and functioning of the body. An essential nutrient is one that cannot be synthesized by the body and must be obtained through food. The functions of nutrients fall into three categories:

- Provision of energy
- Building and repair of tissues
- Regulation and control of metabolic processes
- Metabolism refers to the sum of all body processes that sustain life.

Carbohydrates

Carbohydrates are the body's preferred source of energy. When the diet does not supply an adequate amount of energy from carbohydrate and fat, body protein is used as an energy source. There are two forms of carbohydrate: simple and complex.

Foods that contain complex carbohydrates include breads, cereals, grains, dried peas and legumes, potatoes, and other starchy vegetables. Cakes, candies, pastries, and sweets that contain sugars are examples of simple carbohydrates. For weight-control purposes, they should be limited because they are poor sources of vitamins and minerals.

Protein

Protein is an essential nutrient for every cell in the body. The functions of protein include:
- Maintenance, growth, and repair of tissues.
- Regulation of body processes.
- Regulation of the body's immune system
- Provision of a back-up energy source.

Amino acids are the building blocks of proteins. They are classified as either essential or nonessential. Essential amino acids are ones that cannot be manufactured by the body and must be obtained from one's daily diet. The nine essential amino acids are lysine, methionine, phenylalanine, leucine, isoleucine, valine, tryptophan, threonine, and histidine. Nonessential amino acids can be made in the body from proteins found in foods.

Both animal and plant sources provide protein. Those sources that contain all the essential amino acids are called complete proteins. Those that lack one or more essential amino acids are called incomplete proteins. Meat, poultry, fish, milk, cheese, and eggs are complete protein foods. Plant products provide incomplete proteins, but can be complemented (combined) to provide all essential amino acids. For details on complementing proteins, see the Vegetarianism section.

Fat

Fat functions as the body's secondary energy source. It is an important storage form of energy; when excess calories are consumed, they are converted and stored as fat. The functions of fat include:
- Serving as the carrier for the fat-soluble vitamins A, D, E, and K.
- Regulating body temperature through the layer of fat beneath the skin.
- Supporting the cellular wall structure and padding internal organs (such as kidneys).
- Providing satiety and flavor to the diet.
- Providing essential fatty acids needed by the body for growth and healthy skin.

Fats are found in butter, margarine, shortening, oils, cream, cheeses, nuts, and meat. There are saturated, monounsaturated, and polyunsaturated fatty acids. When polyunsaturated fats replace saturated fats, this aids in the reduction of blood cholesterol levels.

Water

Water is an important nutrient that is often overlooked. Water constitutes approximately two-thirds of the body's weight and is a major component of all cells and tissues. The functions of water include:
- Acting as a solvent to transport nutrients to cells and waste products away from cells.
- Serving as a lubricant for joints and movement along the digestive tract.
- Assisting in chemical reactions.
- Aiding in the regulation of body temperature.
- Building tissues and replacing daily water losses.

Water is found in most foods, including solids. Eight to ten glasses of fluid (non-caffeinated is preferred) each day is recommended for most people.

Vitamins and Minerals

Vitamins and minerals are necessary in regulation and control of metabolic processes. To achieve an adequate intake, a wide variety of foods should be eaten. Except in certain clinical conditions, supplementation of vitamins and minerals is generally unnecessary when the healthy individual is eating adequate amounts of a variety of foods.

Vitamin or mineral supplementation should be done only with the guidance of a dietitian or physician. For further information, see the "Statement on Vitamin and Mineral Supplementation" and the other information on fat-soluble vitamins, water-soluble vitamins, minerals, and trace minerals.

Professional References

1. Albertson AM, Tobelmann RC, Engstrom A, Asp E. Nutrient intakes of 2- to 20-year-old American children: 10 year trends. J Am Dietetic Assoc. 91 (12): 1492-1496, 1992.
2. American Academy of Pediatrics. Pediatric Nutrition Handbook, 3rd Edition, Elk Grove Village, IL: American Academy of pediatrics. 1993.
3. Block G. Dietary Guidelines and the results of food consumption surveys. American Journal of Clinical Nutrition 53: 356S-357S, 1991.
4. An evaluation of dietary guidance alternatives: The evolution of the Eating Right Pyramid. Nutrition Reviews 50(9): 275-282. 1992.
5. Food and Nutrition Board. Recommended Dietary Allowances. 10th Edition. Washington DC: National Academy of Sciences. 1989.
6. Hegarty V. Decisions in Nutrition. St. Louis: Times Mirror/Mosby College Publishing. 1988.
7. Herron D. Strategies for promoting a healthy dietary intake. Nursing Clinics of North America, 26(4): 875-884, 1991.
8. Queen PM, Lang CE, editors. Handbook of Pediatric Nutrition. Gaithersburg, MD: Aspen Publishers, Inc., 1993.

9. Ranade V. Nutritional recommendations for children and adolescents. International Journal of Clinical Pharmacology, Therapy and Toxicology. 31(6): 289-90, 1993.
10. Satter E. Child of Mine: Feeding with Love and Good Sense, 2nd edition. Palo Alto, CA: Bull Publishing, 1986.
11. United States Department of Agriculture and United States Department of Health and Human Services. Nutrition and Your Health: "Dietary Guidelines for Americans", Home and Garden Bulletin No. 232, Hyattsville, MD: USDA Human Nutrition Information Service, 1992. Copies available from: Superintendent of Documents, Consumer Information Center, Department 159-Y, Pueblo, CO 81009.
12. United States Department of Agriculture and United States Department of Health and Human Services. "Food Guide Pyramid", Hyattsville, MD: USDA Human Nutrition Information Service, 1992. Copies available from: Superintendent of Documents, Consumer Information Center, Department 159-Y, Pueblo, CO 81009.
13. Williams SR. Basic Nutrition and Diet Therapy, 9th edition, St. Louis: Mosby-Year Book, Inc., 1992.

Client Resources

1. American Dietetic Association. "What's to Eat? Healthy Foods for Hungry Children" and "Right from the Start: ABC's of Good Nutrition for Young Children", Chicago: American Dietetic Association.
2. National Dairy Council, "Guide to Good Eating", Rosemont, IL: National Dairy Council, 1992.
3. United States Department of Agriculture and United States Department of Health and Human Services, Nutrition and Your Health: "Dietary Guidelines for Americans: Home and Garden Bulletin No. 232, Hyattsville, MD: USDA Human Nutrition Information Service, 1992. Copies available from: Superintendent of Documents, Consumer Information Center, Department 159-Y, Pueblo, CO 81009.
4. United States Department of Agriculture and Food Marketing Institute. "The Food Guide Pyramid…Beyond the Basic 4", Hyattsville, MD: USDA Human Nutrition Information Service, 1992.
5. United States Department of Agriculture and United States Department of Health and Human Services. "Food Guide Pyramid", Hyattsville, MD: USDA Human Nutrition Information Service, 1992. Copies available from: Superintendent of Documents, Consumer Information Center, Department 159-Y, Pueblo, CO 81009.

Evaluating Nutrition Claims

Throughout history myths have grown around the special "curative" or health enhancing powers of certain foods or substances. Over the years, legitimate scientific research has shown that many of the myths have no scientific basis. Yet, the consumer is constantly confronted with many old myths as they are periodically recycled into popularity. New myths are created as public interest changes.

Today, the self-proclaimed nutritionist may promise the unsuspecting consumer "instant" weight loss with a nutritionally inadequate diet or product. Unnecessary and often dangerous uses of food supplements are promoted by promising that they will give freedom from illness, stress, or old age. The legitimate nutrition scientist tests new ideas in the research laboratory for accuracy, safety, and effectiveness before submitting the results to other scientists for review. By contrast, the pseudo-nutrition scientist avoids scientific scrutiny and goes directly to the public for financial gain.

Guidelines for Evaluating Nutrition Claims

Before making any decision about a product or diet promising "magical" results, the consumer should seek answers to the following questions:

1. Does the author or promoter of the book, product, or diet recommend the consumption of a wide variety of foods, or, does the author promote the consumption of food or, is the emphasis on the use of a very limited number of foods? Does the weight reduction program consist of consuming only a special formula with no emphasis on exercise or behavior modification?
2. Does the author or promoter of the book, product, or diet claim to be persecuted by health professionals or the government? (Ethical nutrition scientists actively seek scientific review of their work.)
3. Is the "research" cited to support the claims based on emotional, personal testimonials or anecdotal stories? (Example: "My aunt was crippled with painful arthritis and cured with bee pollen and XYZ supplements.")
4. Are nutrition claims made on accompanying literature, but not on product labels or in advertising? (The Food and Drug Administration has regulatory authority over claims made on labels. The Federal Trade Commission regulates advertising claims.)
5. Does the author or promoter of the book, product, or diet have a financial or personal motive? (Example: A statement saying the proceeds from sales go to a foundation of unknown purpose that carries the author's name.)

Check the Facts

Contact any of the following sources for accurate and reliable nutrition information. Many of these organizations offer a variety of accurate and inexpensive (or often free) nutrition materials for health professionals and consumers.

1. Registered dietitians employed by hospitals, clinics, long-term care facilities, community organizations, or public health departments. To find a registered dietitian in your area, call the American Dietetic Association Consumer Nutrition Hotline at 1-800-366-1655.
2. State, county, and city health departments.
3. Federal, state, or county agriculture extension services.
4. The American Dietetic Association at 216 West Jackson Blvd., Chicago, IL 60606-6995/(312)-899-0040.
5. US Government Consumer Information Center, PO Box 100, Pueblo, CO 81002.
6. Human Nutrition Information Service, US Department of Agriculture, Room 325A - Federal Building, Hyattsville, MN 207

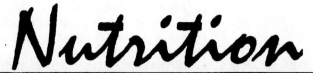

FACT•SHEET

Food Labels for Infants Under Two Years

New infant food labels will look different from adult food labels. While infant food labels also use the Nutrition Facts format, the information provided is different.

Infant Food Label
The label for infant foods contains important information.

Infant Oatmeal Cereal

Nutrition Facts
Serving Size 1/4 cup (15 g)
Serving Per Container About 30

Amount Per Serving		
Calories 60		

Total Fat		1 g
Sodium		0 mg
Potassium		50 mg
Total Carbohydrate		10 mg
Fiber		1 g
Sugars		0 g
Protein		2 g

	Infants	Children
% Daily Value	0-1	1-4
Protein	7%	6%
Vitamin A	0%	0%
Vitamin C	0%	0%
Calcium	15%	10%
Iron	45%	60%
Vitamin E	15%	8%
Thiamin	45%	30%
Riboflavin	45%	30%
Niacin	25%	20%
Phosphorus	15%	10%

Total Fat
Total fat content on the food label shows the amount of total fat in a serving of the food. Unlike adult food labels, infant food labels will not list calories from fat, saturated fat or cholesterol. Since babies under two years need fat, the infant food labels does not include the fat details. Parents should not attempt to limit their infant's fat intake.

Serving Size
Serving sizes for infant foods are based on average amounts that infants under 2 years usually eat at one time. Serving sizes on adult food labels are based on average amounts that adults typically eat at one time.

Daily Values
Food labels for infants and children under four years of age list Daily Value percentages for protein, vitamins and minerals. Unlike adult food labels, daily values for fat, cholesterol, sodium, potassium, carbohydrate, and fiber are not listed because they have not been set for children under four.

Infants and Food
The first 24 months of life is a time of rapid growth and high nutritional demands. The infant's small stomach limits the volume of food that they can reasonably consume. Because of these unique conditions, the main goal of infant feeding is to provide enough calories and nutrients to support optimal growth and development.

Infants Need Fat
Infants have different nutrient and dietary requirements than adults. Adult food labels list calories from fat, amount of saturated fat, and the amount of cholesterol to help adults make healthful food choices. Infant food labels omit the detailed listing of fat information because infants need fat as a concentrated calorie source to fuel their rapid growth. Efforts to limit fat in the infant diet are unwise. Health professionals do not endorse feeding reduced-fat dairy products such as skim milk to infants under two years. Whole milk is an important source of calories for infants who no longer receive breast milk or formula.

Food Choices

Every baby is an individual, with individual food likes. Food choices that lead to dietary variety in the first two years can play an important role in developing lifelong healthy eating patterns. Serving a variety of foods, from all major food groups, provides the balance needed to begin a natural moderation of fat intake after two years of age.

By reading the new infant food label, parents can select a nutritious variety of foods for their baby's healthful diet.

Tips on Variety

Offer infants foods that help establish a lifetime of good eating habits.

■ Fruits and Vegetables

Fruits and vegetables are good sources of vitamin C and beta-carotene. The frequent feeding of these foods at mealtimes helps children become familiar with the flavors of a variety of foods, setting the stage for continued acceptance and enjoyment. A word of caution related to the use of high fiber foods. Some foods, such as high fiber adult cereals or certain raw vegetables, are often low in calories and high in bulk. Avoid feeding these types or large amounts of these foods to infants because they fill an infant's small stomach while providing minimal calories and nutrients that infants need to grow. Infants and young children will get enough fiber for their needs by eating a variety of foods.

■ Breads, Cereals, Grains

Cereals fortified with iron are a good way to provide iron to infants during the first 24 months. Offer foods that contain iron (such as iron-fortified infant cereal) with foods that contain vitamin C (such as fortified infant juices) to help improve iron absorption. Other choices include soft cooked noodles, rice or pasta.

■ Meats and Milk Products

These foods are valuable sources of protein and minerals needed for developing bones and muscles. Offer a variety of soft, pureed meats such as chicken, turkey, or beef to provide nutrients critical for tissue development and growth.

Whole milk is an important source of nutrients such as calcium and fat. Infant bone development requires an adequate intake of calcium from food. Good sources of calcium include cheese, yogurt, milk and cottage cheese.

For more information
The American Dietetic Association/ National Center for Nutrition and Dietetics. Call the Consumer Nutrition Hot Line at (800/366-1655) to listen to a food and nutrition message, speak to a registered dietitian, or for a referral to a registered dietitian in your area.

Gerber Products Company
445 State Street
Fremont, MI 49413
800/4-GERBER

This fact sheet is supported by a grant from Gerber Products Company.

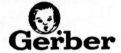

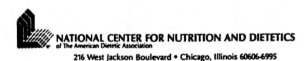

NATIONAL CENTER FOR NUTRITION AND DIETETICS
of The American Dietetic Association
216 West Jackson Boulevard • Chicago, Illinois 60606-6995

Nutrition During Pregnancy

Description

Prenatal nutrition is one of the most important environmental factors affecting the health of pregnant women and their infants. Studies indicate that adequate nutrient intake is necessary for maintaining maternal body tissues and for the growth and development of the fetus.

Nutritional Adequacy

Requirements for energy and for several nutrients are increased during pregnancy. Dietary assessment is recommended for all pregnant women to evaluate the need for dietary changes or for vitamin or mineral supplements (Institute of Medicine, 1990).

Energy and Weight Gain

A 15 percent increase in calories (an average of 300 calories/day) is needed to meet the energy needs of pregnancy. A pregnant woman's age, activity level, pre-pregnancy weight, and rate of weight gain are factors that affect energy needs at any particular time during the pregnancy.

There is strong evidence relating adequate maternal weight gain during pregnancy to increased infant birth weight and a decreased incidence of neonatal death and morbidity. A total weight gain of 25 to 35 pounds for a woman of normal weight at the start of pregnancy is currently recommended by many professionals. The recommended rate of weight gain is 2 to 4 pounds in the first trimester and about 1.0 pound per week during the remainder of the pregnancy.

If a woman is overweight at the start of her pregnancy, she should gain 15 to 25 pounds at a rate of about 0.66 pounds per week during the second and third trimesters. Weight reduction during pregnancy is not recommended. If a woman is underweight at the start of her pregnancy, a weight gain of 30 to 40 pounds is recommended for optimal pregnancy outcome. Weight gain should be at a rate of slightly more than 1 pound per week during the second and third trimesters. Additional weight gain is needed for more than one fetus in gestation, such as twins or triplets; 35 to 45 pounds of total weight gain is suggested for a woman carrying twins. Young adolescents and Black women should try to gain weight toward the upper end of the recommended range. Short women should try to achieve gains at the lower end of the range.

Protein

An additional 10 grams of protein per day is required to provide for fetal needs and to permit required maternal tissue growth and maintenance, such as increase in blood volume and growth of breast and uterine tissue. Since protein is abundant in most diets in the United States, recommendations regarding protein are usually unnecessary.

Calcium

An additional 400 mg of calcium is recommended above non-pregnant needs to prevent demineralization of the maternal skeleton. Pregnant women who are lactose intolerant or who cannot or will not consume at least 4 servings of milk or milk products per day should receive calcium supplements in the gluconate or carbonate form. Pregnant women under age 35 may need additional calcium and vitamin D since bone mineral density is still increasing.

Iron

Owing to the high demands for iron during pregnancy, the normal diet would be supplemented with 30 mg of elemental iron in the form of ferrous salts during the second and third trimesters. Larger amounts are necessary when iron depletion exists. Food sources high in protein and iron, such as liver, other meats, eggs, dried beans and peas, green leafy vegetables, dried fruits, and enriched or whole-grain breads and cereals are recommended in addition to supplementation. To increase absorption of iron, take the prenatal vitamin with beverages high in Vitamin C (such as orange, tomato, vegetable juice or juices fortified with Vitamin C). Eat foods high in Vitamin C at the same time as eating iron-containing foods (i.e., strawberries with iron-fortified breakfast cereal). Cook in an iron skillet.

Folic Acid

The U.S. Public Health Service recommends that all women of childbearing age in the U.S. who are capable of becoming pregnant consume 0.4 mg of folic acid per day to reduce their risk of having a pregnancy affected by neural tube defects (CDC, 1992). This should be as a supplement in addition to consumption of foods high in folic acid (Amer Soc Clin Nutr, 1994). The total should not exceed 1mg of Folic Acid per day (Public Health Service). Women who have had a previous conception with neural tube defects, or are at risk of a pregnancy affected by neural tube defects, should consult their physician before becoming pregnant about taking a supplement of 4.0 mg of folic acid per day.

During pregnancy additional amounts of folic acid are necessary for increased blood volume and maternal tissue syntheses. Supplementation of 0.4 to 0.8 mg of folic acid per day are recommended throughout pregnancy for all women. Women who are at increased risk for a pregnancy affected by a neural tube defect should receive a supplement of 4.0 mg per day as recommended by their physician. In addition, all pregnant women should consume foods that are good sources of folic acid each day, such as green leafy vegetables, organ meats, dried beans and peas, fortified breads and cereals, and peanuts.

Routine supplementation with vitamins and minerals other than folic acid and iron is of uncertain value. However, some supplements may be needed for pregnant women in high-risk categories or who do not routinely consume an adequate diet, such as women carrying more than one fetus, heavy cigarette smokers, alcohol and drug abusers, complete vegetarians, and adolescents.

Food Guide

Daily food intake during pregnancy should include the following:

Milk Group   4 servings
One serving is 1 c. milk, 1 c. yogurt, 1½ oz. cheese, 1 c. pudding, 1¾ c. ice cream or ice milk, or 2 c. cottage cheese.

Meat or Substitute Group   3 servings
One serving is 2-3 oz. lean meat, fish, or poultry; 2 eggs; 2 oz. cheese; ½ c. cottage cheese; 1 c. dried beans or peas; or 4 Tbsp. peanut butter.

Vegetable Group   3 servings
One serving is ½ c. cooked, ¾ c. juice; 1 c. raw, or the portion commonly served, such as a medium-sized potato.

Fruit Group   2-3 servings
One serving is ¾ c. juice; ½ c. chopped, cooked or canned fruit; 1 c. raw; or the portion normally eaten such as 1 medium-sized apple.

Starch/Bread/Grain Group   6-11 servings
One serving is 1 slice bread; 1 c. ready-to-eat cereal; or ½ c. cooked cereal, pasta, rice, or grits.

A good source of vitamin A and one of vitamin C should be included each day. At least one serving of green, leafy vegetables should be eaten each day. Consumption of 8-12 c. fluid per day is recommended; sources should include non-caffeinated beverages with water as the best choice.

Other Considerations
Caffeine

Research on the effects of caffeine on the fetus have not clearly demonstrated adverse effects of caffeine consumption during pregnancy. However, it is recommended that caffeine consumption be limited during pregnancy to reduce the risk of adverse effects. Consuming 500 mg or more daily increases the amount of time a fetus spends in an active, awake state and may cause a decrease in the baby's birth weight and head circumference. No specific limits have been set for caffeine consumption, but generally, caffeine containing beverages should be limited to 2 to 3 per day (no more than 200 mg daily).

Smoking

In addition to the many other hazards of smoking (such as decreased blood flow to the fetus and low-birth-weight infants), it may also decrease the mother's appetite so she may not gain enough weight during pregnancy. If pregnant women do choose to use products with artificial sweeteners, it has been recommended to limit them to 2-3 products per day. Consistent exposure of the pregnant woman to second-hand smoke may also have adverse effects on the fetus.

Sugar Substitutes

The American Diabetes Association recommends that pregnant women limit their intake of saccharin. The use of aspartame by pregnant women is also controversial. Since it adds no nutrients to the diet, it is best to avoid foods containing sugar substitutes and concentrate on more nutrient-dense foods and beverages.

Sodium

Routine restriction of salt during pregnancy is not recommended since sodium is required for the expanded maternal tissue and fluid compartments as well as the needs of the fetus. Sodium restriction may be indicated if the woman develops complications such as excessive fluid retention and swelling of extremities, pre-eclampsia, or toxemia.

Professional References

1. American Society for Clinical Nutrition, Inc. Recent Developments in Maternal Nutrition and Their Implications for Practitioners. Amer J Clin Nutr, Feb 1994; vol. 59(2S).
2. Centers for Disease Control. Recommendations for the Use of Folic Acid to Reduce the Number of Cases of Spina Bifida and Other Neural Tube Defects. Morbidity and Mortality Weekly Reports (MMWR), 1992, 41: 1-7.
3. Institute of Medicine. Subcommittee on Nutritional Status and Weight Gain During Pregnancy. Nutrition During Pregnancy: Part I. Weight Gain. Part II: Nutrient Supplements. Washington DC: National Academy Press, 1990.
4. Worthington-Roberts B, Rodwell-Williams S; Nutrition in Pregnancy and Lactation, 5th Edition, St. Louis: Mosby-Year Book, Inc. 1993.

Client Resources

1. American Dietetic Association. "Blue Ribbon Babies: Eating Well During Pregnancy". Chicago: American Dietetic Association.
2. American Dietetic Association. "How to Have a Healthier Baby: Tips for Pregnant Teens". Chicago: American Dietetic Association.
3. Brown J. Everywoman's Guide to Nutrition, Minneapolis: University of Minnesota Press, 1991.
4. National Dairy Council. "Guide to Good Eating". Rosemount, IL: National Dairy Council, 1992.
5. National Dairy Council. "Great Beginnings". Rosemount, IL: National Dairy Council, 1992.
6. Swinney B. Eating Expectantly: The Essential Guide and Cookbook for Pregnancy. Colorado Springs, CO: Fall River Press, 1993.
7. Johnson, Robert V, Mayo Clinic Complete Book of Pregnancy and Baby's First Year, William Morrow and Company, Inc., 1994

Nutrition During Lactation

Description

During lactation, a good diet is necessary for maternal tissue maintenance and replenishment of nutrient stores. In addition, a high-quality diet helps produce breast milk of sufficient quantity for optimum infant growth and development.

While a good diet is important, some research has suggested that concern over lifestyle restrictions, including diet restrictions or changes, is a barrier which keeps some women from breastfeeding (Best Start, 1989). Because of this, important considerations in providing diet counseling for the breastfeeding woman include: 1) providing individualized diet counseling, which includes assessment of cultural attitudes, food preferences, and lifestyle, 2) positive reinforcement of diet strengths and the woman's ability to consume an adequate diet, and 3) reminding the woman that a good diet is important for her health, whether or not she is breastfeeding (Minnesota WIC Program, 1994).

Nutritional Adequacy

Requirements for most nutrients are increased during lactation. Energy requirements for lactation are proportional to the quantity of milk produced. An additional 500 calories per day above non-pregnant needs is recommended throughout lactation (Food and Nutrition Board, 1989). A lactating woman should drink to satisfy thirst. For specific information on increased needs for other nutrients, see the 1989 RDAs in the appendix of this manual. Nutrient and calorie needs will depend on activity level, amount of breastfeeding, and other factors. General guidelines to meet the recommendations are outlined below:

Milk Group: 4 servings
One serving is 1 cup milk, 1 cup yogurt, 1-1/2 oz. Cheese, 1 cup pudding, 1-3/4 cup ice cream or ice milk, or 2 cups cottage cheese.

Meat or Substitute Group: 2-3 servings
One serving is 2 oz. Lean meat, fish or poultry, 2 eggs, 2 oz. Cheese, ½ cup cottage cheese, 1 cup dried beans or peas, or 4 Tbsp. Peanut butter.

Vegetable Group: 3 servings
One serving is ¾ cup juice, ½ cup cooked; 1 cup raw, or the portion commonly served such as one medium-sized potato.

Fruit Group: 2-3 servings
One serving is ¾ cup juice, ½ cup chopped, cooked or canned fruit, 1 cup raw, or the portion normally eaten such as 1 medium sized apple.

Starch/Bread/Grain Group: 6-11 servings
One serving is 1 slice bread, 1 cup ready-to-eat cereal, ½ cup cooked cereal, pasta, rice or grits.

Other Considerations

Vegetarians. Complete vegetarians should include a source of vitamin B12, as their breastfed infants may show signs of B12 deficiency, even when the mother has no symptoms (Institute of Medicine, 1991).

Cultural issues. As with any dietary counseling, it is important to consider cultural and lifestyle factors, and modify dietary advice accordingly.

Weight Loss. As the average increase in calories of 500 per day assumes that some calories will be provided from the lactating woman energy stores, an average weight loss of about 1 to 2 pounds a month is normal-although not all women lose weight. If an overweight woman would like to lose weight while breastfeeding, a weight loss of up to 4-5 pounds per month is not likely to decrease milk production, however at this level of weight loss indicators that milk supply may have decreased should be carefully monitored. This includes watching for signs the infant is not satisfied, and monitoring the weight of the infant (Food and Nutrition Board, 1991). See also infant breastfeeding section.

Caffeine. Discourage intake of large quantities of coffee and other sources of caffeine including beverages and medications. The intake of one or two cups of coffee per day, or its equivalent, is unlikely to have a negative effect on the infant (Institute of Medicine, 1991).

Nicotine. Nicotine passes into breastmilk and may affect the infant. Smoking can also decrease milk production. The amount of smoking, risks and benefits of breastfeeding should be weighed.

Medications and other substances. Any medication taken by a breastfeeding woman should be under the supervision of a physician, and any physician prescribing a medication for a breastfeeding woman should be reminded that she is breastfeeding. Several references are available to identify the best medications to use while breastfeeding.

Supporting Breastfeeding

Breast milk is the food of choice for the young infant. The American Academy of Pediatrics Committee on Nutrition declared that breast milk is the best food for the newborn infant. The American Dietetic Association "..advocates breastfeeding because of the nutritional and immunologic benefits of human milk for the infant..." (American Dietetic Association, 1993).

Breastfeeding skills are not innate. The first few days of an infant's life, when a new mother is learning the techniques that will allow her to breastfeed successfully, are critical. Health professionals are encouraged to support policies and practices in their work setting that will provide new mothers with the knowledge and skills to be successful at breastfeeding. The Baby Friendly Hospital Initiative (BFHI) outlines steps which can be taken by hospitals to support breastfeeding. (Kyenkya-Isabirye, 1992).

Client Resources: Video
1. Yes, You Can Breastfeed. Texas WIC Program, 1990. $6.00. 7 minutes. MetroPost/501 N IH 35/Austin, Texas 78702, 512-476-3876.
2. Breastfeeding: A Special Relationship. Eagle Video Productions, 1991. $179.00. 24 minutes. Eagle Video Productions, 2201 Woodnell Dr., Raleigh, NC 27603-5240, 919-779-7891 or 800-869-7892.
3. A Healthier Baby by Breastfeeding, Television Innovation Company, 1991, $19.95. 20 minutes. Television Innovation Company, 8349 N. Arrowridge Road, Charlotte, NC 28273, 704-527-0800 or 800-868-4336.

Client Resources: Books
4. Gotsch, Gwen. Breastfeeding Pure and Simple. Franklin Park, IL: La Leche League International, 1994.
5. Huggins, Kathleen. The Nursing Mother's Companion. Massachusetts: Harvard Common Press, 1990.
6. Kitzinger, Sheila. Breastfeeding Your Baby. New York: Knopf. 1991.
7. La Leche League International. The Womanly Art of Breastfeeding. Franklin Park, IL: La Leche League International, 1991.

Client Resources: Pamphlets

1. Breastfeeding: Getting Started in 5 Easy Steps
2. Helpful Hints on Breastfeeding
3. Both pamphlets available in English and Spanish from Childbirth Graphics.

Professional References

1. American academy of Pediatrics Committee on Drugs. The Transfer of Drugs and Other Chemicals Into Human Milk. Pediatrics 93:1, January 1994. Pp 137-150.
2. Briggs, GG, Freeman, RK and Sumner, SJ *Drugs in Pregnancy and Lactation*, third ed. Baltimore: Williams and Wilkins, 1990.
3. Committee on Nutrition, American Academy of Pediatrics. Breastfeeding. *Pediatrics* 1978, 62:591.
4. Food and Nutrition Blard. *Recommended dietary Allowances*, 10th edition, Washington D.DC.: National Academy of Sciences, 1989.
5. Institute of Medicine. *Nutrition During Lactation*. Washington D.C.: National Academy of Sciences, 1991.
6. Kyenkya-Isabirye, M. UNICEF Launches The Baby-Friendly Hospital Initiative. *Am J Matern Child Nurs*, 1992 Jul/Aug, 17: 177-79.
7. Lawrence, Rugh. *Breastfeeding: A Guide for the Medical Profession.* St. Louis: Mosby, 1989.
8. Minnesota WIC Program, Staff Training Materials, 1994.
9. Mohrbacher, Nancy and Julie Stock. *The Breastfeeding Answer Book*. Franklin Park, IL: La Leche League International, 1990.
10. *Nutrition in Pregnancy and Lactation*, 5th edition. St. Louis: Mosby Yearbook, Inc., 1993.
11. Position of the American Dietetic Association: Promotion and Support of Breastfeeding. J Am Diet *Assoc* 1992: 93, 467-469.
12. Seattle-King County Department of Public Health. Breastfeeding Triage Tool. Seattle, Washington: Seattle-King County Department of Public Health, 1990.

Nutrition Through Childhood
(Infant - 12 Years)

General Description

Throughout childhood, nutrition affects a child's growth, development and health. For a child to grow at their genetically predetermined rate, they need to be provided both a variety of nutritious foods and a positive feeding environment. Ellyn Satter(1986)points out that providing a positive feeding environment demands a division of the feeding responsibility. "The parent is responsible for what the child is offered to eat, the child is responsible for how much and even whether, she eats." This "division of responsibility" holds true throughout the childhood years.

Indications For Use

The diet is for children with no special dietary needs.

Nutritional Adequacy

The diet is adequate in all nutrients if a wide variety of foods are included each day and if the amount of food eaten is regulated by the child's appetite, appropriate weight gain and linear growth.

Instruction Sheets
- The Food Guide for Infants
- Baby Bottle Tooth Decay
- Guidelines for Introducing Solid Foods
- Choking Prevention
- Developing Food Preferences
- The Food Guide Pyramid

Professional References

1. American Academy of Pediatrics. Revised First Aid for the Choking Child. *Pediatrics*, 1986; 78:177.
2. Baker D, Henry R. *Parents' Guide to Nutrition: Healthy Eating from Birth Through Adolescence*. Adison-Wesley Publishing Company, 1986.
3. Barnes G, Parker W, Lyon T, Drum MA, Coleman G. Ethnicity, location, age, and fluoridation factors in baby bottle tooth decay and caries prevalence of Head Start children. *Public Health Reports*, 1992:107: 162-173.
4. Berman C, Fromer J. *Meals Without Squeals*. Palo Alto, CA: Bull Publishing, 1991.
5. Birch LL, McPhee L, Steinberg L, Sullivan S. Conditioned flavor preferences in young children. *Physiology and Behavior*, 1990; 47:501-505.
6. Casey R, Rozin D. Changing children's food preferences: Parent opinions. *Appetite*, 1989: 12(3):171-182.
7. Committee on Nutrition, American Academy of Pediatrics. *Pediatric Nutrition Handbook*. 3rd Edition. Elk Grove Village, IL: American Academy of Pediatrics, 1992.
8. Crow D. Baby bottle tooth decay prevention - A new program for the Texas Department of Health. *Texas Dental Journal*, 1992;109(8):141.
9. Debruyne LK, Rolfes SR. *Life Cycle Nutrition Conception Through Adolescence*. St. Paul, MN: West Publishing Company, 1989.
10. Dwyer J. Promoting good nutrition for today and the year 2000. *Pediatric Clinics of North America*, 1986; 33:799-882.
11. Fomon SJ. *Nutrition for Normal Infants*, 3rd Edition. St. Louis: Mosby-Yearbook, Inc., 1993.
12. Harris CS, Baker SP, et al. Childhood Asphyxiation by Food. *Journ Amer Med Assoc*, 1984; 251:2231.
13. Johnsen D. The role of the pediatrician in identifying and treating dental caries. *Pediatric Clinics of North America*, 1991; 38:1;173-1181.
14. Kirks B, Hughes C. Long-term behavioral effects of parent involvement in nutrition education. *Journ Nutr Educ*, 1986; 18:203-206.

15. Pipes PL, Trahms CM. *Nutrition in Infancy and Childhood*, 5th Edition. St. Louis: Mosby-Yearbook, Inc., 1993.

16. Satter E. *How to Get Your Kid to Eat...But Not Too Much.* Palo Alto, CA: Bull Publishing Co., 1987.

17. Satter E. The feeding relationship: Problems and Interventions. *Journal of Pediatrics*, 1990; 117(2): S181-S189.

18. Why children and parents must play while they eat: An interview with T.Berry Brazelton, MD. Commentary. *Journ Amer Dietet Assoc*, 1993; 93(12): 1385-1387.

Infant Feeding: Breastfeeding

Breastfeeding PROVIDES significant benefits for the infant which cannot be duplicated by breastmilk substitutes. Numerous professional associations have identified breastfeeding as the preferred way to feed an infant. (American Academy of Pediatrics, 1978; American Dietetic Association, 1993).

In spite of the benefits, not all women breastfeed. There are numerous societal barriers to breastfeeding, including misinformation and lack of support from family, friends and health professionals.

Because much of the research on the benefits of breastfeeding has been published in the last decade, some health care professionals may not be aware of the benefits of breastfeeding. Benefits of breastfeeding include "Significant reductions in non-gastrointestinal infections, including pneumonia, bacteremia, and meningitis, and with a reduced frequency of certain chronic diseases later in life" (Cunningham, 1991). Research continues to identify additional benefits of breastfeeding (Duncan, 1993; Gerstein, 1994; Goldman, 1993; Harabuchi, 1994; Sullivan, 1994).

Breastfeeding is learned by both mother and infant. The first few hours and days of an infant's life, when a new mother is learning the techniques that will allow her to breastfeed successfully, are critical. Health professionals are encouraged to support policies and practices in their work setting that will provide new mothers with the knowledge and skills to be successful at breastfeeding. Research has demonstrated that breastfeeding success begins immediately after delivery (Righard, 1990). The Baby Friendly Hospital Initiative (BFHI) outlines steps which can be taken by hospitals to support breastfeeding (Kyenkya-Isabirye, 1992). Many women, especially first-time mothers, have many questions in the first weeks at home. Providing information about community support or developing a system of post-discharge follow-up can help assure a good start to breastfeeding (Neifert, 1992).

Health professionals can provide positive reinforcement for breastfeeding and answer questions the mother may have about her own diet or her infant's diet (See Nutrition During Lactation section of this manual.).

Assessment of Breastfeeding

Breastfeeding should not hurt. If it does, correct latch-on and positioning should be reviewed. For assistance with difficult problems contact a lactation consultant.

The breastfeeding experience changes as the infant grows, and as mother and infant get more experience. In assessing the intake of the breastfed infant, keep in mind that there will be variations in frequency and duration of breastfeeding. Indicators of adequate breastfeeding will vary based on the infant's birth weight, feeding style, and developmental stage. The key information to assess includes:

- Mother's perception of breastfeeding and her concerns, if any
- Infant growth and rate of weight gain
- Stooling and urination (wet diapers)
- Feeding based on infant cues rather than a strict schedule
- Alertness of infant/infant's indications of hunger
- Major inadequacies (such as a vegan diet) or excesses in the mother's diet

The young (0 – 6 week) infant will nurse an average of 8 to 12 feedings in 24 hours. Feedings may be every 1½ to 3 hours with one longer period of 4 to 5 hours. Watch for longer periods without feeding for the young infant, and carefully assess the number of feedings in 24 hours, growth, and other indications of breastfeeding. During growth spurts infants will breastfeed more frequently, usually for a 24 hour period, this will lead to additional breastmilk production. Older infants will often feed less frequently, on average 6-10 feedings per 24 hours. Young infants may nurse from 20 to 60 minutes per feeding. The time will vary with infant, and will decrease as the infant gets older. It is important that the infant is actually feeding, which can be determined by observing if the infant is swallowing (Seattle-King County Department of Health, 1990; Minnesota WIC Program 1993). There are many resources which describe patterns and indicators of breastfeeding over the first year of life (Seattle-King County Department of Health, 1990; Mohrbacher and Stock, 1991; Worthington, 1993).

Check with your pediatrician regarding the need for supplementation of Vitamin D (400 IU daily) and iron (ferrous sulfate-7 mg/dl) if an infant is exclusively breastfed.

Young, exclusively breastfed infants (approximately 0-6 weeks) often have three loose stools per day, some more, some less. Most have a minimum of one stool per day. If not, check for other indicators of successful breastfeeding. As they get older, stool frequency will decrease and stool volume will increase. During growth spurts stool volume may decrease. Stooling will also change with the addition of formula or any solid foods. The number of wet diapers per day is sometimes used to assess the adequacy of breastmilk intake. With disposable diapers, this may not be a good indicators.

Six to eight wet diapers per day for young, exclusively breastfed infants, not receiving additional water, can be used to help with assessment, but should not be used as the only indicator. If a breastfed infant is supplemented with formula, the indicators of adequate breastfeeding may change. With supplemental formula stools may be harder, darker, and less frequent, and the time between a formula feeding and the next feeding may be longer. The changes in stooling will vary with the amount of formula provided.

Other Considerations

Jaundice. There are many causes of jaundice, and many misconceptions. The early jaundice which occurs in a breastfed baby has been referred to by some as "lack of breastmilk jaundice". Breastfed babies need to be fed early and often. Supplemental water will not help in reducing serum bilirubin concentrations. A later jaundice, sometimes referred to as "breastmilk jaundice" may develop in a very small percentage of breastfed infants. Freeman (1992) estimates the incidence at one to two percent. Some physicians will temporarily interrupt breastfeeding to assess if serum bilirubin levels decrease, and rule out other causes for the jaundice. If breastfeeding is interrupted, the mother should be given instructions on pumping her milk, and reassurance that she can resume breastfeeding (Aurbach, 1987; Freeman, 1992; Riordan, 1994).

Medications. A breastfeeding woman can continue to breastfeed when taking most medications, but there are a few exceptions. She should inform any physician prescribing medications that she is breastfeeding. There are several resources which discuss prescription medications and breastfeeding (Briggs 1990; AAP Committee on Drugs, 1994).

Smoking. Smoking can decrease milk supply, and nicotine will pass through breastmilk to the baby. Recommendations for breastfeeding in smokers vary. The amount and timing of smoking, risks and benefits need to be weighed. Minchin (1993) provides a review of some of the issues related to breastfeeding and smoking.

Contraindications to breastfeeding. Mothers should be discouraged from breastfeeding when using cocaine, if drinking excessive alcohol, and if positive HIV status. Research continues and recommendations may change in the future.

Professional References

1. AAP Committee on Drugs. The Transfer of Drugs and Other Chemicals Into Human Milk. Pediatrics 93:1, January 1994. Pp 137-150.
2. Aurbach, Kathleen and L. Gartner. Breastfeeding and Human Milk: Their Association with Jaundice in the Neonate, Clinics in Perinatology. 1987 Mar; 14(1): 89-107.
3. Briggs, GG, Freeman, RK and Sumner, SJ. Drugs in Pregnancy and Lactation, third ed. Baltimore: Williams and Wilkins, 1990.
4. Committee on Nutrition, American Academy of Pediatrics. Breastfeeding. Pediatrics 1978: 62:591.
5. Cunningham, A., et al. Breastfeeding and health in the 1980's: A global epidemiologic review. J Pediatr 1991 May; 118(5):659-65.
6. Diet Assessment of the Breastfed Infant, Minnesota WIC Program Operations Manual, Minneapolis: Minnesota WIC Program, 1993.
7. Duncan, et al. Exclusive Breastfeeding for at Least 4 Months Protects Against Otitis Media. Pediatrics. 1993 May; 91(5):867-72.
8. Freeman, Roger and Ronald Poland, ed. Guidelines for Perinatal Care, Third Edition. American Academy of Pediatrics and American College of Obstetricians and Gynecologists, 1992,. Pp 205-11.
9. Gerstein, H. Cow's Milk Exposure and Type 1 Diabetes Mellitus: A critical overview of the clinical literature. Diabetes Care 1994 Jan; 17(1):13-9.
10. Goldman. The immune system of human milk: antimicrobial, antiinflammatory and immunomodulating properties. Pediatr Infect Dis J 1993 Aug:12(8):664-71.
11. Harabuchi, et al. Human Milk Secretory IgA antibody to non-typeable Haemophilus influenzae: Possible protective effects against nasopharyngeal colonization. J Pediatr. 1994 Feb; 124(2):193-8.
12. Institute of Medicine. Nutrition During Lactation. Washington D.C.: National Academy of Sciences, 1991.
13. Kyenkya-Isabirye, M. UNICEF Launches The Baby-Friendly Hospital Initiative. AM J Matern Child Nurs 1992 Jul/Aug;17:177-79.
14. Lawrence, Ruth. Breastfeeding: A Guide for the Medical Profession. St. Louis: Mosby, 1989.
15. Minchin, Maureen K., Smoking and Breastfeeding: An Overview. J Hum Lact 7(4) 1991, 183-188.
16. Mohrbacher, N and J Stock. The Breastfeeding Answer Book. Franklin Park, Ill: La Leche League International, 1991.
17. Neifert, Marianne. Screening Forms: Aid to Breastfeeding. Pediatric Management. 1992 Jul: 24-27.
18. Position of the American Dietetic Association: Promotion and Support of Breastfeeding. J Am Diet Assoc 1993:93, 467-469.
19. Righard, L, et al. Effect of delivery room routines on success of first breast-feed. Lancet 1990 Nov; 336: 1105-07.
20. Riordan, Jan and Kathleen Aurbach. Breastfeeding and Human Lactation. Boston: Jones and Bartlett. 1993. Pp. 333-345.
21. Seattle-King County Department of Public Health. Breastfeeding Triage Tool. Seattle, Washington: Seattle-King County Department of Public Health, 1990.
22. Sullivan, et al. Infant Dietary Experience and Acceptance of Solid Food. Pediatrics 1994 Feb; 93(2):271-77.
23. Worthington, Nutrition in Pregnancy and Lactation, 5th ed., St. Louis: Mosby, 1993.

Client Resources: Video

24. Yes, You Can Breastfeed. Texas WIC Program, 1990. $6.00. 7 minutes. MetroPost/501 N IH 35/Austin, Texas 78702/512-476-3876
25. Breastfeeding: A special Relationship. Eagle Video Productions, 1991. $1790.00. 24 minutes. Eagle Video Productions/2201 Woodnell Dr./Raleigh, NC 27603-5240/919-779-7891 or 800-869-7892.
26. A Healthier Baby by Breastfeeding. Television Innovation Company, 1991. $19.95. 20 minutes. Television Innovation Company/8349-N Arrowridge Road/Charlotte, NC 28273/704-527-0800 or 800-868-4336.

Client Resources: Books

27. Gotsch, Gwen, Breastfeeding Pure and Simple. Franklin Park, Ill: La Leche Legue International, 1994.
28. Huggins Kathleen. The Nursing Mother's Companion. Massachusetts: Harvard Common Press, 1990.
29. Kitzinger, Sheila. Breastfeeding Your Baby. New York: Knopf, 1991.
30. La Leche League International. The Womanly Art of Breastfeeding. Franklin Park, Ill: La Leche League International, 1991.

Client Resources: Pamphlets

1. Breastfeeding: Getting Started in 5 Easy Steps
2. Helpful Hints on Breastfeeding
3. Both pamphlets available in English and Spanish from Childbirth Graphics, A Division of WRS Group, Inc., P.O. Box 21207, Waco, TX 76702-1207. 800-299-3366, ext. 287.

Providing Breast Milk for Hospitalized Infants

Providing breast milk for a hospitalized infant presents challenges, and may require the mother to pump and collect her milk. However, breastfeeding is recognized as the best way to feed an infant, and has special advantages for the pre-term infant, the benefits outweigh the challenges. The support and encouragement that hospital personnel can give to the mother of a hospitalized infant plays a significant role in her success at breastfeeding.

Many infants who were previously thought unable to breastfeed have demonstrated the ability to breastfeed. New methods of supplementing infants at the breast, such as the Supplemental Nursing System (SNS)*, allow infants with a poor or weak suck, or high calorie needs, to meet their needs at the breast. This helps avoid the possibility of nipple confusion.

A woman's milk supply increases and decreases under the influence of prolactin. Nipple stimulation from nursing or pumping stimulates prolactin activity and thus milk production. An electric breastpump will help stimulate prolactin activity, with a double pump more than doubling the prolactin stimulating effect. Infant suckling provides the best nipple stimulation, therefore, the sooner the infant can be put to breast, the better.

Methods of Collecting Milk

Electric pump. For an infant not put to breast, the electric pump will help stimulate breastmilk production. A double electric pump is preferred, especially for the mother of a premature or hospitalized infant who will be collecting milk for a long period of time.

Hand expression or hand pumping. For occasionally expressing milk, expressing for a short period of time, or expressing to provide milk for a regular missed feeding, either manual expression or hand pumping are good options. The preference of the mother should determine the method used. There are printed and audiovisual instructional materials available to learn hand expression.

Guidelines for Expressing and Storing Breastmilk

Guidelines for storing breastmilk for the well infant at home are published in most breastfeeding books. *The La Leche League Answer Book* discusses home storage. The time that breastmilk can be stored is largely dependent on the type of home freezer available.

Pumping and storing breastmilk for the hospitalized infant requires a stricter protocol. Current guidelines for storing breastmilk can be obtained from the Human Milk Banking Association of North America.

* Supplemental Nursing System and SNS are copyrighted by Medela. Information on use of the system can be obtained from Medela.

Professional References

1. Frantz, Kitty. *Breastfeeding Techniques That Work, Volume 6; Hand Expression* (Video), Geddes Productions, 1992, 18 minutes $39.95, Geddes Productions, 10546 McVine, Sunland CA 91040, 818-951-2809.
2. Franz, Kitty. *Breastfeeding Techniques That Work, Volume 7: Supplemental Nursing System* (SNS), Geddes Productions, 1992, 23 minutes. Geddes Productions, 10546 McVine, Sunland, CA 91040, 818-951-2809.

3. The Human Milk Banking Association of North America. Recommendations for Collection, Storage, and Handling of a Mother's Milk for Her Own Infant in the Hospital Setting. The Human Milk banking Association of North America, Inc., P.O. Box 370464, West Hartford, CT 06137-0464, USA, 1993.
4. Mohrbacher, N and J Stock. *The Breastfeeding Answer Book.* Franklin Park, Ill.: La Leche League International, 1991.
5. Riordan, J and K Auerbach. *Breastfeeding and Human Lactation.* Boston: Jones and Bartlett, 1993.
6. Walker, MTI. Breastfeeding the premature infant. NAACOGS *Clin Issu Perninat Womans Health Nurs* 1992; 3(4):620-33.

Infant Formula
General Description

The American Academy of Pediatrics recommends iron-fortified formula as the primary source of nutrients when the infants are not breast-fed.(1) Iron fortified formulas have practically eliminated overt iron deficiency, the most common cause of anemia in children. (3) Controlled studies (2) failed to find significant differences in the symptoms between infants fed iron-fortified formula and those fed low-iron formula.

Indications for Use

The Committee on Nutrition sees no role for the use of low-iron formulas in infant feeding and recommends that iron-fortified formula be used for all formula fed infants.(3) When complaints are received about iron-fortified formula, there are many other causes of GI symptoms to rule out before implicating iron. The following list includes several situations that could lead to GI symptoms and suggested inquiries to determine if the condition exists.

SITUATION	INQUIRY
Parent incorrectly diagnoses diarrhea, vomiting, or constipation.	Ask for specific description of symptoms, such as frequency, color, and consistency of stools in the case of diarrhea. Remember, stools may change when infant's diet changes, for example, from breast milk to formula.
Formula is diluted incorrectly.	Ask or observe how formula is prepared.
Conditions surrounding formula preparation and feeding are unsanitary or unsafe.	Ask how bottles are prepared, how formula is stored, and what happens to partially used bottles of formula.
Water supply is unsafe.	If source of water is a private well, ask if water has been checked for safety.
Feeding practices are inappropriate.	Obtain diet history and check for early introduction of solids and juices or for overfeeding.
Child may be ill.	Ask about other symptoms such as fever, colds, flu, etc.
Home environment may be stressful causing reactions in infant.	Carefully explore with parent how things are going at home, especially how mother feels, and how mother, father, and other children are getting along.

Child may be more sensitive to one form or brand of formula than to another.	Suggest changing from powder to liquid or changing brand of formula to another iron-fortified formula. Allow several days before assessing results.
Child may be intolerant to milk-based formulas.	Suggest iron-fortified soy-based formula or lactose reduced formula.
Infant is not burped during feeding or is handled roughly during or after feeding, causing vomiting.	Ask parent about burping and handling. Recommend burping gently one or two times during feedings and gentle handling of baby immediately after feeding.
Infant may experience symptoms if iron-fortified formula is introduced after infant is accustomed to low-iron formula.	Suggest feeding mixture of iron-fortified and low-iron formula. Start with 1:3 ratio during one week, gradually increase proportion of iron-fortified formula. At end of week, feed 100% fortified formula.
Infant formula may have a constipating effect.	Offer diluted prune juice or supplemental bottles of water.
Child may have either organic or psychologic pathology.	Further evaluation and treatment may be indicated.

Other Considerations

Rare conditions that do preclude the use of iron-fortified formula are congenital hemosiderosis and congenital disorders of hemoglobin.

Professional References

1. Committee on Nutrition, American Academy of Pediatrics. Pediatric Nutrition Handbook. 2nd ed. Elk Grove Village, IL:American Academy of Pediatrics, 1985.
2. Lack of Adverse Reactions to Iron-Fortified Formula. Nutrition Reviews. 47(2):41-43, 1989.
3. Committee on Nutrition, Iron-Fortified Infant Formulas. Pediatrics. 84(6):1114-1115, 1989.
4. Fomon SJ. Nutrition of Normal Infants. St. Louis:Mosby, 1993.
5. Foman SJ. Reflections on Infant Feeding for the 1970's and 1980's. Am J Clin Nut. 1987; 46:171-182.
6. Nelson SE, Ziegler EE, Copeland AM, Edwards BB, Fomon SJ: Lack of Adverse Reactions to Iron-Fortified Formula. Pediatrics. 81(3):360-364, 1988.
7. Tsang RC, Nichols BL: Nutrition During Infancy. Philadelphia: Henley & Belfus, 1988.
8. Bradley CK, Hillman L, Sherman AR, Leedy D, Cordano A: Evaluation of Two Iron-Fortified, Milk-Based Formulas During Infancy. Pediatrics. 91(5):908-914, 1993.

Feeding the Infant/Toddler
Age, Developmental Achievements, and Related Eating Skills and Behaviors

Age	Skill Development	Related Feeding Skills/Behaviors
Birth	Visual preference for human face[1]	Rooting, sucking, swallowing, and extrusion reflex[2] Tearless hunger cry[2]
1 month (4 weeks)	Tonic neck posture predominates[1]	Face brightens on satiety[2] Eye contact when feeding[2,3] Two night feedings[2,3]
2 months (8 weeks)	Smiles on social contact; listens to voice and coos[1] Peak of crying episodes[3]	One nightly feeding[2,3]
3 months (12 weeks)	Early head control with bobbing motion[1] Sustained social contact[1] Reaches toward and misses objects[1]	Choking response to solids[2,3] Extrusion reflux still present[4]
4 months (16 weeks)	Reaches and grasps for objects and brings to mouth[1] Enjoys sitting with full truncal support[1]	May have hands get in the way when feeding[4] Excited at site of food[1] Mouth poises for nipple[2]
5 months (20 weeks)	Able to grasp objects voluntarily in a mitten-like fashion[4]	Can approximate lips to rim of cup[4] Chewing action begins[4] Begins to pat or loosely hold breast or bottle[2,3] Tongue projects after spoon removed[2,3]
6 months (24 weeks)	Brings hand to mouth, with all objects going into mouth[4] Sits in chair when securely supported[2]	Begins drinking from cup[4] Solid food introduction[5] (if not already done in 4th or 5th month) Providing spoon to hold may provide developmental stimulation[3]
7 months (28 weeks)	Bangs objects on table[4] Eye and hands work together[4] Feet to mouth[2] Transfers object from hand to hand[1] Pivots, crawls or creep-crawls[1]	Able to feed self biscuit[4] Takes solids well[2] Can increase texture and stiffness of solids[6]
8 months (32 weeks)	Bits and chews toys[2] Acquires sitting balance Beginning pincer grasp	Guides caregiver's hand during feeding Holds cup or bottle
9 months (36 weeks)	Radial-digital grasp: Grasp object with opposed thumb and fingertips Sits erect without support	Feeds self cracker well Uses tiptoe cup or bottle
9-10 months (40 weeks)	Relates to objects Grasps objects with thumb and forefinger Pokes at things with forefinger Pulls to standing position Combines two toys, utensils	Reaches for food and utensils Can more easily pick up pellet size food (i.e., dry cereal)[3] Can handle pieces of soft, cooked, moderately seasoned family foods[6]
10-11 months (44 weeks)	"Cruises" – walks sideways holding on to furniture[8] Has vocabulary of two or three words[8]	Tries to feed self[2] Tries to use spoon[2]
1 year (52 weeks)	Walks with one hand held[1] Picks up small objects with unassisted pincer movement of forefinger and thumb; releases object to others on request or gesture[1] Importance of mouth as primary sensory organ dimishes[2]	Cessation of drooling[2,3] Grasps cup with both hands[2]

Age	Skill Development	Related Feeding Skills/Behaviors
15 months	Walks alone; crawls upstairs[1] Follows simple commands[1] Indicates some needs and desires by pointing[1]	Bottle discarded[2,3] Sucks through straw[2,3] Able to use spoon with greater skill[3] May start throwing food[2,3]
18 months	Runs stiffly; sits on small chair; walks upstairs with one hand held[1]	Can use spoon and fork, but prefers finger foods[2] Hands empty dish to caregiver[2,3]
21 months	Walks up/down stairs alternating feet Kicks a ball Scribbles	Uses spoon right side up[2,3] Can ask for more[2,3] Handles cup without spilling[2,3]
2 years (24 months)	Runs well; walks up and down stairs; climbs on furniture[1] Puts three words together[1] Fond of repetitive daily structure and routine[2,3] Vocabulary to 300 words; speaks in 2-word combinations[8]	Uses spoon well[2,3] Feeds doll[2,3] Picks same place to eat[2,3] Mature rotary chewing[5]
3 years (36 months)	Rides tricycle	Pours from small pitcher[2,3,4] Feeds self well with little spilling[2,3,4]
4 years (48 months)	Uses scissors to cut out pictures Vocabulary of 1500 words	Can begin to fix simple meals with assistance (i.e., bowl of cereal or sandwich)[3]

Professional References

1. Behrman RE, ed, *Nelson Textbook of Pediatrics, 14th Edition*. Philadelphia: WB Saunders Co; 1992.
2. Ekvall SW, ed, *Pediatric Nutrition in Chronic Diseases and Developmental Disorders*. New York: Oxford University Press; 1993.
3. Padgett D. Behavior Management of Feeding Problems. *Nutrition Focus*; 1992; 7(1):1-6.
4. Hendricks KM, Walker WA. *Pediatric Nutrition, 2nd Edition*. Toronto, Philadelphia: BC Decker Inc.; 1990.
5. Cloud HH, Bergman J. Eating/Feeding Problems of Children: The Team Approach. *Nutrition Focus*; 1991; 6(6):1-8.

Food Guide for Infants

Infants: Birth - 4 Months

Food Group	Recommended Daily Amount **	Rationale
Breast milk and/or iron-fortified formula.	Daily Totals for Formula: 0-1 mo. 18-24 oz. 1-2 mo. 22-28 oz. 2-3 mo. 25-32 oz. 3-4 mo. 28-32 oz.	Infants' well-developed sucking and rooting reflexes allow them to take in breast milk and formula. Infants do not accept semisolid food because their tongues protrude when a spoon is put in their mouths. They are unable to transfer food to the back of the mouth.
Water	Not routinely recommended.	Small amounts may be offered under special circumstances, such as hot weather, diarrhea, vomiting, or constipation. Check with your pediatrician about adding 400 IU Vitamin D as prophylaxis for rickets in exclusively breast-fed infants.

Infants: 4 - 6 Months

Food Group	Recommended Daily Amount **	Rationale
Breast milk and/or iron-fortified formula.	Daily Totals for Formula: 4-5 mo. 27-39 oz. 5-6 mo. 27-45 oz. 6-8 mo. 24-32 oz.	Iron-fortified formula or iron supplementation with breast milk continues to be needed.
* Iron-fortified cereal: Begin with rice cereal (mix cereal with breast milk or iron-fortified formula).	4-8 TBSP (after mixing)	At this age, there is a decrease of the extrusion reflex. The infant is able to depress the tongue and transfer semisolid food from a spoon to the back of the pharynx to swallow it. Infant is also able to support his/her own head and turn away to refuse Cereal adds a source of iron and B vitamins.
Water	As desired.	Do not offer water as a substitute for formula or breast milk, but rather as a source of additional fluids.

*   Indicates new food item for the age group.
**   Serving amounts are general guidelines. Intake will vary depending on the infant's appetite.

Infants 6 - 8 Months

Food Group	Recommended Daily Amount **	Rationale

Breast milk and/or iron-fortified formula.	Daily Totals for Formula: 4-5 mo. 27-39 oz. 5-6 mo. 27-45 oz. 6-8 mo. 24-32 oz.	Iron-fortified formula or iron supplementation with breast milk continues to be needed.
Iron-fortified cereal: Begin with rice cereal (mix cereal with human milk or iron-fortified formula).	4-8 TBSP (after mixing)	At this age, there is a decrease of the extrusion reflex. The infant is able to depress the tongue and transfer semisolid food from a spoon to the back of the pharynx to swallow it. Cereal adds a source of iron and B vitamins.
Water	As desired.	Do not offer water as a substitute for formula or breast milk, but rather as a source of additional fluids.
* Fruits: Plain strained; jarred; or soft, peeled and mashed. * Vegetables: Plain strained; jarred; or soft cooked peeled and mashed.	2-4 TBSP 2-4 TBSP	Fruits and vegetables: Introduce new flavors and textures one at a time Teething is beginning; thus there is an increased ability to bite and chew.
*Unsweetened fruit juices: Plain, Vitamin C fortified. Dilute juices with equal parts of water.	2-4 oz.	Juice should be introduced in a cup. Delay orange, pineapple, grapefruit, or tomato juice until 9-12 months of age.

*   Indicates new food item for the age group.
**   Serving amounts are general guidelines. Intake will vary depending on the infant's appetite.

Infants 9 - 11 Months

Food Group	Recommended Daily Amount **	Rationale
Breast milk and/or iron-fortified formula. Water	24 - 32 oz. As desired.	
Iron-fortified infant cereal	4-6 TBSP	
Fruits: Plain strained; jarred; or soft, peeled and mashed. Vegetables: Plain strained; jarred; or soft cooked, peeled and mashed.	2-4 TBSP 2-4 TBSP	Fruits and vegetables: Introduce new flavors and textures. Teething is beginning; thus there is an increased ability to bite and chew.

Unsweetened fruit juices: Plain, Vitamin C fortified. Dilute juices with equal parts of water.	2-4 oz.	Juice should be introduced in a cup. Delay orange, pineapple, grapefruit, or tomato juice until 9-12 months of age.
* Meats: Plain strained; ground or soft, cooked bite size pieces. Tofu or mashed beans. * Bite-size cheese pieces, cottage cheese, yogurt.	2-4 tsp.	Formula consumption may begin to decrease; thus begin other sources of calcium, riboflavin, and protein.
* Finger foods (dry cereal, graham crackers)	In small servings.	Rhythmic biting movements begin; enhance this development with foods that require chewing. Decrease amounts of mashed foods as amount of finger foods increases.

*   Indicates new food item for the age group.

**   Serving amounts are general guidelines. Intake will vary depending on the infant's appetite.

Infants 11 - 12 Months

Food Group	Recommended Daily Amount **	Rationale
Breast milk and/or iron-fortified formula. Water	24 - 32 oz. As desired.	At 12 months, whole milk may be given instead of breast milk or formula. Introduction of milk prior to this is discouraged due to potential of intestinal blood loss, renal solute load, and potential allergy.
Fruit: Soft canned fruits or ripe banana, cut up. Peeled raw fruit as the infant approaches 12 months. Vegetables: Soft cooked, cut into bite-sized pieces. Meats: Strips of tender, lean meat; cheese, peanut butter.	1/2 cup 1/2 cup 2 oz. or 1/2 cup chopped	Infant is relying less on breast milk or formula for nutrients. A proper selection of a variety of solid foods (fruits, vegetables, starches, protein sources, and dairy products) will continue to meet the young child's needs. Delay peanut butter until one year of age.
Fruit juice	4 oz.	
* Soft table foods as follows: Cereal, and dry unsweetented cereal as a finger food. Breads: Crackers, toast, pasta, zwieback.	4-6 TSBP 1-2 small servings	Motor skills are developing; enhance this with more finger foods. Rotary chewing motion develops; thus child is able to handle whole foods, which require more chewing.

*   Indicates new food item for the age group.

**   Serving amounts are general guidelines. Intake will vary depending on the infant's appetite.

Guidelines for Introducing Solid Foods

There are two main reasons for starting solid foods: 1) to help the infant develop eating skills, 2) to provide additional nutrients. By 4-6 months of age, most infants are ready for solid food. Feeding solid foods before 4 months of age is not recommended because infants are not developmentally ready and the additional food will take the place of the breast milk or formula which is their best source of nutrients.

1. Start solid foods when the infant can:

    - sit up with some support
    - follow spoon with eyes
    - open (or close) mouth when he/she sees food coming

2. Infants eat best when they are the leader.
    Pay close attention to the infant during feeding and let him/her be in control. Wait for the infant to pay attention to the spoon and open his/her mouth. Feed at the infant's speed and stop feeding when the infant is done (turns head, pushes spoon away).

3. Add one new food at a time.

    Wait at least 3 days before adding any other new foods. This allows sufficient time to look for signs of possible food sensitivity such as rashes, vomiting, diarrhea, or wheezing.

4. The infant learns to eat by gradually increasing the thickness and lumpiness of the food.

    Begin with smooth, soft foods and gradually increase the texture as the infant's eating skills progress.

5. Let the infant explore the food with hands or spoon in attempts to self-feed.

    At about 7 months offer easy-to-handle, bite-sized finger foods. Good finger foods include banana pieces, peas, dry cereal, and cracker pieces.

> **TIP**
> When the infant is starting to eat adult cereals, dampen the cereal with formula or breast milk. This softens the cereal and makes it easier to pick up and chew.

6. These foods should be avoided until the child is 1 year old:

    - egg whites (may cause allergies)
    - chocolate (may cause allergies)
    - peanut butter (may cause choking)
    - honey (may cause infant botulism)
    - other small, hard, and round foods, eg. hot dogs, grapes (may cause choking)

Baby Bottle Tooth Decay

Description

Baby bottle tooth decay (BBTD) is extensive decay in the primary or baby teeth. It is a preventable tooth problem. It results from bottle or breast feeding a child incorrectly or for too long. BBTD may develop from giving a baby a bottle of milk, formula, fruit juice, or sweet drink or breastfeeding to pacify or comfort a child throughout the day, or a nap and bedtime. Giving a baby a bottle past one year of age may also cause tooth decay. BBTD has also been called nursing caries, nursing bottle mouth and bottle mouth cavities.

The best way to treat Baby Bottle Tooth Decay is to prevent it.

To prevent Baby Bottle Tooth Decay

Show love with hugs, kisses and attention, not a bottle or sweetened pacifier.
Use bottle or breast feeding to nourish, not to pacify.
Hold children during feeding and place them in bed without a bottle when done.
If a bedtime bottle is needed, it should have only plain water in it.
Give plain pacifiers, not ones dipped in honey, sugar, peanut butter, or anything else.
Begin weaning at six months of age by introducing a cup.
Sweet drinks (including fruit juice) should be given in a cup and never in a bottle.
After teeth come in, wipe teeth daily with a gauze pad or soft cloth until teeth can be brushed.
Begin regular dental care, such as cleaning, fluoride, and sealants between two and three years of age.

Choking Prevention

Choking on food is a common hazard in infancy and childhood. Children cannot chew very effectively until about four years of age. Children may also chew while running, playing, walking, laughing, or in a hurry, and they often don't take the time to chew well.

Children can choke on almost any food, but they are most likely to have trouble with foods that are smooth, hard, slippery and/or just the right size to plug the airway. When the food becomes stuck, it prevents coughing which might expel it. In addition, children cannot make noise to get help from an adult. It is important to know the first aid measures for choking in children. These techniques are different for children than for adults and can be learned from the local Red Cross of American Heart Association. However, it is more important to take measures to prevent choking.

Suggestions to prevent choking in children under four years of age:

- Never leave children unattended while eating.
- Don't allow children to eat in a moving car.
- Serve foods cut into small square pieces.
- Children should only eat while sitting down.
- Keep foods out of children's reach.
- Discourage overstuffing of the child's mouth.
- Serve foods that are appropriate for the child to chew.
- The best prevention is awareness and supervision.

Foods that may cause choking:
Wieners and hot dog-like products, unless cut in quarters lengthwise
Grapes, unless cut in quarters lengthwise
Popcorn
Peanuts and other nuts, unless ground fine
Sunflower, pumpkin and other seeds, unless ground fine
Round, hard, or sticky candies
Chewing gum
Hard, raw vegetables and fruits
Foods with "skin"
"Stringy" foods such as orange segments, unless cut into small pieces

Developing Food Preferences

Generally most food preferences are learned and developed at home throughout childhood. Family members, such as parents and siblings, have a strong influence on which foods children like or dislike and eating patterns. When children are very young, a feeding relationship is begun between parent and child. Parents offer food and the child eats it or doesn't eat it. Sometimes difficulties can result when a child refuses to eat the food that is offered. Maintaining a positive feeding relationship requires a division of responsibilities between parent and child.

Parents are responsible for **what** the child is offered to eat. Regular and nutritious meals and snacks should be provided in a pleasant and supportive fashion. The child, on the other hand, is responsible for deciding whether or not he or she eats the food provided and **how much** of the food will be eaten.

Common Feeding Problems

The child won't try new foods. It is common for preschoolers and school-aged children to be picky about food. Children are suspicious of new foods. It may take several exposures to a new food for them to taste and eventually like it. Offer a new food without comment. Forcing a child to eat or taste food may create a bad association with that food, which can last for years.

Be sensitive to how the food is prepared. Some children may prefer the food prepared in a different way or at a different temperature. Parents should respect their child's food preferences and not try to dictate them.

The child eats the same food over and over. "Food jags" are common among young children. Usually food jags don't last long or cause serious nutrition problems. Offer a variety of food at mealtime including at least one food the child likes. Don't offer substitutes, but let the child pick and choose from what is available. Most likely the child will gradually increase the variety of foods he or she will eat.

The child dislikes vegetables. Many children refuse to eat vegetables. Some children will eat only starchy vegetables such as potatoes or corn. Others will eat only one to two different vegetables. To increase the vegetables children will eat, parents should serve vegetables frequently and eat a variety of vegetables themselves.

Sometimes creative preparation may make vegetables more appealing. Steam fresh vegetables until they are tender-crisp. Serve raw vegetables with a dip for a snack. Shredded vegetables can be added to sandwich spreads. Soups and stews are other ways to serve vegetables. Children who are encouraged to select vegetables at the market or grow them in a garden may be more eager to try them at meals.

The child dislikes fruit. To increase fruits, parents can add it to cereals, gelatin, pudding, custard, or ice cream. Fruit or fruit juice can be blended with milk to make a milk shake. Parents should serve fruits frequently and eat a variety of fruits themselves.

The child does not like meat. Meats are sometimes unappealing to young children due to texture and strong flavor. There are many ways to make sure children get enough high-quality protein. Meats, such as chicken, turkey, tuna and other fish may be easier to chew. Eggs, peanut butter, cooked beans and legumes, milk, and cheese also are excellent sources of protein. Offer your child a variety of meats or meat substitutes.

The child dislikes milk. Milk is an important source of protein and calcium for children. Parents can encourage their child by drinking milk themselves, providing milk at meals, and limiting the amount of other beverages such as juice and soft drinks. Sometimes offering the milk in a new cup or glass or allowing the child to pour it from a small pitcher can revive interest in milk as a beverage. It the child refuses to drink milk try cooking hot cereals and soups with milk, making puddings and custard, and serve yogurt, cottage cheese, and cheese slices.

How to Use the Food Guide Pyramid
What Counts as One Serving?

Age	Breads, cereals, rice, pasta	Vegetables	Fruits	Milk, yogurt, cheese	Meat, poultry, fish, dry beans, eggs, nuts
1 to 3 years	1/2 slice bread, waffle, 5" pancake, muffin, tortilla or taco shell 1/4 bagel, English muffin, or sandwich bun 1/4 cup cooked rice, noodles, cereal, infant cereal, pasta, or grits 1/2 ounce ready-to-eat cereal crackers - 3 soda, 6 wheat thins, 4 triscuit, 1 whole graham (2 squares)	3 ounces juice 1/4 cup cooked or raw 1/2 cup raw leafy	1/4 cup canned or cooked 1/2 medium size fresh 3 ounces juice 2 Tbsp dried	1 cup milk, yogurt, pudding (whole milk should be used until age 2 years) 1 1/2 ounce cheese 1/3 cup grated cheese 2 cups cottage cheese 1 1/2 cups ice cream, ice milk, frozen yogurt	1 ounce meat (chicken, beef, pork, fish) 2 Tbsp ground meat 1 egg 2 Tbsp peanut butter 1/2 cup cooked dried beans, peas, lentils 3 ounces tofu
3 to 6 years	3/4 slice bread, waffle, 5" pancake, muffin, tortilla or taco shell 1/3 bagel, English muffin, or sandwich bun 1/3 cup cooked rice, noodles, cereal, pasta, or grits 3/4 ounce ready-to-eat cereal crackers - 4 soda, 8 wheat thins, 6 triscuit, 1 1/2 whole graham (3 squares) 2 cups popcorn	4 to 6 ounces juice 1/3 to 1/2 cup cooked or raw 3/4 cup raw leafy	1/3 cup canned or cooked 3/4 medium size fresh 1/2 to 3/4 cup juice 2 Tbsp dried	1 cup milk, yogurt, pudding 1 1/2 ounce cheese 1/3 cup grated cheese 2 cups cottage cheese 1 1/2 cups ice cream, ice milk, frozen yogurt *Low -fat choices are good for children over 2 years.	1 1/2 ounce meat (chicken, beef, pork, fish) 3 Tbsp ground meat 1 to 2 eggs 3 Tbsp peanut butter 3/4 cup cooked dried beans, peas, lentils 4 1/2 ounces tofu

| 6 years to adult | 1 slice bread, waffle, 5" pancake, small muffin, tortilla, or taco shell 1/2 bagel or sandwich bun 1/2 cup cooked rice, noodles, cereal, pasta, or grits 1 ounce ready-to-eat cereal crackers - 6 soda, 12 wheat thins, 8 triscuit, 2 whole graham (4 squares) 3 cups popcorn | 6 ounces (3/4 cup) juice 1/2 cup cooked or raw 1 cup raw leafy | 1/2 cup canned or cooked 1 medium size fresh 6 ounces (3/4 cup) juice 1/4 cup dried | 1 cup milk, yogurt, pudding 1 1/2 ounce cheese 1/3 cup grated cheese 2 cups cottage cheese 1 1/2 cups ice cream, ice milk, frozen yogurt *Low -fat choices are good for children over 2 years. | 2 to 3 ounces meat (chicken, beef, pork, fish) 2 eggs 4 Tbsp peanut butter 1 cup cooked dried beans, peas, lentils 8 ounces tofu |

Vitamin A Sources: apricots, asparagus, bok choy, broccoli, brussel sprouts, cantaloupe, carrots, kale, mangos, papaya, peaches, pumpkin, prunes, spinach, squash, sweet potatoes, watermelon - **Recommended 3 or 4 times per week**

Vitamin C Sources: broccoli, raw cabbage, cantaloupe, cauliflower, grapefruit, green pepper, kiwi, orange, baked potato, strawberries, tangerine, tomatoes, watermelon, juices with vitamin C added - **Recommended daily**

The Food Guide PYRAMID

The Food Guide Pyramid is a good example of how to turn the Dietary Guidelines for Americans (issued in 1995 by U.S. Health & Human Services Department) into actual food choices.

The Dietary Guidelines and their relationship to a Food Guide Pyramid are:

- Eat a variety of foods
- Balance the food you eat with physical activity—maintain or improve your weight
- Choose a diet with plenty of grain products, vegetables, and fruits
- Choose a diet low in fat, saturated fat, and cholesterol
- Choose a diet moderate in sugars
- Choose a diet moderate in salt and sodium
- If you drink alcoholic beverages, do so in moderation

The Food Guide Pyramid

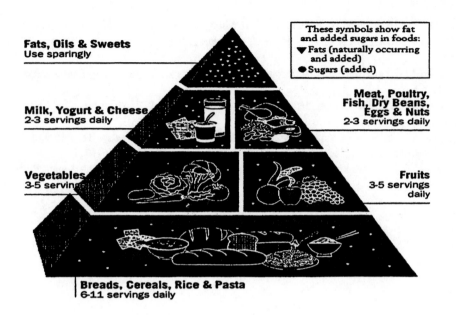

Fats, Oils & Sweets
Use sparingly

These symbols show fat and added sugars in foods:
▼ Fats (naturally occurring and added)
● Sugars (added)

Milk, Yogurt & Cheese
2-3 servings daily

Meat, Poultry, Fish, Dry Beans, Eggs & Nuts
2-3 servings daily

Vegetables
3-5 servings

Fruits
3-5 servings daily

Breads, Cereals, Rice & Pasta
6-11 servings daily

Statement on Vitamin and Mineral Supplementation

Healthy children and adults should obtain adequate nutrient intakes from dietary sources. Meeting nutrient needs by choosing a variety of foods in moderation, rather than by supplementation, reduces the potential risk for nutrient deficiencies and nutrient excesses. Individual recommendations regarding supplements and diets should come from physicians and dietitians.

Except for fluoride supplementation in unfluoridated areas, the American Academy of Pediatrics does not support supplementation for normal, healthy children. The following are some circumstances that may indicate supplement usage:

- Children from deprived families and those who are abused or neglected
- Children with anorexia, poor appetites, and poor eating habits
- Children consuming vegetarian diets without dairy products
- Pregnant teenagers
- Children with food allergies
- Children who omit entire food groups

Certain disorders or diseases and some medications may interfere with nutrient intake, digestion, absorption, metabolism, or excretion and thus change requirements.

Nutrients are potentially toxic when ingested in sufficiently large amounts. Safe intake levels vary widely from nutrient to nutrient and may vary with the age and health of the individual. In addition, high dosage vitamin and mineral supplements can interfere with the normal metabolism of other nutrients and with the therapeutic effects of certain drugs.

The Recommended Dietary Allowances represent the best currently available assessment of safe and adequate intake and serve as the basis for the U.S. Recommended Daily Allowances shown on many product labels. There are no demonstrated benefits of self-supplementation beyond these allowances.

Professional references

1. Alhadeff L, Gulatier CT, Lipton M. Toxic effects of water-soluble vitamins. Nutr Rev 1984: 42(2):33.
2. American Dietetic Association. A clinical guide to nutrition care in end stage renal disease. 2nd edition. Chicago: 1992.
3. Bell LS, Fairchild M. Evaluation of commercial multivitamin supplements. J Am Dietetic Assoc 1987:87(3):341-43.
4. Food and Nutrition Board. Recommended Dietary Allowances. 9th ed. Washington, D.C.: National Academy of Sciences. 1989.
5. Markoff R, PhD. Walker Soluble Vitamin Status in Patients with Renal Disease Treated with Hemodialysis or Peritoneal Dialysis, Review Article. J Ren Nutr, Vol 1, No. 2 (April), 1991: 56-73.
6. Queen PM, Lang CE, editors. Handbook of Pediatric Nutrition. Gaithersburg, MD: Aspen Publishers Inc., 1993.

Vitamins—Water Soluble

See the Recommended Dietary Allowances of the National Research Council for recommendations on specific amounts of vitamins.

Vitamins	Function	Possible Deficiency Symptoms	Source
Vitamin C (ascorbic acid)	Promotes growth & tissue repair. Enhances iron absorption, wound healing, resistance to infection. Functions in body cell structure.	Scurvy, cracked lips, bleeding gums, slow wound healing, easy bruising.	Citrus fruits and juices; strawberries, tomatoes, potatoes, and some green vegetables. Fortified fruit juices.
Thiamin (vitamin B_1)	Promotes normal appetite and digestion; nerve tissue; assist energy release from food.	Beriberi; anorexia; nausea.	Meats, especially pork; enriched or whole grain breads; dried peas and beans. Soybeans, Brewer's yeast.
Riboflavin (vitamin B_2)	Cell utilization of oxygen; integrity of skin, tongue, and lips.	Cheilosis, dermatitis, glossitis, dimness of vision.	Milk; cheese; lean meats; liver. Enriched and whole grain breads. Eggs.
Niacin	Maintains nervous system; integrity of skin, mouth, tongue, digestive tract; helps cells use other nutrients. Energy metabolism.	Pellagra, dermatitis, diarrhea, anorexia, indigestion, mental disorders.	All meat, poultry, fish. Enriched and whole grain cereal products, dried peas and beans; fish, liver, lean meats.
Vitamin B_6 (pyridoxine)	Functions in protein metabolism; chemistry of blood; brain; essential fatty acids.	Convulsions, nausea, vomiting, dermatitis, nervous disorders.	Red meat, potatoes. Green vegetables, yellow corn, organ meats.
Vitamin B_{12} (cyanocobalamin)	Essential for normal function of amino acid production and adequate red blood cell formation.	Megaloblastic anemia, glossitis.	Animal sources-liver, lean meats, eggs, milk, shellfish
Folacin	Breakdown of amino acids; process of red blood cell formation; reproductive system.	Macrocytic anemia, weakness, glossitis, gastrointestinal disturbances.	Dark green, leafy vegetables, nuts, whole wheat products, liver. Brewer's yeast. Navy beans, raw orange.
Pantothenic acid	Component of coenzyme A; metabolism of carbohydrate, fat, and protein.	Dietary deficiency not recognized.	Egg, liver, meats, legumes, wheat, bran, milk.
Biotin	Role in fatty acid synthesis; reactions involving CO_2	Anorexia, nausea, vomiting.	Egg, milk, liver, sardines, salmon, rice, soybeans, yeast.
Choline	Fat metabolism; nervous system function.		Egg yolk, liver, meats, whole grains, legumes, milk.

Vitamins—Fat Soluble

Vitamins	Function	Possible Deficiency Symptoms	Source
Vitamin A (retinol)	Maintains skin, mucous membranes, hormones, bone development & tooth formation; necessary for new cell growth. Chemistry of vision.	Xerophthalmia, faulty bone development, night blindness, keratinized epithelial cells. Dry, rough skin.	Liver, egg yolk, deep green and deep yellow vegetables and fruits. Mixed vegetables, with carrots. Whole or fortified milk; tomatoes; butter; fortified margarine.
Vitamin D (calciferol)	Regulates intestinal absorption of calcium and phosphorus; bone formation.	Rickets (in children); tetany (adults); osteomalacia, delayed dentition.	Fortified milk; cod liver oil. Synthesis in skin by sunlight (in adults).
Vitamin E (alphatocopherols)	Antioxidant in cells.	Increased hemolysis of red blood cells *in vitro*. Macrocytic anemia and dermatitis in infants.	Vegetable oils, green, leafy vegetables, meats, fish, poultry, eggs, whole grain breads.
Vitamin K	Blood coagulation; prothrombin formation.	Hemorrhages; liver injury.	Green, leafy vegetables, liver. Also produced by intestinal bacteria (K_2).

Minerals

See the Recommended Dietary Allowances of the National Research Council for recommended amounts of minerals.

Minerals	Major Function	Possible Deficiency Symptoms	Good Source
Calcium	Formation of bones & teeth; blood clotting. Muscle & nerve function. Utilization of other minerals by the body.	Growth retardation, tetany, bone deformation (rickets), osteomalacia, osteoporosis, muscle cramping.	Milk, cheese, ice cream, yogurt, broccoli, some green vegetables. Salmon, sardines, whole canned fish.
Phosphorus	Deposited with calcium in bone & tooth formation.	Demineralization of bones.	Foods high in calcium; meats, turkey. Cereals, nuts, legumes, whole grains.
Iodine	Integral part of thyroid hormones, thyroxines, and triiodothyronine.	Endemic goiter. Also an increased need in cretinism, thyrotoxicosis.	Seafood, iodized salt (excellent sources). Vegetables, meats, dairy products, breads, & cereals.
Magnesium	Activates enzymes involved in protein synthesis.	Growth failure.	Dried beans; dark green, leafy vegetables. Soybeans, fish & shellfish. Wheat germ; whole wheat bread.
Zinc	Constituent of various metalloenzymes.	Growth failure (hypogonadism and dwarfism).	Pork liver, lean meats, shellfish, poultry, peanuts, cheese, whole grain bread.

Trace Elements

See the Recommended Dietary Allowances of the National Research Council for recommended amounts of specific minerals.

	Major Functions	Possible Toxicity	Sources	Interactions Affecting Absorption or Utilization	Deficiency Signs & Indications of Increased or Decreased Need
Chromium	Cofactor for insulin.	None demonstrated from excess consumption of food.	Brewer's yeast, black pepper, liver, cheese, wheat germ, whole grain breads & cereals.		Reported decline in tissue levels with an increase in age or long-term TPN.
Cobalt	Essential component of vitamin B_{12}.	Excess causes polycythemia, hyperplasia of bone marrow & interferes with cell oxidation.	Beet tops, buckwheat, figs, lettuce, pears, spinach, walnuts, apricots, wax beans, cabbage, corn, onions, potatoes, rice.		Deficiency relevant to strict vegetarians whose intake of preformed vitamin B_{12} severely limited, those solely dependent on bacterial form (e.g., Strict vegetarian).
Copper	Cofactor for erythocytosu-peroxide dismutase.	None demonstrated from excess consumption of food. Primarily as a result of excess parenteral administration of copper.	Shellfish, liver, nuts, seeds, dried legumes.	High Zinc intake depresses absorption and retention. Iron deficiency increases Copper absorption.	Decreased need in Wilson's disease. Increased need in some hypochromic anemias. Deficiency signs include anemia.
Fluoride	Incorporation into tooth enamel whereby susceptibility of solubilization by acid is reduced.	Fluorosis.	Tea, salt pork, seafood, Fluoridated water, potatoes, wheat germ, beef, lamb, kale, cheese, butter, apples.		Beneficial for maintaining teeth and a normal skeleton.

Trace Elements, continued

	Major Functions	Possible Toxicity	Sources	Interactions Affecting Absorption/ Utilization	Deficiency Signs & Indications
Iron	Constituent of hemoglobin, myoglobin and a number of enzymes.	None demonstrated from excess consumption of food.	Liver, organ meats, meat, dried peas & beans, enriched or whole grains.	See High Iron Diet. Absorption capacity of iron.	For increased need see High Iron Diet (indications for use). Decreased need due to genetic defect (e.g., hemo-chromiatosis).
Manganese	Constituent of several enzymes.	None demonstrated from excess consumption of food.	Whole grains, egg yolk, green vegetables, shellfish, liver, and tea.	Less than 5% of ingested Manganese is absorbed.	Deficiency signs are poor reproductive performance, growth retardation, congenerative malformations, impaired glucose tolerance, abnormal formation of the cartilage. Needed in specific enzyme activity, oxidative phosphoryla-tion, cofactor in fatty acid and cholesterol synthesis.
Molybdenum	Constituent of several enzymes.	None demonstrated from excess consumption of food.	Legumes, cereals, grains, leafy vegetables, liver, kidney, milk & public water supply.	Adequate protein intake is needed for elimination of dietary Mo. Toxic levels of Mo antago-nistic to Cu.	
Selenium	Presence at active site of glutathione peroxidase.	None demonstrated from excess consumption of food.	Seafoods, kidney, liver, meats, grains	Functions in close association with vitamin E.	Increased need in prolonged administration of TPN unsup-plemented with selenium.

Vegetarian Diets

General Description

A considerable body of scientific data suggests a positive relationship between vegetarian diets and risk reduction for several chronic diseases. The American Dietetic Association position paper on vegetarian diets (1993) recognizes the vegetarian diet as a healthful and nutritionally adequate dietary alternative for all groups when appropriately planned.

Vegetarian diets can be categorized into several types. The following types are the most common:

- Vegan: People who exclude all foods of animal origin - meat, poultry, fish, eggs, and dairy products such as milk, cheese, and ice cream.
- Lacto-ovo: People who include milk products and eggs, but exclude meat, poultry, and fish.
- Lacto: People who include milk or milk products, but exclude meat, poultry, fish and eggs.

Nutritional Adequacy

A well planned vegetarian diet consisting of a variety of largely unrefined plant foods supplemented with some milk and eggs (lacto-ovo) meets all known nutrient needs for growth.

A total plant diet (vegan) can be made adequate by careful planning and should include reliable sources of B-12, vitamin D and riboflavin. Intake of these vitamins will be adequate if an appropriately supplemented rice or soy beverage is used. Calcium, iron, and zinc intakes may also deserve special attention, although intakes are usually adequate if a variety of foods and adequate energy are consumed.

Energy

In marginally adequate ranges of protein intake, energy levels appear to have a much greater effect on nitrogen balance than does protein. A vegetarian diet (vegan) must be properly planned to provide needed calories. If adequate calories are not planned, dietary protein will be metabolized to provide the energy needed. Dietary protein should be used to maintain tissue protein and other protein functions. Under these circumstances, a protein content equivalent to the Recommended Dietary Allowances (RDAs) may become marginal or even deficient. However, when more food is ingested to meet energy needs, not only is protein spared for protein functions, but the protein content of the diet will also increase.

Protein

Plant sources of protein can provide adequate amounts of the essential amino acids and nonessential amino acids, assuming that dietary protein sources from plants are reasonably varied and that caloric intake is sufficient to meet energy needs and support growth.

It is not necessary to plan combinations of these foods within a given meal. A mixture of plant protein eaten throughout the day will provide enough essential amino acids. Beans, breads, cereals, nuts, peanut butter. tofu, soy milk or cow's milk, and low-fat cheese are some foods which are especially good sources of protein.

Food Combinations Which Provide Complementary Proteins

Carbohydrates

Carbohydrates, especially complex carbohydrates, are the major source of energy. Plant carbohydrates usually provide liberal amounts of dietary fiber.

Fats

Plant fats differ from animal fats in two ways: They are cholesterol free, and many contain a higher percentage of poly- and mono-unsaturated fatty acids compared to animal fats that contain high amounts of saturated fatty acids. (Palm, palm kernel, and coconut oils are the exceptions -- they contain higher percentages of saturated fatty acids than other plant oils.)

Vitamins and Minerals

Vitamin B-12

Vitamin B-12 is found only in animal products. Individuals that consume milk or milk products and eggs are unlikely to be deficient in B12. Vegans should include a reliable source of B-12 in their diets. Previously recommended sources of vitamin B-12, such as unfortified nutritional yeast, seaweed, tempeh and other fermented foods, are not reliable since their vitamin B-12 content is variable and they often contain inactive analogs.

Sources of B-12 include:
- Fortified soy or rice beverage
- Fortified breakfast cereal (Total, Corn Flakes, Grape Nuts, Product 19)
- Fortified meat substitute
- Supplement in which B-12 is present (or cobalamin)
- Red Star T-6635 nutritional yeast (1 Tbsp)

Riboflavin

Milk and meat are among the best sources of riboflavin. Lacto-ovo vegetarians tend to meet the RDA. However, an adequate supply may be difficult to obtain on a vegan diet. Dark green leafy vegetables, legumes, soy foods, and sea vegetables are good plant sources of riboflavin. For children on a vegan diet, fortified soy and rice beverage should be included.

Vitamin D

Vitamin D is vital for absorption of calcium. Those at greatest risk of vitamin D deficiency are infants who are breastfed for more than 6 months without supplementation of the vitamin or adequate exposure to sunlight. Children who have no dietary source of vitamin D and who have limited exposure to sunlight may require supplements.

Calcium

Calcium is needed for strong bones as well as nerve and muscle function and blood clotting. Foods rich in this mineral include beans, soy products (tofu, TVP, soy milk, tempeh), dark green leafy vegetables, sea vegetables, and many nuts and seeds. Consuming four to five servings of these calcium rich foods can meet the RDA.

Calcium requirements may be influenced by high protein intakes. High protein diets seem to increase calcium excretion. Therefore, a vegetarian diet whose protein intake is lower may be associated with better calcium retention.

Each of the following foods supply about 300 mg. calcium, the amount in one cup of milk:
- 1 cup fortified soy milk
- 2 cup cooked broccoli
- 1 1/2 cups cooked bok choy, kale, or mustard greens
- 8 ounces tofu, processed with calcium
- 1 cup calcium-fortified orange juice

Iron

Iron deficiency occurs in both vegetarians and non vegetarians. Heme iron, which is more easily absorbed, is present only in animal tissues. Meat, fish, and poultry contain approximately 40% heme and 60% nonheme iron. Inhibitors and enhancers affect the absorption of nonheme iron, the form of iron found in plants. Factors that inhibit nonheme iron absorption include phytic acid in whole grain cereals, tannic acid in tea, and soy protein. The effects of these inhibitors of iron absorption seem to be overcome when foods rich in vitamin C are consumed at the same meal.

Non-heme Iron Sources
- Legumes, lentils
- Iron-fortified breakfast cereal
- Whole grains
- Nuts
- Green leafy vegetables, spinach, broccoli, collard greens
- Eggs
- Dried fruit
- Tofu

Vitamin C Sources
- Citrus fruits and juice
- Fortified fruit juice
- Potatoes
- Strawberries
- Cantaloupe
- Broccoli
- Tomato and spaghetti sauce

Zinc

Since zinc is essential for growth, tissue repair, and sexual maturation, it is important to include adequate amounts in the diets of children. Good non-meat sources of zinc include:
- Legumes
- Whole grains
- Nuts
- Milk

Special Considerations

1. All vegetarians should choose from a wide variety of foods and consume adequate calories to meet energy needs. Since vegan diets tend to be high in bulk, care should be taken to ensure that infants and children consume sufficient amounts of calories to meet energy needs.
2. Vegetarian (and non-vegetarian) infants who are solely breastfed beyond 4-6 months of age should receive supplements of iron and vitamin D (if exposure to sunlight is limited).
3. Young children should receive milk or fortified soy or rice beverage.

4. Vegans should have a reliable source of vitamin B-12 such as fortified breakfast cereal, fortified soy or rice beverage, or supplement. A vitamin D supplement is recommended if exposure to sunlight is limited.
5. Some meat analogs (textured vegetable protein) have a high sodium content and should not be included in the diets of infants.

Professional References

1. American Dietetic Association. Position paper on vegetarian diets. J Am Dietetic Assoc. 1993;93:13171319.
2. Sabate J, Lindsted K, Harris R, Sanchez A. Attained height of lacto-ovo vegetarian children and adolescents. Eur J Clin Nutr. 1991;45:51-58.
3. O'Connell J, Dibley M, Sierra J, Wallace B, Marks J, Yip R. Growth of vegetarian children: The Farm study. Pediatrics. 1989;84:475-480.
4. Heaney R, Weaver C. Calcium Absorption from Kale. Am J Clin Nutr. 1989;51:656.
5. Dwyer J. Nutritional consequences of vegetarianism. Annual Review of Nutrition. 1991;11:61-91.
6. Marsh A, Sanchez T, Michelsen O, Chaffee F, Fagal S. Vegetarian lifestyle and bone mineral density. Am J Clin Nutr. 1988;48:837-841.
7. Jacobs C, Dwyer J. Vegetarian children: Appropriate and inappropriate diets. Amer J of Clin Nutr. 1988;48(3):811-818.
8. Seventh-Day Adventist Dietetic Association, P.O. Box 75, Loma Linda, CA 92354. (714)824-4593.
9. Vegetarian Nutrition Dietetic Practice Group, American Dietetic Association, 216 West Jackson Blvd., Chicago, IL 60606-6995. (312)899-0400.
10. The Vegetarian Resource Group, P.O. Box 1463, Baltimore, MD 21203. (301)366-8343.

Client Resources

11. Eating Well - The Vegetarian Way. 1992. Available from the American Dietetic Association, 216 West Jackson Blvd., Chicago, IL 60606-6995. (312)899-0400.
12. So you Want to be a Vegetarian? 1990. Available from Vegetarian Education Network, P.O. Box 3347, West Chester, PA 19380. (215)696-VNET.
13. Robbins, John. Diet For A New America. Walpole, NH: Stillpoint Publishing, 1987.
14. Robbins, John. May All Be Fed. New York. William Morrow and Co., 1992.
15. Robertson, Laurel: Flinders, Carol; Ruppenthal, Brian. The New Laurel's Kitchen: Berkeley: Ten Speed Press, 1986.
16. Ballentine, Rudolph MD. Transition to Vegetarianism. Honesdale, PA: The Himalayan International Institute, 1897.
17. Vegetarian Journal's Guide to Natural Foods Restaurants in the U.S. and Canada. The Vegetarian Resource Group. Avery Publishing. 1(800)548-5757.
18. Madison, Deborah. The Greens Cookbook. New York: Bantam Books, 1987.
19. Frances Moore Lappe. Diet For a Small Planet. New York. Ballantine Books, 1982.
20. Messina, Mark and Messina, Virginia. The Vegetarian Way. New York. Crown Trade Paperbacks, 1996.
21. Kriznanic, Judy. A Teen's Guide to Going Vegetarian. Puffin Books. 1994.

Websites

1. http://www.soyfoods.com
2. http://envirolink.orglaws/VRG/home.html
3. http://catless.ncl.ac.uk/veg/Guide
4. World Guide to Vegetarianism
   (lists vegetarian and vegetarian-friendly restaurant, stores, organizations, etc.)

Diet Plan for the Vegan Child[*]

Food Group	Standard Serving Size	Daily Servings		
		6 mo. to 1 year	1 to 4 years	4 to 6 years
Enriched cereals or grains	1 to 5 TBSP	½ (½ to 2½ TBSP) finely ground	1	2
Breads	1 slice	1	3	4
Legumes, meat analogs, soy products, nuts, seeds (grind for toddlers)	1 to 6 TBSP	2 cooked and sieved	3 chopped (1/4 – ½ c)	3 (½ - 1 c)
Fortified soy milk (Isomil, Nursoy, Prosobee, Soyalac, etc.)	1 cup	3	3	3
Fruits (include two servings of citrus fruit or juice each day)	¼ to ½ cup	3 pureed	4 juice or chopped	5
Vegetables, green leafy or deep yellow	¼ to 1/3 cup	¼ (1 to 1½ TBSP)	½ (2 to 2½ TBSP)	1
Other		½ (2 to 2½ TBSP) cooked and pureed	1 chopped	1
Oils	1 tsp	0	3	4
Miscellaneous Red Star (T-6635+) Brewer's yeast Molasses Wheat germ	1 TBSP 1 TBSP 1 TBSP	0 0 0	1 1 optional	1 1 optional

*Truesdell DD, Acosta PB. Feeding the vegan infant and child. Copyright, The American Dietetic Association. Reprinted by permission from JOURNAL OF THE AMERICAN DIETETIC ASSOCIATION 1985;85:837

The Practitioner's Guide to Vegetarian Nutrition

Category	Kcal	Protein	Vitamins/Minerals
Pregnancy	300	60 grams	Calcium: absorbed especially well during pregnancy; calcium needs lower in vegetarians with lower protein intake; consume 4 or more servings of greens, tofu, blackstrap molasses, and Tahini. RDA 600-1200 mg/day

Category	Kcal	Protein	Vitamins/Minerals
			Iron: needed for increased maternal blood volume and formation of baby's blood; sources include whole and enriched grains, legumes, nuts and seeds, and many vegetable and dried meats; RDA 30 mg/day
			B12: needed for tissue synthesis; sources include fortified cereals, soy milk, meat analogues.
			Zinc: needed for growth and development; RDA 2x amount as for non-pregnant; sources include grains and nuts.
			Folic Acid: increased needs during pregnancy; sources include whole grains, nuts, legumes, and oranges.
Lactation	500	65 grams	B12 & Vitamin D
Infants			Iron, vitamin D, vitamin B12
Children	Adequate to meet needs	Soy products (tofu, soy-milk, Tempeh, textured vegetable protein (TVP)), grains (bread, pasta, crackers, rice)	**Calcium:** sources include figs, calcium-fortified orange juice, oranges, tofu, baked beans, raw broccoli, almond butter, Tahini, fortified soymilk, and cow's milk; RDA 800 mg/day
		RDA 0.4-0.5 grams/#	**Iron:** supplement at 6 months.
			Vitamin D: sun exposure (20-30 minutes 2-3 times per week), cow's milk, eggs, fortified soymilks, cereals, and meat analogues.
			B12: sources include fortified soymilk, Red Star T-6635+ nutritional yeast, cereals and meat analogues.
			Iron: sources include iron-fortified infant cereals, enriches grains, soy products, dried fruits, beans, and nuts; serve good sources vitamin C to increase iron absorption.
			Riboflavin: needed for production of energy; sources include cow's milk, fortified milks, whole grains, almonds, almond butter and avocados.
Teens	Needs 50% more kcals than adults	Beans, breads, cereals, nuts, peanut butter, tofu, soy milk, cow's milk, cheese.	**Calcium:** RDA 1200 mg/day; sources include dairy products, tofu, green leafy vegetables.
			Iron: 12(boys)-15(girls) mg/day; consume vitamin C source with iron-rich foods.
			B12: needs 50% more than that for young children; sources include fortified soymilk, cereals, and meat analogues.
			Zinc: crucial for bone growth and sexual maturation; high levels of protein and phosphorus may raise zinc needs; sources include cow's milk, legumes, oatmeal, bran flakes, nuts, and leafy green vegetables.

Cultural Food Ways

When completing the socio-economic assessment of a patient or client, the dietitian should have information about the food practices which different groups of people observe, taking care to avoid generalizations about food practices, while remaining sensitive to the variability of an individual's food preferences. This awareness is basic to successful implementation of a program of general nutrition or medical nutrition therapy.

Cultural food ways may consist of the use or avoidance of various foods for religious practices or celebrations. In addition some people also believe that certain foods are needed for restoring strength, vigor, and longevity. During times of illness or other stress, these foods are particularly important. This food may be as common as chicken noodle soup, or fruit juices, or for a person of Latin heritage, it may be the use of certain "hot" or "cold" foods to restore a healthful balance.

From a professional perspective, most of these food practices may be considered helpful or harmless, while a few may be considered harmful. Emphasizing the positive, the dietitian or nutrition education can maximize the effectiveness of the diet or nutrition education by honoring these practices.

Reference:

1. Jones, DV and M Darling. *Ethnic Foodways in Minnesota: Handbook of Food and Wellness across Cultures.* St. Paul: University of Minnesota, Department of Food Science and Nutrition, 1995/1996.

African-American Food Ways
Typical food habits

- Two or three meals are eaten per day, along with several snacks. The large meal usually is served at midday.
- "Soul food" is thought of as well-seasoned meats and starches that are simple, nourishing, and abundant.
- Rice, potatoes, and hominy grits frequently are eaten. Biscuits, rolls, bread, or corn bread often accompany meals.
- Common meats include chicken, fish, pork chops and ribs, liver, and cured meats such as ham and bacon. Meat may be eaten at all meals and is often breaded and fried.
- Eggs and legumes, especially black-eyed peas and butterbeans, may be eaten frequently.
- Vegetables most often eaten include greens, sweet potatoes or yams, cabbage, green beans, corn, and peas. Vegetables are usually flavored with bacon, sausage, or salt pork, and are cooked for a long time.
- A wide variety of fresh fruits are popular.
- There may be limited use of milk by adults. Lactose intolerance is quite common.
- Pop and other sweetened beverages often are served as a mealtime beverage.
- Snacks and desserts include cookies, pie, fruit cobbler, cake, ice cream, candy, chips, and pop.

Positive diet features

- The traditional diet is quite high in complex carbohydrates and fiber.
- Dark green and yellow vegetables (vitamin A sources) are familiar and popular.
- Small amounts of meat are often "stretched" by serving a large portion of starch, legumes, or vegetables.
- The traditional diet is often high in calcium due to large amounts of turnip greens, collard greens, and kale eaten, including the cooking liquid.
- Food is regarded as a symbol of hospitality and friendliness. Great pride is taken in homestyle cooking.

Nutritional concerns
- High fat cuts of meat often are preferred.
- Many foods are prepared by frying. Lard or bacon fat often is used.
- Calcium intake may be low due to limited use of milk, cheese, and decreased consumption of greens.
- Prolonged cooking time for vegetables destroys much of the vitamin C.
- Sodium intake is potentially quite high due to use of cured meats, salt, and salt-based seasonings.
- Increased use of fast food or convenience versions of traditional foods (such as fried chicken) often increases fat and sodium intake and reduces intake of more nutritious traditional foods (such as greens, sweet potatoes).

Dietary counseling recommendations

- Select lower fat meats. Trim fat and/or drain off any visible fat as needed.

- Prepare foods by boiling, baking, broiling, steaming, or stewing rather than frying. If food is fried, use vegetable oil. Try "oven-frying" to maintain traditional flavor and reduce some fat.

- Cook vegetables for a shorter length of time. Use onions, garlic, vinegar, etc., for seasoning instead of salt.

- Reduce use of salt and cured meats, especially if high blood pressure is present.

- Select low fat milk, such as 1%, skim, or buttermilk. Serve milk at each meal, especially for children. Serve milk in small amounts if needed to avoid symptoms of lactose intolerance.

- Select snacks and desserts lower in fat and sugar, such as ice milk, fruit ice, low fat frozen yogurt, and fresh fruits.

- Suggest trying lower fat versions of traditional foods, such as turkey ham, reduced fat sausage, and using smaller amounts to season foods.

Professional references

1. Black Americans, cultural foods and renal diets. Council on Renal Nutrition of N. California and N. Nevada, 1990.
2. Kaplan, Anne R., Marjorie A. Hoover, Willard B. Moore. *The Minnesota Ethnic Food Book.* St. Paul: Minnesota Historical Society Press, 1986, pp. 235-260.
3. Kittler, Pamela G. and Sucher, Kathryn. *Food and Culture in America* New York: Van Nostrand Reinhold, 1989, pp. 285-311.
4. Minnesota Department of Health WIC Program. *Nutrition a la Culture: Nutrition Education Units for Minority Groups Served by the WIC and MAC Programs.* Minnesota: Minnesota Department of Health WIC Program, 1992.

Client resources

1. Minnesota Department of Health WIC Program. Nutrition a la Culture: Nutrition Education Units for Minority Groups Served by the WIC and MAC Programs. Minnesota: Minnesota Department of Health WIC Program. 1992.
2. National Cancer Institute. Down Home Healthy: Family Recipes of Black American Chefs Leah Chase and Johnny Rivers. Bethesda, MD: National Cancer Institute, Feb. 1993. NIH Publication No. 93-3408.

Ethiopian Food Ways
Typical food habits

- The diet is rich in legumes, beans, grains, and vegetables, with small amounts of meat being used.

- Most foods are turned into stews called "wat." These stews are served on a flat fermented bread called injera or budeena.

- Food is eaten with the right hand only and scooped up with a piece of bread. Utensils are not used.

- Typical vegetables eaten are collard greens, onions, potatoes, cabbage, peppers (both hot and sweet), and carrots.

- Typical grains are wheat, buckwheat, and xaafii (t'ah-fee). Xaafii is a special strain of millet grown in Ethiopia.

- Meat is only an occasional addition. Pork is not eaten due to religious law, and Coptic Christian Ethiopians are vegetarians. Fasting is a frequent occurrence, totaling about 200 days per year. Fasting to Ethiopians involves not eating until midday and then abstaining from any type of animal product for the rest of the day. Consequently, Ethiopians have created many vegetarian substitutes for meat.

- Ethiopians are accustomed to eating raw meat and eggs in their country.

- Dessert is not common. The cuisine has developed completely without white sugar, but honey is used in coffee and wine making.

- There are 72 different nations in Ethiopia, each with its own regional way of cooking. However, the basic food staples remain the same throughout the country. The main difference lies in the way the foods are spiced.

- Blending spices is very important and mixtures are especially HOT. The proper spices are hard to obtain in the United States. Berbere is the common spice mixture used in most stews. It is said that the right spice mixtures are ones "that linger in the mind long after they have faded from the tongue."

- There is usually no fixed routine for eating. Most Ethiopians have two or maybe only one meal per day. Snacking is common.

Positive diet features

- The diet is vegetable-based, with small amounts of meat.

- Refined sugar is traditionally not incorporated into the diet.

- There is a communal dining tradition.

- Bread (injera or budeena) is eaten at every meal—grains are an integral part of the diet. Therefore, complex carbohydrate intake is quite high.

Nutritional concerns

- Large quantities of butter are used in cooking.

- Coffee trees grow wild in Ethiopia and therefore some people are very heavy coffee drinkers.

- Eating raw meat and eggs may be unsafe and therefore is not recommended.

- Ethiopians do not eat a lot of dairy products, except butter. They may be lactose intolerant.

- More men than women have immigrated here. In Ethiopia, women do all the cooking and serving of food. Men may need to learn cooking skills in the United States.

Dietary counseling recommendations

- Reinforce traditional eating habits. Discourage the addition of sugary foods, such as pop, candy and desserts.

- Suggest fats other than butter for cooking, such as margarine or vegetable oil.

- Encourage cooking meat and eggs, rather than eaten raw.

Professional references

Center for Applied Linguistics. Ethiopians Refugee Fact Sheet Series #1. Washington, DC: Center for Applied Linguistics, June 1981.

Jewish Kosher Dietary Guidelines
Description

The term Kosher defines what is fit and proper to eat according to the Jewish Dietary Laws (Kashrath). These laws comprise the written regulations that have been carried down through the centuries. There are three major Jewish groups each with its own degree of adherence to the teachings:

- Orthodox - strict observance of the dietary laws
- Conservative - less rigid, but most follow some of the dietary laws
- Reform - less likely to follow the dietary laws, but some may observe some laws especially regarding holidays.

Adherence to dietary laws is an individual matter. In an acute or long-term care setting, it is best to discuss the matter with the patient or client and their family.

The Jewish dietary laws emphasize three areas:
- Forbidden foods
- Selection and slaughter of food
- Mixing of foods.

- <u>Forbidden foods (*treif*)</u>: In general meat (*fleishig*) must be the forequarters of cloven-hoofed animals which chew the cud. This allows cattle, sheep, goats and deer to be eaten, but eliminates pigs and rabbits. In addition domestic chicken, turkey, goose, pheasant or duck are allowed; wild game, wild game birds and birds of prey are not allowed. Only meat which has been properly raised and slaughtered is allowed (i.e. Kosher meat). Fish with fins and removable scales are allowed. Lobster, shrimp and crab are not allowed. Fish does not need the Koshering process, as does other meat. Blood from any animal may not be eaten, including an egg with a blood spot in the yolk. Some dairy foods are not allowed because they are made with non-Kosher meat derivatives such as rennin in cheese, gelatin in ice cream or yogurt, and other derivatives. Usually Kosher alternatives are available.

- <u>Selection and slaughter of food</u>: Slaughtering of animals must be done by a shocket, a observant Jew who is specially trained to do Kosher slaughtering. Slaughter is conducted in a very precise manner and the carcass must be inspected and stamped with the place, date and hour of slaughter, the city and name of the shocket. The Koshering process must follow within 72 hours after slaughter. It is a specific process which includes salting the carcass with coarse salt, then draining and rinsing the meat. It is not known how much salt remains in the meat, thus Kosher meat may have a higher sodium content than non-Kosher meat and may not be appropriate for children on sodium restricted diets.

- <u>Mixing foods</u>: Dairy and meat products may not be mixed together or eaten at the same meal. Dairy (or *milchig*) is considered any milk or milk products including lactose, nonfat dry milk solids, and casein. Dairy foods may be consumed before a meat meal, but some believe the milk must be consumed at least an hour before the meat. Rules vary as to the amount of time that must pass after eating meat before milk or milk products can be eaten, but is usually 72 minutes to 6 hours. Neutral (*pareve*) foods may be eaten with fish or dairy foods. This includes eggs, fish, fruits, vegetables, grains, and some margarine (margarine may not be neutral if it is made with lactose, lactic acid, sodium caseinate or whey). Fish is considered pareve and can be eaten at the same meal as meat, but can not be mixed with meat. It is traditionally eaten before the meat. Traditional orthodox Jews often keep two separate sets of dishes, silverware, and cooking equipment (including ovens, dishwasher racks, etc.) for meat and dairy. They may not accept foods prepared in utensils or equipment used for both meat and milk products.

Jewish Holidays

Many Jewish holidays or holy days are associated with specific food-related practices. Individual Jews' practices will vary, but the most common practices are mentioned here. The Jewish Sabbath (Shabbat) begins each Friday at sundown until sundown on Saturday. Some Jewish families consume special foods (most frequently wine and challah bread) as part of their celebration.

HOLIDAY	WHEN CELEBRATED	PRACTICES
Rosh Hashanah*	September or October	Usually prepare special sweet foods such as apples dipped in honey and honey cakes. No bitter or sour foods. Challah baked in a round shape.
Tzom Gedaliah	Day after Rosh Hashanah	Fast
Yom Kippur*	Ten days after Rosh Hashanah	Fast sunset to sunset, followed by a light meal usually dairy foods or fish, fruit and vegetable.
Sukkot	September or October, lasts one week	Festival of thanksgiving, usually consume special foods associated with harvest such as fruits and fall vegetables.
Hanukkah	Late November or December, lasts for 8 days	Foods fried in oil, especially potato pancakes (latkes)
Purim	February or March	Some fast the day before. A special fruit- or poppy seed- filled cookie, called hamentashen, is often eaten.
Passover*	March or April, lasts for 8 days, first 2 days are primary celebration	Unleavened bread and foods "Kosher for Passover" eaten throughout. Many commercial products are available. Many other special traditional foods are usually eaten during the first two days during a ritual meal. Observant Jews often have a special set of dishes specifically for Passover. Some fast the day before Passover.

*Indicates major holidays observed by almost all Jewish families.

A few other fast days are observed by some Jews. Most fast days are from sunrise to sunset (except Yom Kippur and Tisha b' Av which are from sunset to sunset). On days of fast no food or water are allowed for all boys 13 years and older and girls 12 and older except those who are seriously ill and pregnant or breastfeeding women. Medications are allowed.

Label Reading

A system of labeling exists to help identify if food products are Kosher including therapeutic dietary formulas). The marking (or symbol) is referred to as a hechster. Processed foods are only considered Kosher if they have been certified by a rabbinical authority. Some foods may be referred to as Kosher-style, but these may not be truly Kosher. The symbols must be observed carefully. Common symbols are:

U   Indicates a food is Kosher and is administered by the Union of Orthodox Jewish Congregation of America.

K   Indicates a food is Kosher and is administered by the Organized Kasrus Laboratories.

K   Indicates the company has rabbinical supervision. Some observant Jews may not accept foods with this symbol as it can be misused.

Pareve Indicates a food is considered neutral.

Indications for Use

Any patient that indicates they practice Judaism should be asked about dietary practices and beliefs. Practices vary greatly and it is important to work out a feeding plan that meets the medical needs of the patient, is acceptable to the family and manageable for your facility. Important issues to discuss include:

- Use of Kosher foods, especially meat
- Mixing of meat and dairy, specific rules they follow regarding time between serving meat and dairy
- Practices and preferences for food preparation and serving
- Sabbath foods
- Holidays or holy days, specifically if any will fall during the patient's stay and if they will require any special foods or changes in eating habits.

Nutritional Adequacy

A Kosher diet is nutritionally adequate. Considerations include:

1. Evaluating any need for sodium restriction in which case consumption of Kosher meats may need to be limited.
2. Meal patterns may need to be modified to avoid serving meat and dairy at the same meal. Children may need to be served milk or dairy products as snacks to assure adequate consumption.
3. Holy days which require fasting. Fasting may not be appropriate for a pediatric patient and some type of agreement may need to be worked out with the family.

Other Considerations

In a hospital or long term facility, strict adherence to Jewish dietary laws requires the installation of special facilities and equipment. Some modifications are often possible to meet the needs and wishes of the Jewish family, such as preparing foods in foil, using disposable dishes and silverware, using prepackaged frozen Kosher dinners, or having the family provide some foods.

Professional references

1. American Dietetic Association. *Regional Food Practice Series: Jewish Food Practices, Customs, and Holidays*. Chicago: American Dietetic Association, 1990.
2. Kittler, Pamela G. and Kathryn Sucher. *Food and Culture in America*. New York: Van Nostrand Reinhold, 1989, pages 20-28.
3. Local Rabbinical Association in larger metropolitan areas (consult phone directory under Rabbinical Association or Jewish Community Center); local Rabbi or Synagogue

Client resources

1. American Dietetic Association. *Meal Planning With Jewish Foods*. Chicago: American Dietetic Association, 1990.

Mexican-American Food Ways

Typical Food Habits

- Three or four meals are eaten per day, with the noon, or early afternoon meal traditionally being the largest. Early breakfast and/or early evening supper may consist of only sweetened coffee with milk and a sweet yeast bread or sweet roll (pan dulce).
- Tortillas, beans, rice and chili sauce (salsa) are basic staple foods and may be eaten several times per day.
- Beans, usually pinto, may be served boiled (de olla) or refried (refritos).
- Tortillas may be corn or flour. The choice is often dependent on what region of Mexico a person is from, with persons from northern Mexico using more flour tortillas. An adult can quite easily consume 5-10 tortillas per meal, as tortillas are often used as an eating utensil to scoop up other food.
- A variety of meats are eaten, with the amount and kind often dependent on income. Meats include beef, pork, chicken, fish, and variety meats, such as tongue, liver, brains, and intestine. Meat seldom is served alone, but often extended by addition of potatoes, chilis, tomatoes, or other foods.
- Eggs are eaten often, and are prepared in a variety of ways.
- Common vegetables include red and green chili peppers, tomatoes, tomatillas, lettuce, avocados, corn, green beans, peas, potatoes, squash, carrots, sweet potatoes, cabbage, cactus leaves (nopales), and jicama. Vegetables generally are purchased fresh.
- Fresh fruits include oranges, lemons, limes, bananas, watermelon, cantaloupe, mangoes, papaya, guavas, pineapple, apples, grapes, peaches, and plantains. Choices and frequency of consumption often are dependent on income and availability.
- Milk is more commonly consumed as a beverage by children than adults, with whole milk preferred. Adults may drink various beverages which include milk, such as cafe con leche, hot chocolate, atole, avena, liquados, and maizena. Milk is also used in preparing custard (flan) and rice with milk (arroz con leche). Various cheeses are often used in cooking including cheddar, Monterey Jack, American, and Mexican cheese (queso fresco).
- Traditional seasonings include chilis, cumin, cilantro, onion, garlic, oregano, vanilla, and cinnamon.
- Snack foods include pop, Kool-Aid®, ice cream, popsicles, cookies, cakes, donuts, chips, fresh fruit, fruit juices, candy, and chicharrones (fried pork rind).

Positive Diet Features

- The traditional diet is high in complex carbohydrates.
- Fruits and vegetables frequently eaten are rich in vitamins A and C.
- There is little traditional use of processed foods.
- Corn tortillas and beans, eaten together, provide high quality protein.
  Corn tortillas contribute calcium to the diet due to the lime treatment of corn. Six to eight corn tortillas provide the same amount of calcium as one 8-ounce glass of milk (300 mg).

Nutritional Concerns

- There is liberal use of fat, especially lard, in food preparation. Much food is fried, including meat, beans, rice, and potatoes. Lard is traditionally used to make flour tortillas.
- High-fat meats often are preferred. The skin of chicken is considered delectable. Chorizo, a spicy sausage, and chicharrones (fried pork rind) are eaten often, as are bologna, hot dogs, sausage, and bacon.

- A large number of tortillas frequently are eaten, contributing many calories. Often used as an "eating utensil", they may not be included in food recall.
- High egg consumption (2-3 eggs daily) is common.
- Refined sugar intake may be high due to inclusions of many sweet foods and beverages. Sugar is usually added to coffee. Kool-Aid or soda pop are often served as a mealtime beverage. Cookies, donuts, sweet rolls, and candy are common snacks.
- Fat children are considered healthy and parents may be unreceptive to limiting the intake of high calorie foods for children.
- Children are often allowed to have a bottle for an extended time, often beyond two years of age.

Dietary Counseling Recommendations

- Reinforce traditional use of beans, rice and tortillas as "good" and nutritious.
- Encourage corn tortillas for increased fiber and calcium intake and lower fat intake.
- Encourage eating more boiled beans rather than refried beans to decrease fat intake, or preparing refried beans without added fat.
- Suggest boiling, baking, or broiling meats instead of frying.
- Promote vegetable oils instead of lard for cooking.
- For adequate calcium intake, encourage low-fat cheeses, traditional beverages containing milk, and corn tortillas.
- Encourage 1% or 2% milks instead of whole milks (Skim milk is generally avoided, being viewed as "watered-down" and inferior).
- Encourage reduced egg consumption.
- Encourage weaning babies from the bottle at one year of age. Always ask about bottle feeding for young children.

References

1. American Dietetic Association and American Diabetes Association. *Mexican-American Food Practices, Customs, and Holidays.* Chicago: American Dietetic Association, 1989.
2. Cultural influences on dietary patterns, in *Nutrition during Pregnancy and the Postpartum Period: A Manual for Health Care Professionals.* California: WIC, California Department of Health Services, 1990, ,pp. 187-226.
3. Food habits of newly emigrated Hispanics to San Francisco Area. University of California at Berkeley, Cooperative Extension. 1989.
4. *Handbook of Mexican-American food: Recipes, Nutritional Analysis, Diabetic Exchanges, and Common Practices.* San Antonio, TX: Intercultural Dev. Research Assoc, 1982.
5. Hull, M.A., and D.H. Runyan. *The Migrant Farm Worker Nutrition Manual.* Washington, DC: Child Development Center, Georgetown University, 1990.
6. Kaplan, A.R., M.A. Hoover, W.B. Moore. *The Minnesota Ethnic Food Book.* St. Paul: Minnesota Historical Society Press, 1986, pp. 235-260.
7. Kittler, P.G. and K. Sucher. *Food and Culture in America.* New York: Van Nostrand Reinhold, 1989, pp. 285-311.
8. Mexican-American traditional foods, in *Cultural Foods and Renal Diets for Clinical Dietitians.* Council on Renal Nutrition of N. California and N. Nevada, 1990
9. Minnesota Department of Health WIC Program. *Nutrition a la Culture: Nutrition Education Units for Minority Groups Served by the WIC and MAC Programs.* Minnesota: Minnesota Department of Health WIC Program, 1992.

Native American Food Ways

Typical Food Habits

- The diet contains traditional foods such as wild rice, corn, game, such as venison and rabbit, fish, as well as federal commodities and foods purchased at grocery stores.
- Family meal times, snacking, eating on the run, and reliance on convenience and fast foods follow typical American patterns.
- Everyone shares whatever foods are available in the household.
- One person in the extended family often prepares food for everyone in the household.
- Foods commonly are made into soups or stews, or are fried.

Positive Diet Features

- Native Americans take pride in their food customs, although traditional foods may be expensive and difficult to obtain. The traditional diet is lean, green, rich in vitamins, and high in fiber. Traditional foods are still often preferred by adults when available and affordable and eaten at celebrations.
- Venison is seasonally available to families and well liked. It can be used like beef and is quite lean.

Nutritional Concerns

- Food choices and cooking methods may be high in fat.
- Sources of fat are butter, margarine, fatty meats, lard, oil, shortening, salad dressing, and cream.
- Sources of hidden fat, such as milk fat, chips, gravy, sauces, and ice cream, may not be recognized.
- Sugary beverages and foods provide many calories.
- Fruits and vegetables are used infrequently, especially fresh fruits.
- There is a high prevalence of alcohol use.
- Diabetes and obesity are common, and this incidence is increasing among Native Americans.

Dietary Counseling Recommendations

- Suggest boiling, baking, broiling, or microwaving instead of frying.
- Remind clients to remove visible fat and skin from meat or poultry before eating.
- Suggest refrigerating soups and stews before serving and removing the hardened fat.
- Suggest boiling potatoes and squash instead of frying.
- Suggest cooking beans with onions instead of pork fat.
- Compromise on 2% milk if families have overweight adults and children under 2 years old in the same household. Adult households should try to consume 1% or skim milk
- Suggest use of milk, water, or juices without added sugar, instead of sweetened beverages or pop.
- Suggest buying fruit canned without sugar.

Remind families that everything does not have to be fresh. Canned or frozen fruits and vegetables can provide good nutrition.

Southeast Asian Food Ways
Description

Southeast Asians come to the United States with a rich cultural tradition that includes food preferences and practices distinct from those in the United States. Southeast Asians tend to maintain many of their traditional practices rather than adopting those more common in the United States. Since many of these food habits are healthy it is important to support and encourage these practices. Following is a brief description of the practices. Individual practices vary greatly and are changing rapidly with longer acculturation in the United States.

Staple Foods

Southeast Asian people rely on rice and other starch-rich foods to provide most of their energy needs and a significant amount of protein. Traditionally, rice is served at every meal. Portion sizes of starch-rich foods are large--one to one-and-a-half cups for children, and one to three cups for adults. The type of rice a person prefers depends on his or her origin in Indochina. Hmong prefer short-grain rice; Vietnamese and Cambodians like long-grain rice; and Laotians favor glutinous rice and short-grain rice.

Rice is often washed two or three times before cooking. This practice was necessary in Southeast Asia because most rice was coated with talc, an inedible mineral substance. Most rice in the United States, however, including that sold in Oriental groceries does not contain talc. Thus, rinsing is not necessary nor is it recommended because it causes a loss of the vitamins and iron used for enrichment.

Other forms of rice that are commonly used include rice noodles and rice sticks, often cooked in soup, and rice papers, used to wrap meat and noodles into egg rolls. Other types of staple foods that have come to be popular in the United States are French bread, ready-to-eat cereals, and noodle products made from wheat, such as ramen and spaghetti.

Protein Foods

The types of protein foods consumed frequently by Southeast Asians in the United States are not a true reflection of their traditional diet. Pork, chicken, eggs, tofu, organ meats, and peanuts are frequent choices for those living in the United States. Milk and other dairy products are new to the Southeast Asian diet. Dairy foods were not produced in Southeast Asia and were rarely consumed after infancy. The dairy food most familiar to Southeast Asians is sweetened condensed milk. Adults may have difficulty tolerating lactose-containing foods, but children can often consume these products with little difficulty. Sometimes older children share their parents' dislike of these foods, especially cheese, because they have an unfamiliar taste, texture, and smell. However, acceptance is increasing among school-age children especially for cheese in popular American mixed foods such as pizza, macaroni and cheese, and cheeseburgers.

Fish, fish paste, and many types of seafood were used daily by many Cambodians, Vietnamese, and some Laotians in their native countries. Fish paste, fermented fish, dried fish, and high-quality fish sauce are rich sources of calcium and protein. These foods supply much of the calcium in the diet for Cambodians, Hmong, and Vietnamese. Other high-protein foods which may contribute to calcium intake include tofu, sardines, mung beans, and soybeans.

Fruits and Vegetables

A wide variety of fruits and vegetables were enjoyed by Southeast Asian people in their homeland. Because many of these are not available in the United States or because they are very expensive, the types and amounts of produce used have changed significantly. Vegetables that resemble traditional favorites and are relatively inexpensive have become popular and include a type of cabbage, dark leafy greens, broccoli, and green beans.

Several vegetables and fruits also contribute calcium to the diet. Dark leafy greens, broccoli, bok choy, other cabbages, and oranges all contribute significant calcium to the Southeast Asian diet.

Normally, produce is bought fresh, then chopped and stir-fried with meat and seasonings. Rarely does a single vegetable appear on a plate as a side dish. Portion sizes may be small because vegetables are mixed with other ingredients during preparation.

Fruits are purchased fresh and used mainly as snack items or as dessert, patterns learned in the United States. Fruits were not as plentiful in Southeast Asia compared to the United States and therefore were quite expensive. Because of this, fruits are thought of as high-status foods. Many Southeast Asian families in the United States buy fruits only occasionally, as their budgets permit. Among the favorites in the United States are oranges, bananas, apples, grapes, and melons. Sweet fruit juices such as pineapple, grape, and apple are preferred to those that are tart such as orange and grapefruit juices. There is a common misconception that fruit-flavored drinks are the same as fruit juice.

Seasonings

The cuisine of each region of Southeast Asia has its own style and flavor. Cambodian and Vietnamese food is often elaborately seasoned and quite spicy. The Hmong style of cooking is relatively plain, but some dishes are spiced with red peppers.

Fish sauce, soy sauce, monosodium glutamate, salt, red peppers, black pepper, garlic, and vinegar are used by all ethnic groups from Southeast Asia. The Vietnamese pride themselves on the unique cooking style of every family. The cuisine has undoubtedly been influenced by the ethnic Chinese who live in Vietnam and by the French. Indian cuisine has influenced Cambodian cooking, and some dishes are spiced much like curries. Herbs that are used frequently by Southeast Asians in the United States include coriander (Chinese parsley), lemon grass, and mint, as well as a large variety of herbs that are available in Oriental specialty shops.

Other Foods

Almost as soon as they arrive, Southeast Asians become familiar with American sweets and snacks (empty-calorie foods). They equate these foods with high social status and affluence because such foods were very expensive in their native countries. Carbonated beverages and other soft drinks are consumed by almost all individuals, sometimes to the exclusion of fruit, juice, milk, and water. These beverages are used as a refreshment when visitors call and for festive occasions. Also popular are doughnuts, sweet rolls, cookies, candy, ice cream, and chips, especially among children.

With longer residence in the United States children are beginning to prefer some "American" foods such as hot dogs, cereal, pizza, and chocolate milk. School-age children may eat "American" foods for breakfast (such as cold cereal) and lunch (especially when at school), but traditional foods are generally still eaten and enjoyed for the evening meal.

Meal Patterns

Two types of meal patterns have been observed. The most common pattern is that a family eats two meals each day. The first meal of the day is usually eaten at 9:00 or 10:00 a.m., and the other meal is served late in the afternoon at 3:00 or 4:00 p.m. Other Southeast Asian families follow a three-meal per day pattern, having breakfast at 6:00 or 7:00 a.m., dinner at 12:00 or 1:00 p.m., and supper at 6:00 or 7:00 p.m. The midday meal (1:00 or 3:00 p.m.) is by tradition the largest, most elaborate, and most important meal of the day.

Many Southeast Asian families may not always sit down together at the same time to eat a meal, especially for the morning or evening meals. The food may be prepared and made available at meal time, allowing each family member to serve themselves over a period of one to two hours. Thus, some Southeast Asian families may not place a high value on family togetherness at every meal and may be more flexible than Americans in the timing of meals for their children.

Food Preferences

Staple Foods	Vegetables	Seasonings and Others
Rice	Cabbage	Soy sauce
short grain (Hmong, Laotian)	Bok choy	Fish sauce
long grain(Cambodian, Vietnamese)	Chinese cabbage	Salt
glutenous or sweet(Laotian)	Chinese spinach	Monosodium glutamate
Rice noodles	Mustard greens	Black pepper
Rice sticks	Broccoli	Red peppers
Rice papers	Green beans	Coriander leaves
Wheat noodles	Winter squash	Lemon grass
Ramen	Cucumber	Mint
Bean threads	Tomato	Garlic
Bread(French type)	Green Onions	Ginger
Cereals(ready-to-eat or cooked)	Chinese parsley(coriander)	Vinegar
	Peppers(sweet and hot)	Sesame oil
Protein	Bean sprouts	Peanut oil
Pork	Bitter melon	Lard
Chicken	Turnips	
Fish(Cambodian, Laotian, Vietnamese)	Carrots	Snack Foods
Fish paste(Vietnamese, Cambodian, Laotian)	Mushrooms	Pop
Eggs	Leaf Lettuce	Fruit drinks
Beef(Vietnamese, Cambodian)		Kool-aid®
Tofu	Fruit	Doughnuts
Peanuts	Oranges	Sweet rolls
Sesame seeds	Bananas	Cookies
Mung beans	Apples	Ice cream
Soybeans	Grapes	Candy
Milk(children)	Peaches	Potato chips
Organ meats	Cantaloupes	Corn chips
liver	Strawberries	
heart	Pears	
kidney	Papayas	

	Staple Foods	Vegetables	Seasonings and Others
pork stomach		Pineapples	
Seafood(Cambodian, Vietnamese)		Orange juice	
		Apple juice	
		Pineapple juice	

Meal Patterns Typical of Southeast Asians

HMONG	CAMBODIAN	VIETNAMESE	LAOTIAN
MORNING MEAL Rice or rice noodles Chicken (boiled or stir-fried) Broccoli, stir-fried with seasonings OR Egg (boiled or fried) Cereal Milk Orange juice	Rice soup Fried Meat OR Rice Sardines or dried fish OR French bread Meat or egg Water, juice, or milk	Beef soup with rice noodles and bean sprouts OR French bread Boiled eggs Milk or juice	Sweet rice Boiled egg or roast meat Fish sauce
MIDDAY MEAL Rice Pork (stir-fried) Tofu (stir-fried) Cabbage (stir-fried) Juice or water	Soup with meat, cabbage, turnip, and carrot Rice Pork stir-fried with beans and tomato Fish sauce Water or juice	Clear beef noodle soup Rice Chicken cooked with ginger Carrots, broccoli, onion (stir-fried) Fish sauce Water or juice	Clear chicken soup with noodles Rice Sardines Cucumber salad Juice or water
EVENING MEAL Rice Chicken (stir-fried) Spinach Juice or water	Soup with meat and vegetables Rice Fish, fried with fish sauce, garlic, pepper	Clear soup with vegetables Rice Beef stir-fried with bean sprouts and chives Fish sauce Fresh fruit Water or juice	Pork stew with spinach, onion, hot pepper Rice Juice or water
SNACK Fruit, cookie, pop, juice	Fruit , juice, crackers cookie, pop, chips	Fruit	Fruit, juice

Indications for Use

Children from families of Southeast Asian descent should be asked about food preferences. Timing of meals and foods served may need to be adjusted to meet preferences.

Nutritional Adequacy

- <u>Milk and milk products, calcium and vitamin D</u> intake may be low. Consumption of milk and milk products may vary among Southeast Asian children, but usually decreases with age since it is traditionally not consumed. Many traditional foods may be good sources of calcium (greens, fish sauce, tofu) and these should be encouraged.
- <u>Iron</u> intake may be low for some. Small amounts of meat and few other good sources of iron may be consumed. Encourage use of enriched rice and instruct patient's families not to rinse the rice before cooking to improve iron intake. Young children may benefit from iron-rich snacks.
- <u>Fat and saturated fat intake</u> varies greatly. Most Southeast Asians consume less fat than the average person in the United States. However food preparation practices of some groups may contribute to high saturated fat intakes. Many noodles are made with palm oil or lard and may be consumed in large quantities. Some Southeast Asians, especially the Hmong, prefer to cook with lard. Easier access to high fat foods in the United States seems to lead to higher intakes.
- <u>Sodium</u> intake may be high since many of the preferred seasonings are high in sodium (fish sauce and paste, monosodium glutamate, salt, soy sauce). Often several of these seasonings may be used in one dish. Encourage use of more of the other traditional seasonings and smaller amounts of high sodium seasonings.

Other Considerations
General Guidelines

1. Support traditional food choices and patterns.
2. Encourage economical food practices such as buying fruits and vegetables in season, gardening, and making use of locally grown produce.
3. Point out the difference between enriched rice and talc-coated rice. Encourage use of enriched rice and explain that it should not be washed. Most bags have this information on the label in English. This is particularly important for anemic patients.
4. Encourage traditional foods containing calcium, especially when milk and cheese are not tolerated or liked. Encourage milk for children.
5. Accurate dietary assessment is difficult to do because of language and culture differences. Using an interpreter when the client speaks limited English is advised. Using pictures of food or food groups and food models is very helpful, with or without an interpreter.

When Instructing Parents Of Infants

6. Encourage introduction of solid foods to infants beginning at 6 months of age. Follow the guidelines recommended by the American Academy of Pediatrics. Many Southeast Asian parents delay introduction of solids until 9 to 12 months. This may contribute to the commonly observed pattern of deviation from the usual growth curve.
7. Encourage use of iron-fortified infant rice cereal as a replacement for soft, boiled rice in the infant diet.

8. Encourage breastfeeding. Women traditionally breastfed in their native land. Discuss how breastfeeding can be done while the mother goes to school or work by giving supplemental bottles of breast milk or formula.

9. When parents choose to bottle feed, give instructions on sanitary preparation, proper dilution, and refrigeration of formula.

10. Encourage parents to discontinue giving the bottle to their infant by 12 months of age. To do this, caregivers need to be encouraged to introduce the cup to their infant beginning at 6 or 7 months of age. Assess for use of bottle for older children and instruct to discontinue as needed.

11. Instruct parents on proper feeding techniques such as not propping bottles, never put juice or other drinks in bottle, not putting children to bed with a bottle, and not letting a child have a bottle ad lib through the day.

When Instructing Parents Of Children Or The Children Themselves

1. Encourage two or more nutritious snacks for young children each day. When a family eats two meals per day, three substantial snacks per day for young children can be suggested. Snack time may be a good time to encourage milk consumption. Ask parents to carry snacks for children when they are away from home over meal or snack times.

2. Explain the difference between pop, fruit drinks, and 100 percent fruit juice. Identify empty-calorie foods, and suggest that their use be limited to social occasions.

3. It is appropriate to use the standard growth curves developed by the National Center for Health Statistics to assess growth. Deviation of growth from established percentiles on the stature/age and weight/stature grids alerts the health professional to possible dietary or medical problems.

4. Over- and underweight can be assessed best by using the weight-for-length or stature grid. Using this method eliminates errors when a child is of short stature, since the weight is compared to a standard for the child's actual height rather than age.

Professional References

1. Carlson E, Kipps M, Thomson J. Feeding the Vietnamese refugees in the United Kingdom. *J Am Dietetic Assoc* 1982; 81: 164-67.

2. Finn JE. The food practices of the Vietnamese population in Los Angeles County. Los Angeles: University of California, 1978.

3. Fishman,C, Evans R, Jenks E. Warm bodies, cool milk: Conflicts in post postpartum food choice for Indochinese women in California, *Social Science Medicine,*, 26 (11): 1125-1132, 1988.

4. Go K, Moore I. The food habits and practices of Southeast Asians. Alameda County Health Care Services Agency, 1979.

5. Hull MA, Runyan DH. *The Migrant Farm Worker Nutrition Manual.* Washington, DC: Child Development Center, Georgetown University, 1990.

6. Ikeda JP. *Hmong American Food Practices, Customs, and Holidays.* U.S.A.: The American Dietetic Association and the American Diabetes Association, 1992.

7. Ikeda JP, Ceja DR, Glass RS, Hardwood JO, Lucke KA, Sutherlin JM. Food habits of the Hmong living in central California, *Journal of Nutrition Education*, 23: 168-175, 1991.

8. Kaplan AR, Hoover MA, Moore WB. *The Minnesota Ethnic Food Book.* St. Paul: Minnesota Historical Society Press, 1986, pp. 235-260.

9. Kittler PG, Sucher K. *Food and Culture in America.* New York: Van Nostrand Reinhold, 1989, pp. 285-311.

10. Cultural influences on dietary patterns, in *Nutrition During Pregnancy and the Postpartum Period: A Manual for Health Care Professionals.* California: WIC, California Department of Health Services, 1990, pp. 187-226.

11. Minnesota Department of Health WIC Program. *Nutrition a la Culture: Nutrition Education Units for Minority Groups Served by the WIC and MAC Programs.* Minnesota: Minnesota Department of Health WIC Program, 1992.

Client Resources

1. Asian food guide for teachers. Dairy Council of California, 1981.
2. Ikeda J. *Food Habits of the Hmong in California-Information Kit.* Berkeley, CA: University of California. Order from Joanne Ikeda, MA, RD, Morgan Hall, Room 9A, University of California, Berkeley, CA 94720, $10.
3. Lew L. *Healthy Foods.* Los Angeles: California Dietetic Association, 1987. Available in Cambodian, Lao and Vietnamese with English translation.
4. Minnesota Department of Health WIC Program. *Nutrition a la Culture: Nutrition Education Units for Minority Groups Served by the WIC and MAC programs.* Minnesota: Minnesota Department of Health WIC Program, 1992.
5. Parent-Child Health Services. *Southeast Asian Food Posters.* Olympia, WA: Parent-Child Health Services, 1986.
6. Patient Education Resource Center (PERC). *Health Education Materials in Many Languages.* San Francisco: San Francisco General Hospital, 1001 Potrero Avenue, San Francisco, CA 94110, (415)206-5400.
7. Southeast Asians, cultural foods and renal diets for the clinical dietitian. Council on Renal Nutrition of Northern California and Northern Nevada, 1990.

Reference List of Cultural Food Ways

African American food ways
Professional references

1. Black Americans, cultural foods and renal diets. Council on Renal Nutrition of N. California and N. Nevada, 1990.
2. Kaplan, Anne R., Marjorie A. Hoover, Willard B. Moore. *The Minnesota Ethnic Food Book.* St. Paul: Minnesota Historical Society Press, 1986, pp. 235-260.
3. Kittler, Pamela G. and Sucher, Kathryn. *Food and Culture in America.* New York: Van Nostrand Reinhold, 1989, pp. 285-311.
4. Minnesota Department of Health WIC Program. *Nutrition a la Culture: Nutrition Education Units for Minority Groups Served by the WIC and MAC Programs.* Minnesota: Minnesota Department of Health WIC Program, 1992.

Client resources

Minnesota Department of Health WIC Program. *Nutrition a la Culture: Nutrition Education Units for Minority Groups Served by the WIC and MAC Programs.* Minnesota: Minnesota Department of Health WIC Program, 1992.

National Cancer Institute. *Down Home Healthy: Family Recipes of Black American Chefs Leah Chase and Johnny Rivers.* Bethesda, MD: National Cancer Institute, Feb. 1993. NIH Publication No. 93-3408.

Ethiopian food ways
Professional references

1. Center for Applied Linguistics. Ethiopians Refugee Fact Sheet Series #1. Washington, DC: Center for Applied Linguistics, June 1981.

Mexican American food ways
Professional references

2. American Dietetic Association and American Diabetes Association. Mexican-American food practices, customs, and holidays. Chicago: American Dietetic Association, 1989.
3. Cultural influences on dietary patterns, in Nutrition During Pregnancy and the Postpartum Period: A Manual for Health Care Professionals. California: WIC, California Department of Health Services, 1990, pp. 187-226.
4. Food habits of newly emigrated Hispanics to San Francisco area. University of California at Berkeley, Cooperative Extension, 1989.
5. Handbook of Mexican-American food: recipes, nutritional analysis, diabetic exchanges, and common practices. San Antonio, TX: Intercultural Dev. Research Assoc, 1982.
6. Hull, M.A., and Runyan, D.H. The Migrant Farm Worker Nutrition Manual. Washington, DC: Child Development Center, Georgetown University, 1990.
7. Kaplan, Anne R., Marjorie A. Hoover, Willard B. Moore. The Minnesota Ethnic Food Book. St. Paul: Minnesota Historical Society Press, 1986, pp. 235-260.
8. Kittler, Pamela G. and Sucher, Kathryn. Food and Culture in America. New York: Van Nostrand Reinhold, 1989, pp. 285-311.
9. Mexican-American traditional foods in cultural foods and renal diets for clinical dietitians. Council on renal Nutrition of N. California and N. Nevada, 1990.
10. Minnesota Department of Health WIC Program. Nutrition a la Culture: Nutrition Education Units for Minority Groups Served by the WIC and MAC Programs. Minnesota: Minnesota Department of Health WIC Program, 1992.

Native American food ways

Professional references

1. Kaplan, Anne R., Marjorie A. Hoover, Willard B. Moore. The Minnesota Ethnic Food Book. St. Paul: Minnesota Historical Society Press, 1986, pp. 235-260.
2. Kittler, Pamela G. and Sucher, Kathryn. Food and Culture in America. New York: Van Nostrand Reinhold, 1989, pp. 285-311.
3. Minnesota Department of Health WIC Program. Nutrition a la Culture: Nutrition Education Units for Minority Groups Served by the WIC and MAC Programs. Minnesota: Minnesota Department of Health WIC Program, 1992.

Client resources

1. "Family food choices: a guide to weight and diabetes control". Indian Health Service Diabetic Program, U.S. Government Printing Office, 1989.
2. "Eat less fat". Omaha, NE: Swanson Center for Nutrition, Inc., 1980.
3. Minnesota Department of Health WIC Program. *Nutrition a la Culture: Nutrition Education Units for Minority Groups Served by the WIC and MAC Programs*. Minnesota: Minnesota Department of Health WIC Program, 1992.
4. "Taking care of your heart". Bellingham, WA: Portland Area Diabetes Program.

NUTRITION ASSESSMENT

General Description

Evaluating a child's nutritional status has application both in clinical and ambulatory care. Assessment of nutritional status includes evaluation of dietary intake as well as anthropometric and biochemical measurements. Correct assess of nutritional status can be one of the major tools for evaluating risks of certain diseases.

Assessment of nutritional status is basic in developing appropriate care plans for children in clinics, hospitals, and other healthcare settings. Growth, weight changes, eating behavior changes, and blood and urine test measurements are useful in monitoring the effectiveness of care plans.

Pregnant or lactating women, children, and severely stresses patients are especially vulnerable groups of which ongoing nutritional assessments are essential.

Procedures

Certain basic procedures are recommended for a minimum level of assessment. More extensive testing may be recommended for specific cases. Procedures for gathering data should be standardized, and people gathering the data should be carefully trained.

Many screening tools are more appropriately applied to large populations rather than to specific individuals. An example of such a tool is the use of the Recommended Dietary Allowances to evaluate individual diets. For lack of a better tool, this guide is applied to evaluating individual diets, at the discretion of an appropriately trained health professional.

The following are some basic procedures used to assess nutritional status, with references for details on the procedure and/or the appropriate table(s) to be used in the procedures. Specific directions on weighing and measuring techniques follows this overview.

Anthropometric measurements

1. Height/length

   Measuring height and/or length is essential for evaluating both growth and weight for stature. Infants and children from birth to age two years are measured recumbent, preferably on a measuring board. At age two, children may be measured in the standing position, again using a measuring device designed specifically for this purpose or a measuring tape against a walk in an uncarpeted area. Use of height bar on a clinic scale is not recommended since this does not give consistently accurate results. See the NCHS Growth Grids in the appendix for details on appropriate heights and weights for children.

2. Weight

   Weight should be determined on a regular basis, using a good beam or direct-reading electronic scale rather than an ordinary bathroom scale. All scales should be zero-balanced before each weighing (see Guidelines for Weighing and Measuring). Growth rate slows during the first year of life. Average growth rates are listed below:

Average Growth Rates

0-3 months	23-39 gm/day
3-6 months	20 gm/day
6-12 months	15 gm/day
12-18 months	8 gm/day
18-24 months	6 gm/day
2-7 years	38 gm/month
7-9 years	56-62 gm/month
9-11 years	67-77 gm/month
11-13 years	85-110 gm/month

3. Weight for height

This measurement, using the growth grids in the appendix, is appropriate only for prepubescent children. The Weight for Height Ratio is computed as follows:

-locate patient's height on the 50th percentile weight

-determine corresponding 50th percentile weight

-Wt/Ht Ratio = Actual Weight / 50th Percentile Weight

-Interpretation

0.9 -1.1	normal
0.8 -0.9	mild malnutrition
0.7 -0.8	moderate malnutrition
0.7 or less	severe malnutrition

(Adapted form: Waterlow JC. British Medical Journal, 1972.)

4. Tables of standard weights and heights for older adolescents

The Metropolitan Life tables from 1983 and other tables for assessing body frame can be used. The choice of which set of tables to use is determined by the policies of the various institutions since no consensus has been reached on the controversy surrounding the tables.

5. Head circumference

This is particularly important when assessing infants and young children (24 to 36 months of age).

6. Skin fold thickness evaluation

This measurement provides a more direct measurement of body fat, but varies considerably between observances. it also takes a great deal of practice to realize consistent measurements, and preferably, should be done by the same person each time.

7. Arm circumference

This is less useful for assessment of individuals. Coupled with skin fold measurement, it can give and indication of arm muscle area.

8. Clinical examination

Evaluating skin, hair, lips, gums, eyes, teeth and tongue can give an idea of overall health.

9. Laboratory evaluation

Hematocrit, hemoglobin, transferrin, saturation percent, and many other laboratory indices can be very helpful in determining nutritional status.

Dietary Assessment

There are several ways to look at a child's food intake. These methods may be used singly or in combination.

1. Food record or food diary—these may cover one or several days.
2. 24-hr food recall—this has the disadvantage of relying on memory for both food items and portion sizes.
3. Diet history—this usually takes more time, but gathers information on usual eating practices rather than on practices in one time period.
4. Food Frequency—usually does not give information on quantity of food eaten.

Comparing intake to the Recommended Dietary Allowances (RDA) must be used with caution since the RDA's levels are intended to cover the largest group of the population: they do not, however, take into consideration special stress considerations such as surgery.

Potential Nutritional Risk Factors

Condition which limits or impairs oral intake: Enteral or parenteral nutrition Chewing/swallowing problems Problems with feeding self Dental caries Periodontal Disease	Inadequate intake as assessed by caregiver/patient.
Weight below 5th %ile or above 95th %ile	Food Allergies Food Sensitivities Food Intolerances Food Aversions
Flat growth curve Acute Weight loss of 10% or more History of LBW, and under 2 years of age.	Medications with potential diet/drug interactions.
Clinical Data such as low Hgb/Hct.	Admission for treatment which may interfere with oral intake, digestion, and/or absorption, or condition which may alter nutrient requirements.
Bowel/Bladder management program required. Identification of special dietary restrictions or concerns	Medical condition including: Eating disorder Malabsorption Burns Liver disease Cancer Congenital heart disease Prematurity Inborn errors of metabolism Unusual losses (diarrhea, emesis) Failure to thrive Malnutrition

References

1. Healthy by choice: the Minnesota plan for nutrition and health. Minneapolis: Minnesota Department of Health 1986.
2. Recommended daily dietary allowances. 10th ed. Washington, DC: National Academy of Sciences, 1989.
3. Schulz LO. obese, overweight, desirable: where to draw the line in 1986. J Am Dietetic Assoc 1986:86:1702-4.
4. How to measure obesity. International Obesity Newsletter 1987; 1(7):6-7
5. Smith S, Cowell C, Hreha MS. Practical Nutrition. Rockville, MD: Aspen Publications, 1989.

Nutritional Assessment

Professional References

The following list of resources provides good information on nutritional assessment.

1. Alpers DH, Clause RE, Stenson WF. Assessments and management of macronutrient deficiency. In: Manual of Nutrition therapeutics. Boston: Little, Brown & Company, 1983:131-270.
2. Austin J. The perilous journey of nutrition evaluation. Am J Clin Nutrition 1978; 12:232-8.
3. Berkowitz CD. Nutritional assessment of the child with failure to thrive. Nutrition and the MD 1987;3.
4. Body composition assessment in youth and adults: report of the sixth Ross Conference on medical Research. Columbus, Ohio; Ross Laboratories, 1985
5. Christakis G. Nutritional assessment in health programs. Washington DC: American Public Health Association, 1973.
6. Glassman RG. Nutrition Assessment: a critical review. Topics in Clinical Nutrition 1986: (Oct)
7. Gethell EL. Estimating energy and protein needs for the hospitalized child. Am J IV Ther Clin Nutr 1983; April 7-15.
8. Grant A, DeHoog S. Nutritional assessment and support. 3rd ed. Seattle: published by authors, 1985.
9. Healthy by choice: the Minnesota plan for nutrition and health. Minneapolis: Minnesota Department of Health, 1986.
10. Himes JH, Bouchard C. Do the new Metropolitan Life Insurance height-weight tables correctly assess body frame and body fat relationships? American J Public Health 1985:9:1076-9.
11. Jensen G, Englert DM, Dudrick SF. Nutritional assessment: a manual for practitioners. Norwalk, Conn.: Appleton-Century-Crofts, 1983.   57
12. LeLeika NS, Stawski C, Benkov K, Luder E, McNierney M. The Nutritional assessment of the pediatric patient. as found in: Grand RJ, Stuphen JL, Dietz WH, eds. Pediatric Nutrition: Theory and Practice. Boston, MA: Butterworths, 1987.
13. Metropolitan Life Foundation. Statistical Bulletin. New York: 1983; 64:1-10.
14. Minnesota WIC Program operations manual. Minneapolis: Minnesota Department of health , 1982.
15. Minnesota WIC Program training manual for nutrition educators. Minneapolis: Minnesota Department of Health, 1987.
16. Ney D. Nutritional assessment . In: Kelts DG, Jones EG. Manual of pediatric nutrition. Boston: Little, Brown & Company, 1984.
17. Nutritional screening of children: a manual for screening & follow-up. Washington, DC: US Department of Health and Human Services, 1981.
18. Queen PM, Boatright SL, McNamara MM, Henry RR. Nutritional Assessment of pediatric patients. Nutr Sup Serv 1983;3(5):23-34.
19. Recommended daily dietary allowances. 10th ed. Washington DC, National Academy of Sciences, 1989.
20. Ross P. A new chart to monitor weight gain during pregnancy. Am J Clin Nutr 1985; 3:644-52.
21. Simko MD, . Gilbride JA. Nutritional assessment: a comprehensive guide for planning intervention. Rockville, Md.: Aspen Systems Publications, 1984.
22. Smith S, Cowell C, Hreha MS. Practical nutrition. Rockville, MD: Aspen Publications, 1989.
23. Solomons NW. Assessment of nutritional status: Functional indicators of pediatric nutriture. Ped Clin Nut Am 1985: 32(2):319-334.
24. Task Force on Nutrition. Assessment of maternal nutrition. Chicago: American College of Obstetricians and Gynecologists and the American Dietetic Association, 1978.
25. Weigley ES. Average? ideal? desirable? A brief overview of height-weight tables in the United States. J Am Dietetic Assoc 1984;4:417-23.
26. Weinsier RL, Butterworth CE. Handbook of clinical nutrition: clinician's manual for the diagnosis and management of nutritional problems. St. Louis: C.V. Mosby, 1981.

Guidelines for Weighing and Measuring
Infants through Adults

Measurement of height (or length) and weight provide important clues for identifying persons at risk for nutrition problems. It is essential to follow correct procedures to ensure that this information is accurate and reliable. The following paragraphs will give instructions for taking accurate length, height, and weight data on ambulatory patients.

Use the proper measuring equipment

Use measuring boards to measure length for infants and children up to age two. The boards should have immobile ends and a moveable foot board. A metal tape should be permanently attached with zero at the fixed end and the largest number at the moveable end.

For older children and adults, use a measuring board or a metal tape affixed to a flat wall that has no baseboard or molding. This should be in an uncarpeted area. Use a headpiece that is wide enough to cover the top of the head and long enough to reach the wall. It should have a flat edge at 90 degrees to the headpiece to rest flush with the wall. A wood triangle works well.

Weight should be measured on a beam balance scale that is checked for accuracy every three to four months. Infants should be weighed on a table-model beam balance scale, and adults and older children should be weighed on a floor-model beam balance scale.

Use the proper techniques

Measurements should be taken without shoes and in minimum indoor clothing. Infants should be measured in diaper only. Measurements should be repeated until two separate readings are in agreement.

Measuring length from birth to age two
1. During the first two years, children should be measured laying down on a measuring board. Place the child face up on the measuring board. The body must be straight, and lined up with the measuring board.
2. Have an assistant or the parent hold the infant's head firmly against the headboard until the measuring is complete.
3. With one hand, hold the infant's ankles, completely straightening the infant's hips and knees.
4. With the other hand, move the footboard until it is resting firmly against the infant's heels. The toes should point directly up.
5. Read the measurement to the nearest 1/8 inch and write it down.
6 Slide the footboard away from the infant's heels and start again. To be sure the measurement is correct, measure the length and write it down as many times as necessary until you get two readings that agree within 1/4 inch.
7. Record the final measurement on the chart.

Measuring standing height

1. Measurements should be made without shoes or hats and with minimum indoor clothing. Children between 2 and 3 years may be measured either recumbent or standing.
2. Have the person stand on a bare, flat surface with heels slightly apart and their back as straight as possible. Heels, buttocks, and shoulder blades should touch the wall or measuring surface. Eyes should be straight ahead, arms at sides, and shoulders relaxed. Be sure that knees are not bent and that heels are not lifted from the floor.
3. Place the headpiece firmly on top of head, parallel to the floor. Make sure the headpiece makes contact with the wall or measuring surface and that it is not just resting on the hair but is firmly on the crown of the head.
4. Read the height measurement to the nearest 1/8 inch and write it down.
5. Take the headpiece away, check the patient's position, and repeat the measurement as many times as necessary until you get two readings that agree within 1/4 inch.
6. Record the second measurement that agrees within 1/4 inch in the chart.
7. For measuring elderly adults, see "Nutritional Anthropometric Assessment Records" for elderly women and for elderly men.

Weighing infants

1. Zero-balance the scale before each weighing.
2. Weigh the infant nude or in diaper only.
3. Place the infant in the center of the scale.
4. Move the larger (pound) weight until beam is almost in balance. Move the smaller (ounce) weight until the beam is in final balance.
6. Read the weight to the nearest 1/2 ounce.
7. Repeat this process until you get two measurements that agree within 1/2 ounce. Record the second measurement in the chart.
8. Return the weights to zero.

Weighing adults and children older than two years

1. Zero-balance the scale.
2. Weigh the person in minimum indoor clothing and without shoes.
3. The person should stand in the center of the scale platform.
4. Move the lower weight until the beam is almost in balance. Move the upper weight until the beam is in final balance.
6. Read the weight to the nearest 1/4 pound.
7. Repeat this process until you get two measurements that agree within 1/4 pound. Record the second measurement in the chart.
8. Return the weights to zero.

Plotting measurements on growth charts

Age

The growth charts for infants and children were developed for age and sex. Infants and children under two years **must** be recorded on the 0-36 month chart for the appropriate sex. Children between the ages of two and three years may be plotted on the 0-36 month chart if they have been measured recumbent. If they have been measured standing, plot their measurements on the 2-18 year chart. These growth charts should become a permanent part of the health record. At each visit, the measurements should be added to the chart to enable proper monitoring of growth over time.

First, calculate the correct age and round it accurately. To do this, take the date of screening and subtract the date of birth. For example:

	year	month	day
Date of screening 6/25/94	1994	6	25
Date of birth 3/27/91	1991	3	27
	3	2	28

Correct age: 3-1/4 years

	year	month	day
Date of screening 6/25/94	1994	6	25
Date of birth 10/21/93	1993	10	21
	0	8	4

Correct age: 8 months

To round off an infant's or child's age, follow these rules:

0-15 days	round to the previous month
16-31 days	round off to the next highest month
0-1 month	round to the previous whole year
2-4 months	round off to 1/4 year
5-7 months	round off to 1/2 year
8-10 months	round off to 3/4 year
11-12 months	round off to the next whole year

The Percentile Curve

The curved lines on the charts are percentiles from the 5th to the 95th. This indicates where a specific child is in height and/or weight for age when compared to other children of the same age. Measurements above and below these outer limit percentiles should be carefully followed, and the child may need to be referred for followup.

Height

Plot the height in appropriate units (feet and inches or meters and centimeters) in the correct age category. Use a ruler or other straight edge to draw a line from the age category through both the height and the weight curves. Using the straight edge again, draw a short line where the age and height lines cross. The percentile for age-specific height will be a rough determination of where the weight should be. Children outside the 5th to 95th percentiles of age-specific height should be carefully followed or referred for a more definitive diagnosis. This is especially true for children who appear to be falling away from their established percentile curve.

Weight

Plot the weight in appropriate units (pounds and fractions of pounds or kilograms and fractions of kilograms). Use the same plotting procedure as for height. The percentile established by the height should be about the same percentile for weight if weight is ideal. To check for under-and overweight, use the weight-for-stature chart. **The weight-for-stature chart should only be used for the prepubescent child.**

Weight-for-Stature

This chart is used to determine whether weight is appropriate for height. Underweight is at the 5th percentile or below, and overweight is at the 95th percentile or above. **This chart should only be used for the prepubescent child.**

Professional references

1. Nutritional Screening of Children: a manual for screening & followup. Washington, D.C.: U.S. Department of Health and Human Services, 1981.
2. Minnesota WIC Program operations manual. Minneapolis: Minnesota Department of Health, 1993.
3. Minnesota WIC Program training manual for nutrition educators. Minneapolis: Minnesota Department of Health, 1987.
4. Nutrition evaluation: a self instruction program for nurses: in screening, a self-instruction manual for child and teen check up. MCH, 1993.
5. Anthropoemetry, a video on weighing and measuring infants and children; Minnesota.

Estimating Nutrient Requirements Of Children
Recommended Dietary Allowances

The Recommended Dietary Allowances of the National Research Council contain the most complete information for estimating nutrient requirements. These recommended allowances are intended for healthy populations and represent the average intake of nutrients needed to maintain good health over an extended period. Except for energy, the Recommended Dietary Allowances exceed actual requirements in order to allow for individual variation in needs and for the ability to use the nutrients supplied.

Energy Requirements of Children

There are several formulas for estimating the energy requirements of children:

1. Recommended Daily Dietary Allowances- see the next page in this section and the appendix.

2. Nomogram for use with children 5 years and older--see appendix.

3. Surface area method--1,200 kilocalories per square meter for basal metabolism, plus 40-to 50 percent for growth and activity.

Determine the surface area as follows:
1.5 kg	m2=0.05 x kg + 0.05
6-10kg	m2=0.04 x kg. + 0.10
11-20kg	m2=0.03 x kg + 0.20
21-40kg	m2=0.02 x kg + 0.40

4. Basal Energy Expenditure (for use with patients over 25kg and/or 5 years of age)

Males: $BEE = 66 + (13.7 \times W) + (5 \times H) - (6.8 \times A)$
Females: $BEE = 655 + (9.6 \times W) + (1.7 \times H) - (4.7 \times A)$

W= Weight in kilograms
H= Height in centimeters
A= Age in years

Add: 10% of the BEE for growth
10% of the BEE to promote weight gain

Multiply: The above equation should be multiplied by an activity/stress factor.
Suggested activity/stress factors are:
130%- moderate activity stress level
150%- high activity/stress level

Example of caloric needs for pediatric patient with normal growth and moderate activity level: 130% (BEE + 10%).

Caloric Distribution for Infants

The recommended caloric distribution for the full-term, normal infant is:
Carbohydrates:	33 to 65% of total kilocalories
Protein:	7 to 16% of total kilocalories
Fat:	30 to 55% of total calories

Energy and Protein Requirements

In pediatric practice, it has been traditional to estimate protein requirements per kilogram of body weight, rather than as a percentage of total kilocalories. The Recommended Daily Dietary Allowances for protein are listed in the following table and in the appendix:

Age	Calories Per Kg	Calories Per lb	Protein gm/Kg
0.0-0.5	108	49	2.2
0.5-1.0	98	44.5	1.6
1-3	102	46	1.3
4-6	90	40.9	1.2
7-10	70	31.8	1.0
11-14			
male	55	25	1.0
female	47	21.3	1.0
15-18			
male	45	20.4	0.9
female	40	18	0.8
19-24			
male	40	18	0.8
female	38	17	0.8

Fluid

There are several formulas for estimating fluid requirements. Most result in requirements similar to the guidelines listed in the following table of maintenance fluid requirements.

Weight (kg)	Water Requirement
1-10	100 ml/Kg/day
11-20	1000 plus 50 ml/kg for each Kg > 10 Kg
Above 20	1000 plus 20 ml/Kg for each Kg> 20 Kg

Professional References

1. Committee on Dietary Allowances, National Academy of Sciences. Recommended Dietary Allowances. 10th ed. Washington, DC National Academy of Sciences, 1989.
2. Committee on Nutrition, American Academy of Pediatrics. Pediatric Nutrition handbook. 2nd ed. Elk Grove Village, Ill.: American Academy of Pediatrics, 1985.
3. Cone TE, Graef JW. Manual of Pediatric Therapeutics. 2nd ed. Boston: Little, Brown, and Company, 1980: 186-90.
4. Fomon SJ. Infant nutrition. 2nd ed. Philadelphia: W.B. Saunders, 1974: 376.
5. National Dairy Council. How to eat for good health. Rosemount, Ill.: National Dairy Council, 1986.
6. Robbins S. Thorp JN, Wadsworth C. Tube feeding of infants and children (monograph). American Society of Parenteral and Enteral Nutrition, 1981:4.
7. Rolewicz TF. Fluids and electrolytes in pediatrics. Personal Communication, 1982.
8. Walker WA, Hendrecks KM. manual of Pediatric Nutrition. Philadelphia: W.B. Saunders Company, 1985.
9. Queen, Patricia M., Lang, Carol E., Handbook of Pediatric Nutrition: Aspen Publishers, 1993.

CONSISTENCY MODIFICATIONS

Introduction

The following principles are presented as guidelines only. Although there are some general principles that apply to specific disease states, nutritional care for all patients with diseases of the intestines must be individualized.

Some of the diets presented have evolved to meet special needs and/or a clinical practice's specific requirements. Some are combinations of diets used in individual area hospitals.

CLEAR LIQUID DIET

Description

The Clear Liquid Diet is restricted to

- Those foods that are liquid or will become liquid at body temperature
- Liquids that leave little or no residue and that may be absorbed easily with a minimum of digestive activity

Because the Clear Liquid Diet is so restrictive (see Adequacy below), it does not meet the Recommended Dietary Allowances of the National Research Council. The Clear Liquid Diet provides some electrolytes, mainly sodium and potassium, and a limited number of calories. Kilocalories are primarily from carbohydrate, even though the recommended foods provide minimal amounts of protein and fat.

The Clear Liquid diet can be useful, in specified situations, in providing hydration and in keeping calorie residue to a minimum.

A high-protein, low- or no-residue supplement should be used to meet an individual's nutritional requirements when the Clear Liquid Diet is continued for more than 2 to 3 days. In a malnourished patient, supplementation should be initiated promptly.

A Surgical Clear Liquid Diet is similar to the Clear Liquid Diet. The exceptions are the avoidance of (1) any fruit juices, and (2) any red gelatin, fruit ice, etc. Low-residue supplements are also omitted.

Indications for Use

1. In acute conditions for the presurgical and/or postsurgical patient
2. As the first step in oral feeding
3. For fluid and electrolyte replacement in diarrheal diseases
4. As a test diet

Adequacy

The Clear Liquid Diet is adequate only in ascorbic acid, according to the Recommended Dietary Allowances of the National Research Council. (Refer to the Enteral section in this manual for appropriate supplements to use.)

Professional references

The professional references for the Clear Liquid, Full Liquid, Soft, Mechanical Soft, Surgical Soft, and Six Small Feedings Diets are found later in this section.

CLEAR LIQUID DIET

This diet is very restrictive and cannot meet the Recommended Dietary Allowances of the National Research Council. Its use should be limited to a very short period of time and only under the advice or supervision of your physician or dietitian.

FOOD GROUP	ALLOWED/RECOMMENDED	AVOID/USE SPARINGLY
BREADS/STARCHES	None are allowed.	All are avoided.
VEGETABLES	Strained tomato or vegetable juice.	Any others.
FRUIT	Strained fruit juices and fruit drinks; include one serving of citrus or vitamin C-enriched fruit juice daily.	Any others.
MEAT & SUBSTITUTES	None are allowed.	All are avoided.
MILK	None are allowed.	All are avoided.
SOUPS & COMBINATION FOODS	Clear bouillon, broth, or strained, broth-based soups. High-protein broth.	Any others.
DESSERTS & SWEETS	Flavored gelatin, ices or popsicles that do not contain milk. Sugar, honey. High-protein gelatin.	Any others.
FATS & OILS	None are allowed.	Any others.
BEVERAGES	Carbonated beverages	Any others
CONDIMENTS	Iodized salt. pepper.	Any others, including
SUPPLEMENTS*	Residue-free, see Enteral Section of this manual for supplements.	Any others that contain lactose, residue, or are not palatable orally.

* Use of supplements on a Clear Liquid Diet is controversial. Policies for their use is decided by each institution or according to individual circumstances. A sample meal pattern for the Clear Liquid Diet is available from your dietitian.

CLEAR LIQUID DIET
Sample Meal Pattern

SAMPLE MEAL PATTERN*

Breakfast	4 oz. strained orange juice 1/2-1 cup gelatin (plain or fortified)
Midmorning Snack	1/2 cup gelatin (plain or fortified)
Noon Meal	1 cup broth or consommé 4 oz. strained grapefruit juice 1/2 cup gelatin (plain or fortified)
Midafternoon Snack	1/2 cup fruit ice and/or 1/2 cup strained fruit juice
Evening Meal	1 cup broth or consommé 1/2 cup cranberry juice 1/2 cup flavored gelatin (plain or fortified)
Evening Snack	4 oz. strained apple juice (vitamin C-fortified) 1/2 cup flavored gelatin (plain or fortified)

* The above sample meal pattern cannot meet the Recommended Dietary Allowances of the National Research Council, except for vitamin C.

FULL LIQUID DIET

Description

The Full Liquid Diet includes those foods that are liquid or will become liquid at body temperature. It provides easily absorbed nourishment with very little stimulation to the gastrointestinal tract.

A high-calorie, high-protein supplement should be used to meet the individual's nutritional requirements when the Full Liquid Diet is continued for more than 2 or 3 days (see Adequacy below). In an already debilitated patient, supplementation should be initiated promptly.

Indications for use

1.   As a transition diet between the Clear Liquid Diet and solid foods
2.   When patients cannot tolerate solid foods

Adequacy

The Full Liquid diet is nutritionally inadequate, according to the Recommended Dietary Allowances of the National Research Council, except in ascorbic acid and calcium. Protein requirements can be met if adequate amounts of dairy products are consumed daily.

The Full Liquid Diet can be nutritionally adequate if it is fortified with a nutritional supplement. (Refer to the Enteral section in this manual for appropriate supplements to use.)

FULL LIQUID DIET

Special notes

This diet is very restrictive and does not meet the Recommended Dietary Allowances of the National Research Council. Its use should be limited to a short period of time and only under the advice or supervision of your physician or dietitian.

FOOD GROUP	ALLOWED/RECOMMENDED	AVOID/USE SPARINGLY
BREADS/STARCHES	None are allowed.	All are avoided.
Crackers:	None except pureed in soup.	Any others.
Cereals:	Cooked, refined corn, oat, rice, rye, and wheat cereals.	Any others.
Potatoes/Pasta/Rice:	None except pureed in soup.	Any others.
VEGETABLES	Strained tomato or vegetable juice. Vegetables pureed in soup.	Any others.
FRUIT	Any strained fruit juices and fruit drinks. Include one serving of citrus or vitamin C-enriched fruit juice daily.	Any others.
MEAT & SUBSTITUTES	Eggs in custard; eggnog mix; eggs used in ice cream or pudding (e.g., New York vanilla ice cream). eggs.	Any meat, fish, or fowl. All cheese. All other cooked or raw
MILK	Milk and milk-based beverages, including milk shakes and instant breakfast mixes. Smooth yogurt.	Any others.
SOUPS & COMBINATION FOODS	Broth, strained cream soups. Strained, broth-based soups. Fortified broth or cream soup.	Any others.
DESSERTS & SWEETS	Custard, flavored gelatin, tapioca, plain ice cream, sherbet, smooth pudding, junket (Danish dessert), fruit ices, popsicles, pudding pops. Other frozen bars with cream; fudgsicles; chocolate syrup. Sugar, honey, jelly, syrup.	Any others.

FOOD GROUP	ALLOWED/RECOMMENDED	AVOID/USE SPARINGLY
FATS & OILS	Margarine, butter, cream, sour cream, oils.	Any others.
BEVERAGES	All.	None.
CONDIMENTS/ MISCELLANEOUS	Iodized salt, pepper, spices, flavorings. Cocoa powder.	Any others.
SUPPLEMENTS	High-protein/calorie supplements designed for enteral use may be used to improve nutritional adequacy. See Enteral Section of this manual.	Any others that are not intended for enteral use are not palatable orally.

SAMPLE MEAL PATTERN*

Breakfast
1/2 cup orange juice
1 cup cream of wheat
1 cup milk
Sugar if desired

Noon Meal
1 cup cream soup
1/2 cup fruit juice
Sugar if desired

Evening Meal
1 cup cream soup
1/2 cup fruit juice
1/2 cup custard   1/2 cup

Midmorning Snack
1 cup pasteurized eggnog**

Midafternoon Snack
1 cup milk shake

Evening Snack
1 cup allowed supplement

To increase calories, sugar, cream, butter, or margarine should be added if possible.
Nutritional supplements will also increase the total calories.

*   The above sample meal pattern cannot meet the Recommended Dietary Allowances of the National Research Council without appropriate supplementation under the guidance of your physician or dietitian.

**   One that is made from powdered eggs mixed with milk; avoid the use of raw eggs.

POST-TONSILLECTOMY DIET (T & A)

Description

Clear, cold liquids are given on the day of surgery as soon as the patient is able to tolerate them. The diet is progressed to full, cold liquids as tolerated. The next progression is to soft, smooth, cold, or lukewarm, non-irritating foods. The use of straws is not permitted on this diet. Foods containing red coloring are usually excluded so that if the patient vomits, parents can be certain that red streaks in the emesis are indeed blood.

Indications for use

It is prescribed postoperatively for patients undergoing tonsillectomy or adenoidectomy surgery.

Adequacy

This diet is inadequate in iron, niacin, folacin, and thiamin, according to the Recommended Dietary Allowances of the National Research Council. Unless citrus or enriched juices are used, the diet is also inadequate in ascorbic acid.

Professional references

1.   American Dietetic Association. Manual of Clinical Dietetics. Chicago: ADA, 1988.

2.   Nelson, JK, et al. Mayo Clinic Diet Manual 7th Ed.Chicago: Mosby, 1994.

POST-TONSILLECTOMY DIET

Special notes

1. It is common to experience nausea and vomiting during the first 24 hours after surgery.

2. Encourage liquids that are cool in temperature. This will keep the child's throat moist and lessen the discomfort felt when swallowing. Offer liquids such as juice, water and pop that has lost its fizz.

3. Continue liquids and soft foods for about one week and then begin to add different foods to the child's diet.

4. Avoid foods that are hot in temperature and spicy-hot.

5. Avoid foods that may irritate the throat such as crackers, toast, chips, pretzels and raw vegetables. Citrus fruits and juices, including orange juice, may sting the child's throat, but they do not need to be avoided.

6. Foods and liquids that are red in color should be avoided because they can be mistaken for blood if the child vomits.

CLEAR LIQUID T & A

Foods Allowed/Recommended:	Lemon/lime soft drinks or gingerale. Popsicles, fruit ice, plain gelatin. Nectars, apple juice, non-citrus fruit punches. Juices that contain ascorbic acid (vitamin C) should be included at least once a day.
Do not use straws.	**Avoid Red Foods.**

FULL LIQUID T & A

To the Clear Liquid T & A diet, add:	Plain ice cream, pudding, custard, eggnog*, milk, milk drinks, smooth sherbet, and smooth yogurt.

*Eggnog made from powdered eggs and mixed with milk - avoid the use of raw eggs.

SOFT T & A

To the Full Liquid T & A diet, add soft foods such as:

White bread, not toasted (milk toast is allowed).
Margarine or butter.
Lukewarm cooked cereals, mashed potatoes and gravy.
Cooled macaroni and cheese.
Ripe bananas and other soft or canned fruits.
Vegetable purees or vegetable juices.
Soft eggs, moist ground meat.
High-protein, high-calorie oral supplements, if desired.
Avoid highly spiced foods.

NUTRITIONAL CARE FOR CRANIOFACIAL SURGERY

Description

This diet allows foods that are liquid or semiliquid and require little or no chewing. High-calorie, high-protein foods are encouraged.

Indications for use

1. Following craniofacial surgery.
2. Following temperomandibular joint (TMJ) surgery.
3. When patients cannot tolerate solid foods and require increased calories and protein.

Adequacy

This diet can be nutritionally adequate, according to the Recommended Dietary Allowances of the National Research Council. Care should be taken to include a variety of foods and/or supplements in order to meet these requirements.

Professional references

1. Daly KM, Boyne PJ. Nutrition and eating problems of head and neck surgeries: a guide to soft and liquid meals. Springfield, Ill.: Charles C. Thomas, 1985.

2. Wolford DL. Drink to your health. Arlington, Tx.: Arlington Century Printing, 1982.

3. Krause MV, Mahan LK, eds. Food, Nutrition and Diet Therapy. 7th ed. Philadelphia: H.B. Saunders, 1984:539-43.

DIET FOR CRANIOFACIAL SURGERY

Special notes

1. Eating well will make you feel better and will aid your healing. To ensure good healing, a high-protein diet is essential. A high-calorie diet is also needed to meet your energy requirements. If enough calories are not consumed, protein is used for energy rather than for repairing your tissues.

2. It is necessary to avoid chewing for the length of time specified by your physician. The diet should consist of liquid and pureed foods that will flow easily through a syringe or tube.

3. Weight maintenance or a slight weight gain is encouraged. Weight loss is contraindicated at this time, because weight loss does not allow for good healing. Weigh yourself every other day. If you are losing weight, you **must** add more high-calorie, high-protein foods.

4. Small, more frequent feedings are better tolerated than large meals in enabling you to meet your protein and calorie needs.

5. When one or more food group is not included in your diet, a liquid vitamin/mineral supplement should be included to ensure that 100 percent of the Recommended Dietary Allowances are met. If this is not available, a fortified nutritional liquid supplement should be given daily. (See the Enteral Section of this manual for choices.)

6. **DO NOT USE STRAWS** for the first seven days. Use of straws could cause bleeding, wound breakdown, extra stress on muscles, or stomach bloating. Instead, use a large syringe or an infant training cup.

FOOD GROUP	ALLOWED/RECOMMENDED	AVOID/USE SPARINGLY
BREADS/STARCHES *6 -11 servings or more**	No breads are allowed.	All breads.
Crackers:	Crackers pureed into soup.	Any others.
Cereals:	Smooth, refined hot cereals, including cream of wheat, cream of rice, and Malt-O-Meal®. (Note: Thin the hot cereals with milk.)	Oatmeal, pettijohns, Ralston®, and dry cereals.
Potatoes/Pasta/Rice:	Thin, mashed potatoes with butter and/or gravy. Pureed and thinned rice or pasta.	Any others.
VEGETABLES *3 servings or more*	Cooked and pureed vegetables or strained baby vegetables (thinned with cooking liquid or added to soups). Strained vegetable juices.	Any others.
FRUIT *2 servings or more*	Pureed fruits or strained baby fruits (thinned with fruit juice).	Any others.

FOOD GROUP	ALLOWED/RECOMMENDED	AVOID/USE SPARINGLY
MEAT & SUBSTITUTES *2 servings or more*	Pureed meats thinned with broth or added to strained cream soups. Cubed, cooked meat, poultry, or egg pureed with broth or cream soup. Melted cheese (added to cream soup, pureed casseroles, etc.). Powdered eggs used in puddings or eggnogs. (Avoid the use of raw eggs).	Any others.
MILK *2 -3 cups or the equivalent*	Milk, cocoa, chocolate milk, milk shakes, eggnog, malts, instant breakfast mixes, nutritional supplements.** Thinned yogurt; thinned puddings. (These are all good protein sources.)	None.
SOUPS & COMBINATION FOODS	Pureed broth soups and strained cream soups. Combination baby foods, thinned to flow readily through a large syringe. Pureed spaghetti sauce thinned with tomato juice or sauce; other pureed, thinned casseroles.	Any others.
DESSERTS & SWEETS	Melted gelatin; fruit ice; sherbet; flavored ice cream; ice milk. Popsicles, pudding pops, frozen fruit bars, fudgsicles, creamsicles. Strained baby desserts (thinned). Sugar, honey, syrup, ice cream toppings, jelly.	Products containing pieces of fruit, nuts, candy, or chips.
FATS & OILS	Butter, margarine, Half & Half, whipping cream, and gravy, sour cream.	Any others.
BEVERAGES	Any are allowed. Use fruit juices, vegetable juices. Limit use of drinks that supply only calories: carbonated beverages fruit drinks, Koolaid, other drink mixes, diet drinks, and lemonade.	None.
CONDIMENTS	Ground spices and seasonings.	Any others.

** Nutritional supplements should be used with the guidance of your physician or dietitian.

DIET FOR CRANIOFACIAL SURGERY

PRACTICAL TIPS

1. You can prepare Fortified Milk and use it to increase the protein content of milk-based foods. Use it, for example, in cream soups, puddings, milk shakes, malts, hot cereal, and mashed potatoes. It can also be used to thin puddings, cereals, and soups.

FORTIFIED MILK
1 quart whole milk
plus
1 cup powdered (nonfat dry) milk

2. Powdered (nonfat dry) milk can be added directly to soups, beverages, instant puddings, casseroles, scrambled eggs, or any other food item in which it would mix well.

3. Nutritional supplements (as recommended by your dietitian or physician) may be used as needed.

SAMPLE MEAL PATTERN

Breakfast
1 cup instant breakfast drink
1/2 cup pureed fruit thinned with juice
1/2 cup hot cereal thinned with
    1/2 cup milk

Noon Meal
1 cup cream soup made with
    Fortified Milk
1/2 cup juice
1/2 cup thinned pudding
1/2 cup blenderized fruit
    thinned with juice
1/2 cup pureed vegetable
    with butter/margarine

Evening Meal
1 cup cream soup made
    with Fortified Milk
2 oz. pureed meat
1/2 cup thinned mashed
potatoes with
    butter/margarine
1/2 cup pureed vegetables
    with butter/margarine
1 cup milk

Morning Snack
1 cup milkshake

Afternoon Snack
Sport Shake®

Evening Snack
1 cup malted milk

Brand names are used for clarity only and do not constitute an endorsement of any particular product.

* The amounts noted on the food listing indicate the **minimum** number of servings needed from the basic food groups to provide a variety of nutrients essential to good health. Combination foods may count as full or partial servings from the food groups. Dark green, leafy or orange vegetables are recommended 3 or 4 times weekly to provide vitamin A. A good source of vitamin C is recommended daily. Potatoes may be included as a serving of vegetables. The menu above is provided as a sample; your daily menus will vary.

CALORIE AND PROTEIN CONTENT OF VARIOUS FOODS*
(TO USE ON A LIQUID DIET FOLLOWING CRANIOFACIAL SURGERY)

	Calories	Grams of Protein
BEVERAGES		
Milk [all servings are 1 cup (8 oz.)]		
Whole	150	8
2%	120	8
1%	100	8
Skim	90	8
Chocolate Skim	145	8
Cocoa/hot chocolate (sweetened)		
Made with whole milk	220	9
From mix, water added	110	4
Fortified milk - made with whole milk	210	14
Instant breakfast mix - made with whole milk	280	15
Milk shake - Homemade	420	11
Sport Shake®	270	11
Great Shake®	307	12
Carbonated beverages (sweetened)	105	-
Koolaid, lemonade, other sweetened		
drink mixes	95	-
Nutritional supplements/manufacturer	See Enteral Section of this manual	
CEREAL, HOT		
3/4 cup or 1 packet	100	3
1 packet, flavored	155	4
DESSERTS		
Creamsicle	105	1
Custard, 1/2 cup	155	7
Fruit ice, 1/2 cup	125	trace
Fudgsicle	90	4
Ice cream, 1/2 cup	160	2
Ice milk, 1/2 cup	100	3
Jell-O®, 1/2 cup	80	2
Popsicle, twin bar	95	trace
Pudding made with whole milk	170	4
Pudding pop	95	3
Sherbet, 1/2 cup	125	1
Strained baby desserts/jar	95	1
Yogurt, 8 oz. (1 cup)		
Plain, made with whole milk	140	8
Fruit-flavored, made with whole milk	240	10

FATS (Tablespoons)	Calories	Grams of Protein
Butter or margarine	110	trace
Cream		
Half and Half	20	trace
Whipping	50	trace
Sour	25	trace
Gravy		
Homemade	40	trace
Mix, made with water	4	trace
Whipped toppings	10	trace

FRUITS

	Calories	Grams of Protein
Baby fruit, strained, 1 jar	75	trace
Canned fruit, sweetened and pureed, 1/2 cup	95	trace
Juices, 1/2 cup	60	trace

MEAT AND SUBSTITUTES

	Calories	Grams of Protein
Baby meat, strained, 1 jar	115	13
Baby dinners, strained, 1 jar	65	3
Baby high-protein meat/cheese dinners, strained, 1 jar	110	8
Cheese		
Melted, 1 oz.	105	7
Sauce, 1/4 cup	130	6
Spread, 1 oz.	80	5
Egg, 1	80	6

POTATOES

	Calories	Grams of Protein
Baked, 1 medium	95	3
Mashed, 1/2 cup	95	2

SOUPS (1 cup)

	Calories	Grams of Protein
Broth soups, pureed	65	4
Cream soups		
Made with water	100	3
Made with whole milk	175	7

VEGETABLES

	Calories	Grams of Protein
Baby vegetables, strained, 1 jar	50	2
Cooked vegetables, pureed, 1/2 cup	30	2
Vegetable juices, 1/2 cup	25	1

Brand names are used for clarity and do not constitute an endorsement or recommendation of any particular product. Products may change formulation or values may vary depending on the brand of product used.

* The values provided are average values compiled from the following sources:

1. Adams CF, ed. Nutritive values of American foods in common units. Agricultural handbook #456. Washington, D.C.: Agriculture Research Service, USDA, 1975.

2. Pennington JAT. Bowes and Church's Food Values of Portions Commonly Used. 15th ed. New York: HarperPerennial, 1989.

3. Actual product labeling.

DYSPHAGIA IN CHILDREN

Description and indications for use

Dysphagia, or the inability to swallow effectively, may limit adequate oral intake and impair nutritional status. It may occur in any of the three phases of swallowing: oral, pharyngeal, or esophageal. For this discussion, only the oral and pharyngeal phases will be addressed.

Causes may be:
- Mechanical--the result of surgical resection or modification of one or more of the organs of swallowing, due to trauma, cancer, or other disease.
- Neurological--results from a lesion in the cerebral cortex or the cranial nerves of the brain stem, in particular the medulla oblongata. The most common causes are: cerebral palsy, head trauma, oral aversion &/or sensitivity, rehabilitation following or permanent impairment from surgery for brain tumor, tracheallaryngomalacia, and cerebral vascular accident (CVA).

Swallowing difficulties are characterized by
- Weak or uncoordinated muscles of the mouth and/or throat
- Hypo- and/or Hyper- sensitivity of the mouth and/or throat
- Motor and sensory deficits restricting chewing and/or swallowing

The goals of therapy should include:
- Preventing choking and aspiration
- Weight maintenance
- Maintenance of good nutritional and hydration status
- Facilitating independent feeding and swallowing, adjusting feeding schedule as needed to optimize intake
- Patient and family education for transition to home

The management of the dysphagia patient should include a team approach. Members of the health care team should include the patient's physician, nurse, swallowing therapist (usually a speech/language pathologist or occupational therapist), and clinical dietitian. Consultants from other medical specialties including neurology, psychiatry, otolaryngology, and radiology may also be called upon to advise team members. In general, any health care worker or family member who participates in the feeding of a dysphagic patient should be considered a team member.

The **role of the dietitian** should include:

1. Assessing the patient's nutritional status, incorporating duration of illness, medical diagnosis and treatment, related health problems, medications, weight changes, laboratory indices, previous use of parenteral or enteral methods of nutritional support, swallowing ability, and appetite.

2. Determining the patient's nutritional needs and assessing the need for nutrition support if it is determined that the patient is unable to consume adequate amounts of oral intake to maintain nutrition and hydration.

3. Monitoring the nutritional status and intake of the patient through observation, calorie counts, and other methods.

4. Providing an appropriate diet; factors to be considered include the medical status of the patient, swallowing capability, nutrient needs, tolerance, and food preferences.

5. Coordinating efforts with the swallowing specialist for the purpose of providing the appropriate food texture and liquid consistency.

6. Communicating with other team members regarding the patient's nutritional treatment and progress.

7. Providing dietary counseling to the patient and family members.

NUTRITIONAL MANAGEMENT OF THE DYSPHAGIC PATIENT

Introduction of foods

Initially, small amounts of smooth purees that form a cohesive, homogeneous bolus (pudding consistency) are best. Other pureed foods may be mixed with a commercial food thickener or dry infant cereal to achieve the desired consistency. Gelatins, fruit ices and other foods that melt in the mouth become thin liquids and should not be given.

Progression of foods

If the dysphagic patient can demonstrate the oral motor skills of ability to chew with fairly good tongue motion and control, the food texture can be advanced as tolerated. Avoid dry, crumbly, sticky, chewy, and particulate foods until good oral motor skills are present.

Fluids

Fluids are difficult for most patients and should be avoided until it is determined that the patient can adequately tolerate them. Thin liquids, including ice chips, are most difficult to manage. They should be introduced only after the patient can tolerate pureed textures. Patients who exhibit pharyngeal dysfunction are at the highest risk for liquids to be aspirated. The safest way to offer liquids is in controlled amounts using a spoon. Commercial food thickeners can mixed with liquids, if needed. They do not decrease the amount of free water in the thickened liquids.

Professional references

1. Hynak-Hankinson MT, Again M, Gardner C, Jones PL, et al. Dysphagia evaluation and treatment: the team approach, part I. Nutritional Support Services 1984; 4(5):33-41.

2. Margie JD, ed. Nutrition and the stroke patient. Dialogues in Nutrition 1979; 3(4):1-6.

3. Hargrove R. Feeding the severely dysphagic patient. Am Assoc Neurosurgical Nurses 1980; 12(2):102-7.

4. Chencharick JD, Mossman KL. Nutritional consequences of the radiotherapy of head and neck cancer. Cancer 1983; 51:811-15.

5. Diet management in dysphagia. American Dietetic Association National Conference, 1983.

6. Anderson CP, Bussa DW, Felt P. Dysphagia management program. Abbott Northwestern Hospital/Sister Kenny Institute, 1986.

7. Ruttenberg N. Maloney FP, Burks JS, Ringel SP, eds. Assessment and treatment of speech and swallowing problems in patients with multiple sclerosis in interdisciplinary rehabilitation of multiple sclerosis and neuromuscular disorders. Philadelphia: J.B. Lippincott, 1985:129-39, 341-51.

BULBAR, OR FIRST PHASE, DYSPHAGIA DIET

Description

This diet includes foods that are easy to chew and swallow. Foods should be mildly seasoned, of moderate temperature, and moist.

Liquids should be avoided, as they are most difficult for individuals to tolerate and may lead to aspiration. Fluid needs of the patient should not be overlooked. Fluid intake and output should be carefully monitored in order to assure adequate hydration for the patient, especially in the initial phases of management.

Initially, the patient may not be able to take anything by mouth. If this period is prolonged, enteral or parenteral feedings, as appropriate, may be necessary to provide adequate nutrition and hydration. A gastrostomy may be an appropriate means of providing supplemental feedings and still allow the patient socialization at meal times and the emotional satisfaction of an oral intake.

Indications for use

The diet is used for individuals with dysphagia due to: bulbar palsy, complications from radiation therapy or surgery to the head and neck, a cerebral vascular accident, head injury, brain tumor, or other conditions or diseases causing neurologic impairment.

Patients are individual and vary in their degree of difficulty in swallowing as well as their progression rate. Therefore, a patient's intake should be monitored closely and the diet advanced accordingly. In addition, calorie counts will assist in determining the adequacy of a patient's intake.

Patient tolerance and progression of liquids, milk, and dairy products should be monitored. The addition of these food items is dependent upon individual patient tolerance.

Adequacy

This diet is potentially inadequate in calcium and phosphorus, according to the Recommended Dietary Allowances of the National Research Council, especially initially, and in those individual who are unable to tolerate milk and dairy products.

BULBAR, OR FIRST PHASE, DYSPHAGIA DIET

Special notes

This food list will not usually be given to patients, but used as a guideline for dietitians in preparing menus and counseling clients.

FOOD GROUP	ALLOWED/RECOMMENDED	AVOID/USE SPARINGLY
BREADS/STARCHES **Cereals:**	None. Smooth, cooked cereals, moistened as needed.	All. Whole grain, coarse cereals. Any that contain nuts, seeds, dried fruit, or coconut. All others. Any dry cereals.
Potato or Substitute:	Thin, mashed potatoes, especially if moistened with gravy, margarine, or butter. Blended or pureed pasta with gravy, butter, margarine, or sauce.	All other potatoes, rice, noodles, etc.
VEGETABLES	Pureed or mashed vegetables.	All others. Tomato sauce.
FRUIT	Pureed or mashed fruit without skins or seeds. Fruit juice thickened with unflavored gelatin or commercial thickening product.	All others.
MEAT & SUBSTITUTES	Pureed beef, poultry, veal, or pork, moistened with broth or gravy. Eggs-- soft-cooked, or soft scrambled.	Fish, cottage cheese, cheese, peanut butter, fried or smoked meats. Fried or hard-cooked eggs.
MILK	1/2 cup cream or milk for cereal or potatoes. Plain yogurt without pieces of fruit. (Milk and dairy products are allowed or limited according to individual tolerance.)	All others.

FOOD GROUP	ALLOWED/RECOMMENDED	AVOID/USE SPARINGLY
SOUPS & COMBINATION FOODS	Thickened, blenderized soups. Pureed or blenderized casseroles without small pieces or chunks. Soufflés.	All others.
FATS & OILS	Butter, margarine, gravy, small amounts of cream.	All others.
DESSERTS & SWEETS	Plain custard, pudding, or Danish dessert. Ice cream (as tolerated), sherbet, popsicles. Cream pies without nuts or coconut (as tolerated). Sugar, jelly, honey.	Any containing nuts, seeds, dried fruit, or coconut. All others.
BEVERAGES	Thickened liquids as tolerated. Commercial thickeners such as Thick-ItTM or NutraThickTM may be used to thicken liquids.	All others.
CONDIMENTS/ MISCELLANEOUS	Salt, pepper, catsup.	Strong flavors and seasonings. Seeds, nuts, coconut. Fried or sticky foods.

SAMPLE MEAL PATTERN

Breakfast
1/2-1 c. pureed fruit
1 c. hot cereal with sugar
1/4 c. cream
1 egg with margarine
1/2 c. custard

Noon and Evening Meals
3 oz. pureed meat
2 oz. gravy
1/2-3/4 c. mashed potatoes with margarine
1/2 c. pureed vegetable with margarine
1/2-1 c. pureed fruit
1/2-1 c. pudding

SOFT DIET

Description

The Soft Diet has traditionally been used as a transitional diet for patients progressing from liquids to a regular diet. Its use is based on the premise that moderate fiber, mild seasonings, and avoiding gas-producing foods will diminish GI irritation and formation of excess gas and distention.
There is no clinical evidence to support the use of the soft diet, but it may be helpful for those patients who are not physically or psychologically able to tolerate a regular diet.

Indications for use

The Soft Diet is used as a transitional diet between the Full Liquid and the Regular (General) diets or for patients with mild gastrointestinal problems.

Adequacy

The Soft Diet is nutritionally adequate, according to the Recommended Dietary Allowances of the National Research Council.

SURGICAL SOFT DIET

Description

The Surgical Soft Diet has been used as a transitional diet between full liquid and general diets following surgery. It omits those foods that may be gas producing or those that may be gastrointestinal irritants. Restriction of citrus fruits and juices may be beneficial immediately following surgery and in selected patients with gastroesophageal reflux.

Indications for use

The Surgical Soft Diet is used as a transitional diet between the Full Liquid and the Regular Diet, particularly following gallbladder or other gastrointestinal surgery.

Adequacy

The Surgical Soft Diet is nutritionally adequate in all nutrients according to the Recommended Dietary Allowances of the National Research Council.

MECHANICAL SOFT DIET

Description

Any diet can be made a Mechanical Soft Diet by substituting ground or chopped meats to minimize chewing or swallowing difficulties. Fruits, vegetables, and other foods should be allowed, based on the ability of the patient to masticate and/or swallow the food.

Indications for use

The Mechanical Soft Diet should be used for patients who have difficulty chewing or swallowing.

Adequacy

The adequacy of the Mechanical Soft Diet depends upon the adequacy of the original diet being modified.

SIX SMALL FEEDINGS

Description

Any diet can be made into Six Feedings of approximately equal size. It is frequently combined with another restriction such as Bland, Six Small; or Soft, Six Small Feedings.

Indications for use

1. When only small volumes are tolerated due to a specific disease condition.

2. When the appetite is depressed and only small quantities of food are tolerated at a time such as in fever, anorexia nervosa, chemotherapy, cystic fibrosis, etc.

3. When increased calories are needed and cannot be consumed in only three meals per day.

Adequacy

The adequacy of the Six Small Feedings Diet depends upon the adequacy of the original diet being modified.

Professional references

These references are for the Clear Liquid, Full Liquid, Soft, Mechanical Soft, Surgical Soft, and Six Small Feeding diets.

1. American Dietetic Association. Manual of Clinical Dietetics. Chicago: The American Dietetic Association, 1988.

2. Shils ME, Olson JA, Shike M: Modern Nutrition in Health and Disease, 8th ed. Philadelphia: Lea & Febiger, 1994.

3. Twin Cities District Dietetic Association. Manual of Clinical Nutrition. Minneapolis: DCI Publishing, 1994.

SOFT DIET
SURGICAL SOFT DIET

Special notes

The Soft Diet can be used as a transitional diet between the Full Liquid and the Regular (or General) Diets.

The Surgical Soft Diet avoids the use of straws for drinking and citrus fruits.

FOOD GROUP	ALLOWED/RECOMMENDED	AVOID/USE SPARINGLY
BREADS/STARCHES *6 -11 servings or more*	Bread or rolls: white, fine rye, graham, or refined wheat. Plain sweet rolls, doughnuts, waffles, pancakes, French toast, or bagels. Sweet breads without nuts.	Breads, rolls, or crackers made with whole wheat, cracked wheat, bran, seeds, nuts, or coconut.
Crackers:	Soda, saltine, or graham crackers. Pretzels. Plain crackers: melba toast, rusks, or zwieback.	See above
Cereals:	Cooked cereals: cornmeal, farina, cream of wheat, cream of rice, Malt-O-Meal®, Coco Wheats®. Well cooked oatmeal . Dry cereals: corn, rice, oat, and refined wheat cereals.	
Potatoes/Pasta/Rice:	Potatoes without skin. Macaroni, spaghetti, noodles, refined flour pasta, refined rice, hominy.	Fried potatoes, potato skins, Potato chips or other fried snack items. Whole-grain pasta. Wild or brown rice. Popcorn.
VEGETABLES *3-5 servings or more*	Cooked vegetables except those listed to avoid. Tomato and other vegetable juices. Small amounts of lettuce as tolerated.	Raw vegetables. Gas-producing vegetables such as broccoli, Brussels sprouts, cabbage, sauerkraut, cauliflower, green pepper, cucumber, onion, rutabaga, turnips, radishes, parsnips. Corn, peas, and Lima beans. Artichokes and okra. Tomato seeds.
FRUIT *2 -4 servings or more*	All fruit juices. Peeled peach, pear, apricot, nectarine, or plums. Citrus fruit without tough membrane. Canned or cooked fruits without tough skins, membranes, or seeds.	All other fresh fruits and berries Canned fruit with tough skins, membranes, or seeds. Dried fruits.
MEAT & SUBSTITUTES *2 servings or more*	Lean tender meat, fish, or poultry Eggs, mild cheeses such as colby, mozzarella, monterey jack, and cottage	Fried, smoked or highly seasoned meat, fish, or poultry. Fried eggs. Strong or spiced cheeses. Peanut butter. Dried peas & beans. Nuts.

101

FOOD GROUP	ALLOWED/RECOMMENDED	AVOID/USE SPARINGLY
MILK *2-3 cups or the equivalent*	Milk and milk-based drinks. Yogurt.	Yogurt that contains nuts or seeds.
SOUPS & **COMBINATION** **FOODS**	Bouillon, broth, or cream soups made from allowed foods. Casseroles or mixed dishes made with allowed foods.	Any others.
DESSERTS & **SWEETS** *in moderation*	Plain cakes and cookies; gelatin; fruit ice; sherbet; ice cream or ice milk; pudding or custard; cream pie; pie made with allowed fruits. Plain candy, plain chocolate, honey, jelly, molasses, marshmallows, syrup, sugar, chocolate syrup.	Desserts containing nuts, coconut, or dried fruits. Candy with fruit, nuts, or coconut. Jam, preserves, or marmalade.
FATS & OILS *in moderation*	Margarine, butter, cream, mayonnaise, salad oils, French dressing, gravy. Mildly seasoned salad dressings. Crisp bacon.	Fried foods; any other fat source. Highly seasoned salad dressing or dressing containing seeds.
BEVERAGES	All.	None
CONDIMENTS/ **MISCELLANEOUS**	Catsup, mustard, cream sauce, iodized salt, allowed spices and vinegar in moderation.	Garlic, pickles, strong spices, red pepper, chili powder, horseradish, curry, and cayenne. Coconut.

SOFT AND SURGICAL SOFT DIETS
Sample Menus

SAMPLE MENU--SOFT DIET

Breakfast
1/2 cup orange juice
1/2 cup cream of wheat cereal
1 egg
1 slice toast with margarine
1 cup milk
Sugar if desired

Noon Meal
1/2 cup cream of tomato soup or
   tomato consommé, Crackers
1/2-3/4 cup macaroni & cheese
1/2 cup green beans
1 dinner roll (without seeds),
jelly, margarine or butter
1/2 cup canned peaches
   or peach cobbler
1 cup milk

Evening Meal
2-3 oz. baked chicken
1/2 cup mashed potatoes
   with margarine or butter
1/2 cup cooked beets
1 slice light rye bread
   (without seeds)
1 slice yellow cake with
   chocolate frosting
1 cup milk

SAMPLE MENU--SURGICAL SOFT DIET

Breakfast
1/2 cup canned peaches
1/2 cup cream of wheat cereal
1 egg
1 slice toast with small amount
   of margarine, butter, and/or jelly
1 cup milk
Sugar if desired

Noon Meal
1/2 cup strained cream soup
Plain crackers
Sliced turkey sandwich on
2 slices white bread
1/2 cup wax beans
1/2 cup applesauce
1 sugar cookie
1 cup milk

Evening Meal
2-3 oz. tender roast beef
1/2 cup mashed potatoes
   with margarine or butter
1/2 cup cooked carrots
1 slice white bread
1/2 cup vanilla ice cream
1 cup milk

SIX SMALL FEEDINGS

SAMPLE MENU*

Breakfast

1 scrambled egg
1 slice toast with butter or margarine/jelly
1/2 cup orange juice

Morning Snack

1/2 cup milk
3/4 cup dry cereal
1/2 banana

Noon Meal

1/2 cup cream soup
1/2 sandwich (1 slice bread, 1 oz. meat)
Butter, margarine, or mayonnaise as desired
1/4-1/2 cup wax beans
1/2 cup canned pears
1 cup milk

Afternoon Snack

1/2 cup juice
1 tbsp. peanut butter
2 graham crackers

Evening Meal

2-3 oz. roast chicken
1/2 cup rice
1/2 cup cooked carrots
1 cup milk

Evening Snack

1/2 cup ice cream
2 plain cookies

* The above menu is provided as a sample; your daily meal plans will vary. Fats, desserts, and sweets may be added to the meal plan after the requirements for essential nutrients are met.

BLAND DIET

Description

The Bland Diet omits only those foods for which sufficient scientific evidence is available to show that they cause gastric irritation. A diet may relieve distress of an ulcer but does not prevent an ulcer from forming or heal an existing one. Individual diets may need to be adjusted with consideration of specific food intolerances: it can be liberalized according to patient tolerance.

The use of milk and dairy products has been shown to increase gastric acid secretion; therefore, exclusive use is not recommended as the sole nutritional support in the treatment of ulcer disease.

The practice of providing six small feedings has been popular because large meals stimulate acid secretion through gastric distention. Small, frequent feedings have not been shown to be more effective. Such a state of almost continuous feeding, however, may result in prolonged gastric acid stimulation. Therefore, some of the literature suggests a pattern of three meals per day. It is further suggested that the acid secretion response to each meal is then be controlled by medication (e.g., Cimetidine to be given with meals and antacids 1 to 3 hours after the meal).

Acidic fruit juices are contraindicated only for individuals with oral or esophageal lesions and possibly for those individuals with gastric lesions.

Indications for use

- Treatment of peptic ulcer disease
- Other gastrointestinal disorders
- Transitional diet following gastric upset in an individual

Adequacy

The Bland Diet is nutritionally adequate, according to the Recommended Dietary Allowances of the National Research Council. It may become inadequate in certain nutrients if certain groups of foods are omitted owing to individual intolerances.

Special instructions for those with hiatal hernia and/or reflux esophagitis

Individuals with hiatal hernia and/or reflux esophagitis should avoid the following foods in addition to following the Bland Diet restrictions. These foods cause decreased lower esophageal sphincter pressure and/or have an irritating effect on the esophageal mucosa:

Tomatoes	Citrus juice
Tomato juice	Excessively fatty foods
Chocolate	Peppermint

A high-fat diet tends to lower sphincter pressure, which can result in reflux. Limiting the intake of fat (both visible and as a component in foods) helps to reduce the discomfort associated with reflux esophagitis.

Professional references

1. Achkar E. Peptic ulcer disease: current management in the elderly. Geriatrics. 1985; 40(9):77-83.

2. Hollander D. Diet therapy of peptic ulcer disease. Nutrition & the M.D. 1988; 14(2):1-2.

3. Marotta RB and Floch MH. Diet and Nutrition in Ulcer Disease. Medical Clinics of North America. 1991; 75(4): 967-979.

4. Hold KL, Hollander D. Gastric Mucosal Injury. Ann. Rev. Med.1986; 37:107.

5. Graham DY, Smith JL, Opekun AR. Spicy Food and the Stomach. JAMA. 1988; 260(23):3473-33475.

6. Myers BM, et al. Effect of red pepper and black pepper on the stomach. Am J Gastroenterol. 1987; 82(3): 211-214.

7. American Dietetic Association position paper on bland diet in the treatment of chronic duodenal ulcer disease. In: American Dietetic Association. Handbook of clinical dietetics. New Haven, Conn.: Yale University Press, 1981:B23-B25.

BLAND DIET

1. Eat meals slowly, in a relaxed atmosphere.
2. If a food causes distress, eliminate it for a period of time.

FOOD GROUP	ALLOWED/RECOMMENDED	AVOID/USE SPARINGLY
BREADS/STARCHES *6-11 servings or more*	Most breads, rolls, crackers, quick breads, pancakes, waffles.	Any that contain cocoa or chocolate.
Cereals:	All cooked or dry cereals, except as indicated.	Cereals which are cocoa- or chocolate-flavored.
Potatoes/Pasta/Rice:	All prepared without spices that are to be omitted.	Those prepared with spices that are to be omitted. Check labels on convenience potato, rice, or pasta products, especially those prepared with sauces.
VEGETABLES *3-5 servings or more*	All vegetables except as indicated.	Vegetables prepared with spices that are to be omitted. Check labels on frozen vegetables, prepared in or with a sauce.
FRUIT *2-4 servings or more*	All fruits and fruit juices.	None are omitted.
MEAT & SUBSTITUTES *5 to 7 oz. total/day*	All meat, fish, or poultry . Eggs. Cheeses.	Any meat or meat product that is prepared with or that contains spices that are to be omitted; for example, hot dogs, sausage, lunch meat, pickled herring, pepper cheese.
MILK *2-3 cups or the equivalent*	All except those listed to avoid.	Milk, milk-based beverages, or yogurt that contain cocoa or chocolate.
SOUPS & COMBINATION FOODS	Bouillon, broth, or cream soups which do not contain spices that are to be omitted. Casseroles or mixed dishes that do not contain spices that are to be omitted.	Soups prepared with spices that are to be omitted. Combination foods that are prepared with spices that are to be omitted; for example, TV dinners, pot pies, skillet casserole mixes.

FOOD GROUP	ALLOWED/RECOMMENDED	AVOID/USE SPARINGLY
DESSERTS & SWEETS	All except those listed to omit.	Desserts that contain cocoa or chocolate.
FATS & OILS *in moderation*	Margarine, butter, cooking oils, shortening, mayonnaise and mayonnaise-type salad dressing. Gravy prepared without spices that are to be omitted.	Salad dressing or gravy prepared with spices that are to be omitted.
BEVERAGES	Cereal beverages, carbonated beverages that do not contain caffeine; fruit drinks.	Coffee, tea, decaffeinated coffee, carbonated beverages containing caffeine, cola, cocoa, alcoholic beverages.
CONDIMENTS/ MISCELLANEOUS	Salt; vinegar; herbs and spices, except those indicated to avoid. Catsup as tolerated.	Black pepper, white pepper, red pepper, cayenne, curry powder, chili powder. Foods that contain spices to be omitted; for example, BBQ sauce, steak sauce, Tabasco sauce, Worcestershire sauce, and combination seasonings containing pepper.

SAMPLE MENU FOR THE BLAND DIET

Breakfast
1/2 cup orange juice
1/2 cup cornflakes
1 egg
1 slice toast, lightly buttered
1 cup milk
Sugar, as desired

Noon Meal
1/2 cup cream of tomato soup
Crackers
Sliced roast beef sandwich
1 tsp. mayonnaise
1/2 cup canned fruit
1 cup milk

Evening Meal
2-3 oz. chicken
1/2 cup buttered rice
1/2 cup cooked carrots
1 dinner roll
1 tsp. margarine
1/2 cup ice cream
1 cup milk

GASTRITIS

Description

Gastritis is an inflammation of the gastric mucosa. Symptoms may include nausea, vomiting, hemorrhage, pain, malaise, anorexia, or headache.

Attacks may follow episodes of eating too rapidly, eating when overtired or emotionally upset, or after eating a food to which the individual is sensitive.

It is important to identify those foods and/or situations that result in discomfort in order to prescribe individualized therapy.

Indications for use

- Acute gastritis
- Chronic gastritis

Radiation therapy, trauma, burns, surgery, hypoxia, shock, fever, jaundice, or renal failure may all precipitate acute gastritis. In atrophic gastritis, which results in atrophy and loss of stomach oxyntic cells, there is achlorhydria (a loss of gastric secretion) and possible vitamin B_{12} malabsorption. For this reason, vitamin B_{12} needs should be assessed.

Treatment

Initial treatment is to remove the cause, or to eliminate the irritating substance(s), which may include highly seasoned or caffeinated foods.

Nutritional Care in Acute Gastritis

1. A period of nothing by mouth for 24 to 48 hours is needed, or longer if necessary, (especially in the presence of bleeding), to allow the stomach to rest and heal.
2. Liquids may be introduced, as tolerated, after the initial rest period.
3. The volume and number of feedings may be increased according to patient tolerance.
4. Highly seasoned foods should be avoided (refer to the Bland Diet in this section).

Nutritional Care in Chronic Gastritis

The same dietary guidelines as for acute gastritis apply, with the addition of the following recommendations:

1. The diet should be adequate in calories and in other nutrients.
2. A soft consistency should be provided as needed.
3. Meals should be eaten at regular intervals, and food should be chewed well; foods that cause distress should be avoided.
4. Excessive amounts of liquids with a meal should be avoided because they tend to cause discomfort due to stomach distention and increased acid secretion.

HIATAL HERNIA

Description

A hiatal hernia is an outpouching of a portion of the stomach into the chest cavity through the esophageal hiatus of the diaphragm. It is usually congenital in children and is frequently associated with gastroesophageal reflux. Major symptoms include a reflux of the gastric contents and esophagitis.

Nutritional care

Treatment is similar to the treatment for esophagitis. Treatment is directed not at the hernia but at the gastroesophageal reflux.

ESOPHAGITIS

Description

Esophagitis, also referred to as reflux esophagitis, is a burning, epigastric, substernal pain resulting from the irritating effect of acidic gastric reflux on the esophageal mucosa. It has two phases:

- Acute--results from the ingestion of an irritation agent, viral inflammation, or intubation.
- Chronic--results from recurrent gastroesophageal reflux due to hiatal hernia, reduced lower esophageal sphincter (LES) pressure, recurrent vomiting, or other factors.

Nutritional care

The goals of nutritional care are to:

- Prevent irritation of the esophageal mucosa
- Reduce or prevent esophageal reflux
- Reduce the acidity of the gastric juices

In the acute phase, liquids may be preferred, as they are less abrasive to the esophagus. Citrus and tomato products should be omitted. In addition, the following foods and factors decrease LES pressure and should be avoided:

- Fatty meals
- Chocolate which contains caffeine and stimulates gastric acid secretion
- Peppermint and spearmint oils (carminatives)

In addition, the following may be helpful:

- Avoid foods known to cause heartburn.
- Avoid lying down, bending over, or straining immediately after a meal.
- Avoid eating within 2 to 3 hours of going to bed. (Sleeping on a bed with the head raised 4 to 6 inches may also be helpful.)
- Avoid tight-fitting clothes, especially after a meal.
- Lose weight if overweight.

Professional references

1. Krause MV, Mahan LK. Nutritional care in esophageal or gastric disease. In: Food, nutrition and diet therapy. 7th ed. Philadelphia: W.B. Saunders Company, 1984:427-8.

2. Krause MV, Mahan LK. Nutritional care in intestinal disease. In: Food, nutrition and diet therapy. 7th ed. Philadelphia: W.B. Saunders Company, 1984:438-62.

3. Behrman RE, Vaughan VC, Nelson WE. Nelson Textbook of Pediatrics. 13th ed. W.B.Saunders Company, 1987: 773-4.

NUTRITIONAL MANAGEMENT IN THE TREATMENT OF INFLAMMATORY BOWEL DISEASE

I. Definition

Inflammatory bowel disease (IBD) can be defined as a disturbed state of intestinal motility from which no anatomical cause can be found. It includes Crohn's disease (also referred to a ileitis and regional enteritis) and chronic ulcerative colitis: diverticulosis and infectious diarrhea can also be included. Dietary recommendations are dependent on the location and severity of disease, the type of treatment modality, and the nutritional status of the patient. Nutritional deficiencies are frequently noted among the complications since these diseases are characterized by symptoms that contribute to losses of protein, fat, carbohydrate, water, vitamins and minerals. Malnutrition occurs with chronic disease: protein-calorie malnutrition is the most common deficiency.

Symptoms include
- abdominal pain
- diarrhea
- anorexia
- gastrointestinal blood and protein loss
- weight loss
- anemia
- the tendency for fistula formation

By definition, ulcerative colitis is limited to the colon, with minimal, if any, involvement of the terminal ileum. In contrast, Crohn's disease may occur in any portion of the gastrointestinal tract. Crohn's is also referred to as regional enteritis, because healthy areas of the bowel may alternate with diseased ones (this is why fistulas sometimes develop). Diverticulosis occurs primarily in the sigmoid colon. It is characterized by herniations of colonic mucosa through the muscular layer of the bowel wall.

Children and adolescents with IBD experience poor linear growth and delay in sexual maturation in addition to other symptoms. Goals of therapy are to stabilize the patient in the acute phase and to control the disease in the chronic phase to achieve normal growth and sexual maturation.

II. Diet therapy

Dietary therapy is supportive rather than curative.

A. Guidelines for Nutritional Therapy

1. **Energy.** Optimum intake is 120-130% of RDA. This is difficult to achieve without some form of supplementation as many children with IBD consume considerably fewer calories, about 40-60% of RDA for age.

2. **Protein.** Many patients are in protein deficient states or low protein status due to protein-losing enteropathies, 150% of RDA for age can be viewed as a goal for protein intake.

3. **Vitamins/Minerals.** Nutrients of particular note are Vitamins A, D, K, C, and B12, Folic Acid, Biotin, Zinc, Calcium, and Magnesium. If adequate intake of calories can be achieved, adequate amounts of these nutrients may be supplied as well. However, monitoring serum concentration of protein, albumin, Folate, B12, Iron, Calcium and Magnesium is helpful in determining the need for additional supplementation.

4. **Fat.** Malabsorption of fat with resulting steatorrhea may require moderation of fat intake in the diet with possible use of medium chain triglycerides (MCT) oil for additional calories as fat.

5. **Fiber.** There still appears to be considerable debate about whether a high-fiber diet is appropriate therapy for patients with inflammatory bowel disease. The research data gathered remains inconclusive. Many other variables are involved, including environment, stress, and genetics; therefore, dietary factors cannot be as the single effective therapy.

B. Feeding modalities

1. **TPN.** In the critically ill patient, total parenteral nutrition may be used to rest the bowel 0 or to nutritionally rehabilitate the patient pre- and post operatively. The frequency of the stools, degree of bleeding, degree of ulceration, and extent of exacerbation in the patient will determine the feeding modality to be used.

2. **Enteral Feedings.** Enteral liquid food supplements are convenient, can be well tolerated, can be administered via nasogastric (NG) tube during sleep, and may not increase diarrhea or abdominal pain in patients. Both elemental as well as non-elemental supplements have been used with equal success. Enteral feedings can be given as continuous drip or bolus feeds.

3. **Low-Residue Diet.** A low-residue diet is suitable for the very ill inflammatory bowel disease patient. Omitting roughage prevents irritation of the inflamed bowel (refer to the Low-Residue Diet).

4. **Regular Diet.** As the patient recovers, he or she can return to a more or less normal diet. From the research available, there is no evidence that eating or avoiding specific foods influences the severity or frequency of relapses in inflammatory bowel disease on a long-term basis.

Professional references

1. Fuchs GJ. Malnutrition and nutritional support in inflammatory bowel disease. Nutr. Support Serv. 1985; 5:28-32.

2. Shills ME, Olson JA, Moshe Shike. Modern Nutrition in Health and Disease, 8th ed. Philadelphia: Lea & Febiger, 1994.

3. Hendricks KM, Walker WA. Manual of Pediatric Nutrition, 2nd ed. Philadelphia: B.C. Decker Inc., 1990.

4. Hodges P, et al. Protein-energy intake and malnutrition in Crohn's disease. J Am Dietetic Assoc 1984; 84:1460-4.

5. Suskind RM, Lewinter-Suskink L. Textbook of Pediatric Nutrition, 2nd ed. New York: Raven Press, 1993.

6. Jones A, et al. Crohn's disease: Maintenance of remission by diet. Lancet 1985; (July 27):177-80.

NUTRITIONAL MANAGEMENT IN THE TREATMENT OF SHORT-BOWEL SYNDROME DUE TO SURGERY

The term short-bowel syndrome is used to describe the metabolic and nutritional consequences that may occur in individuals following small-bowel resection, gastric surgery, intestinal bypass, or diseases of the small bowel.

Clinical features of the short-bowel syndrome include diarrhea, intestinal malabsorption, nutritional deficiencies, gallstones, and hypersecretion of acid. Knowledge of the following factors is important in assessing an individual's nutritional status and in planning goals for nutritional support.

- Amount of intestine resected
- Site of resection
- Function of intestine left
- Removal of ileocecal valve
- Adaptation of the remaining intestine

It takes 6 to 12 months for the bowel to adapt in most individuals. For simplification, management of short-bowel syndrome will be divided into three stages.

I. First Stage - Parenteral

The first stage starts in the immediate post-operative period and usually lasts from 3 to 6 weeks. Clinical manifestations include diarrhea, electrolyte and fluid disturbances, and limited (or absent) peristalsis. Nutritional support is aimed at resting the gut, utilizing parenteral nutrition.

II. Second Stage - Parenteral to Enteral

The second stage is recognized by the slow return of bowel function, peristalsis, and decreased diarrhea. Nutritional support should change from parenteral to an elemental formula or other enteral feeding per patient tolerance. Use of medium-chain triglycerides should be considered.

The shortened bowel must be continually challenged with increasing nutrient densities (elemental/chemically defined/enteral) as intestinal adaptation occurs. Without this challenge, the bowel will not develop the enzymes nor the hypertrophied bowel villi necessary for effective nutrient absorption.

III. Third Stage - Oral feeding

As stated before, diet is unique for each patient and will be dependent on the cause of the short-bowel syndrome and on individual tolerances to food. Each patient should be followed closely, and the diet advanced as tolerated from Clear Liquid to Full Liquid to Low-Residue, Six Small Feedings to Regular Diet.

A. Six small meals per day

In an attempt to avoid excessive distention of the stomach and resulting discomfort, six meals of small to moderate volume are recommended instead of three large meals.

B. **Avoid excessive simple carbohydrate, especially in a concentrated form.**

Carbohydrates (starches and sugars) tend to pass through the stomach quickly, and may result in diarrhea (unless they are mixed with protein and fat). This is especially true of concentrated carbohydrates such as candy, desserts, soda pop, jams, and syrups. Eventually, one may tolerate small amounts of sweets, but these should be introduced into the diet slowly.

C. **Milk and dairy products**

Limit intake of milk and dairy products (containing lactose) if the patient is experiencing diarrhea. Alternative sources of calcium need to be found. These may be in the form of lactose reduced milk, a calcium fortified soy formula or pharmaceutical sources prescribed by a physician.

D. **Fiber**

Until bowel status is under control, a Low-Fiber Diet is recommended. There is no evidence supporting long-term use of a Low-Fiber Diet.

E. **Supplementation**

1. Include a wide variety of food within the Food Guide Pyramid in your meal planning.

2. Vitamin and mineral deficiencies have occurred in patients with short-bowel syndrome. Deficiencies in vitamins A, D, K, B_{12}, and folacin have been noted, as have deficiencies in the minerals calcium, magnesium, and zinc. A multivitamin/mineral supplement (with iron) is recommended. Consider calcium supplementation, with vitamin D added.

Professional references

1. Rees RGP, Hare WR, Grimble GK, et al. Do patients with moderately impaired gastrointestinal function requiring enteral nutrition need a predigested nitrogen source? A prospective crossover controlled clinical trial. Gut. 1992; 333:877-881.

2. Rumessen JJ, Gudmand-Hoyer EG. Functional bowel disease: malabsorption and abdominal distress after ingestion of fructose, sorbitol and fructose-sorbitol mixtures. Gastroenterology. 1988; 95:694-700.

3. Allard J, Jejeebhoy K. Nutritional support and therapy in the short bowel syndrome. GI Clin North Am. 1989; 18:589-601.

4. Dudrick SJ, Latifi R, Fosnocht DE. Management of the short-bowel syndrome. Surg Clin North Am. 1991; 71(3):625-643.

COLOSTOMY AND ILEOSTOMY

Description and general dietary considerations

Surgical treatment of persons with severe ulcerative colitis, Crohn's disease, colon cancer, or intestinal trauma may result in an opening from the surface of the body to the intestinal tract. This opening is referred to as a stoma; it will eventually become about the size of a nickel. The purpose of the stoma is to allow defecation. Location (along the intestinal tract) will determine the consistency of the output.

An ileostomy is an opening into the ileum, performed if the entire colon, rectum, and anus must be removed. Output is liquid. Chronic dehydration and sodium depletion may be a problem.

A colostomy is an opening into the colon, performed if only the rectum and anus are removed. Output can range from mushy to fairly well formed, as determined by the location along the colon.

In some instances, a temporary ostomy may be created to allow surgery and healing in a more distal portion of the intestinal tract.

For many individuals with either a colostomy or an ileostomy, diet as it relates to the ostomy is a concern. Although it is a concern, most individuals consume a Regular Diet. Others experience problems with only certain foods. Too often foods may be omitted out of fear and not because of a need to do so.

Gas and odor are often concerns with ostomies and depend on the individual's own body chemistry, as well as the foods consumed. Gas and changes in odor cannot always be attributed to foods eaten. A sudden change in odor should be treated cautiously as it may be a signal for an unexpected disease. Oral antibiotics and other drugs may change the odor as well.

A Low-Residue Diet is recommended postoperatively. This can then be liberalized as tolerated. Some people choose to continue to follow a low-residue diet permanently, but most often a regular diet is tolerated. Dietary management does influence bowel regularity and malodorous flatus.

For patients with ileostomies, it is important to encourage increased water and fluid intake. Because of the large water losses through the ileostomy, these patients have small urine outputs, making them susceptible to renal calculi. An increased salt intake (up to 8 to 10 grams per day) is also important to avoid sodium depletion. Patients with ileal resections may have an output two to five times greater than if they only had an ileostomy. Vitamin B12 supplementation may also be necessary.

Adequacy

Diets for colostomy or ileostomy are adequate in all nutrients, according to the Recommended Dietary Allowances of the National Research Council.

Professional references

1.   Phillips RH. Coping with an Ostomy. New Jersey: Avery Publishing Co., 1986: 175-85, 265-69.

2.   Colostomy: A Guide. 1991. (Client resource) American Cancer Society.

3.   St Paul Ostomy Association, Inc., P.O. Box 75365, St. Paul, MN 55175.

4.   Managing your ostomy. 1985. Hollister, Inc., 2000 Hollister Drive, Libertyville, IL 60048.

DIETARY CONSIDERATIONS FOR OSTOMY CONCERNS

Special notes

Ostomy is a general term referring to a surgically created opening in the abdominal wall. The most common type is the colostomy, followed by the ileostomy. Each type of surgery is performed for different reasons, but a common reason is inflammatory bowel disease. Individuals are generally able to eat most of the foods afterward that were enjoyed prior to surgery.

Your physician may order a Low-Residue Diet after surgery. This will help avoid irritation, which is important for proper healing, and control the ostomy output. Unless you are advised to continue the Low-Residue Diet, however, you can take steps to return to a Regular Diet over time. The small intestine is still functioning efficiently. The consistency of your output will depend upon the location of your colostomy along the colon.

One of the colon's primary functions is the absorption of water and minerals from intestinal matter. When the colon is removed, as it is in ileostomy surgery, a greater volume of water passes out of the body. Because ileostomy drainage is fairly continuous, it is very important to drink plenty of fluids to avoid dehydration (especially during hot weather). Diarrhea and blockage are serious complications for the person with an ileostomy since dehydration often accompanies them. Since potassium, sodium, and other electrolytes are also lost, it is important to replace them with foods and drinks. A general rule is to drink three more glasses of beverages a day (especially those with potassium) than you did before the operation.

Remember that no single diet will do all it is supposed to for everyone. The same foods may effect people very differently. Food choices are affected by many factors, including occupation, ethnic background, life and dietary habits, and emotional status. You will soon discover which foods to eat and which to avoid.

**Experimenting and individualizing are the keys to your diet.
Try new foods in small amounts, and one at a time.**

Emotional upsets can alter bowel habits. Therefore, if you notice a change, try foods that may have been a problem at a later time in order to determine if it was the food or the situation that caused the change. Chewing food thoroughly, especially high-fiber foods, will help you digest them. Most people report that if they did not tolerate certain foods before their surgery, they cannot tolerate them after. For example, if the cabbage family of foods caused too much gas before the operation, the same will probably be true afterwards.

HELPFUL FOOD GUIDELINES FOR INDIVIDUALS WITH OSTOMIES

Blockage

Foods high in fiber, especially those with seeds and hard-to-digest kernels, may block the stoma.

It is very important to try foods one at a time, in small quantities, and to chew them thoroughly.

Foods more likely to cause blockage include

corn on the cob*	grapefruit	dried fruits
celery	coleslaw	wild rice
popcorn	coconut	meat in casings (lunch meat)
nuts	Chinese vegetables	

*slit the corn kernels with a knife before eating them.

If food becomes lodged and does not move forward, you can become dehydrated. This happens as water transfers from your body cells to the small intestine in an effort to relieve the obstruction. Many blockages relieve themselves. Getting in a knee-chest position for a few minutes or taking a hot shower to relax may help. If the blockage persists for more than three hours, however, contact your physician.

The following are symptoms of which you should be aware:

1. Discharge--changing from semisolid to thin liquid
2. Output volume increases and discharge is continuous
3. Objectionable odor
4. Cramping, usually followed by thin, liquid output
5. Distended abdomen (bloating)
6. Vomiting
7. No ileostomy output (sign of complete blockage)

Constipation

For mild constipation, increase fluids, especially fruit juices (including prune juice). Also, increase intake of fresh fruits and vegetables, and whole grain foods.

Gas and odor

The degree of odor and gas depends on each person's unique body chemistry. Scheduling your social activities around the consumption of problem foods helps to avoid embarrassment. Although they may be troublesome, they are not harmful.

Potential odor-causing foods and substances include:

onions	broccoli	Brussels sprouts
cabbage	cauliflower	fish
eggs	asparagus	antibiotics
dried beans	baked beans	strong cheeses
garlic and some other spices		

Foods that may be helpful in preventing odor include:

cranberry juice	yogurt	buttermilk

Potential gas-forming foods include:

cabbage	broccoli	cauliflower
Brussels sprouts	spinach	peas (split or black-eyed)
corn	cucumbers	green peppers
honeydew melon	watermelon	raw apples
avocados	cantaloupe	
mushrooms	radishes	carbonated beverages
kohlrabi	lentils	rutabagas
sauerkraut	garlic	soybeans
kale	onions (including shallots,	prunes
raisins	scallions, leeks, chives)	dried beans (kidney, lima,
	navy, garbanzo, chickpeas)	

Avoid carbonated beverages

Gas is often due to swallowed air. This may occur while eating, drinking, chewing gum, or using straws, or from illness, pain, nervousness, or anxiety. Eating slowly, chewing with the mouth closed, and avoiding gulping of food can decrease or eliminate swallowed air.

Some patients think they can cut down on foods to decrease their ostomy output. The result, however, may be gas and dehydration.

Diarrhea

You are still subject to diarrhea caused by flu and other causes. The following foods may cause loose stools, and you may wish to avoid them when diarrhea occurs:

cabbage	meat broth	milk
green beans	vegetable soup	fried foods
broccoli	green beans	spinach
highly-spiced foods	raw fruits	
legumes		

You may wish to return to a Low-Residue Diet or try the following foods, which often help bind the stools together, and therefore may be helpful if diarrhea occurs:

strained bananas	buttermilk	applesauce
tapioca	boiled, refined rice	creamy peanut butter
boiled milk	yogurt	

Because you are losing even more fluid in your diarrheal discharge, there is the tendency to become dehydrated. It's very important that you replace lost water and electrolytes (electrolytes are minerals that are involved in your body's water balance; sodium and potassium salts are the most important electrolytes).

A dehydrated person will feel weak, thirsty, and cold; will perspire freely; and may feel rapid heartbeats or experience muscle cramping.

To prevent dehydration and to replace lost water and electrolytes, alternate the following drinks each hour:

1 cup sweetened tea or orange juice

or

1 cup broth (canned or made from a bouillon cube)

or

1 cup fruit juice

If the diarrhea is still present after 12 hours, contact your physician.

Miscellaneous notes

You will experience an increased need for fluids upon exercising or during hot weather. Drink extra fluids when you begin to feel thirsty in order to avoid becoming dehydrated.

After eating beets, you may notice red fecal matter. This is **not** bleeding. Beets do not lose their color during digestion and therefore color the ostomy output.

Professional references

1. Colostomy: A Guide. 1991. (Client resource) American Cancer Society.

2. St Paul Ostomy Association, Inc., P.O. Box 75365, St. Paul, MN 55175.

3. Managing your ostomy. 1985. Hollister, Inc., 2000 Hollister Drive, Libertyville, IL 60048.

DIETARY FIBER

Dietary fiber is a term for the components of plant foods that are not digested by human enzymes This definition includes a variety of compounds-cellulose, hemicellulose, pectin, gums and lignin, and, to some, any substance that escapes digestion in the small intestine. Fiber has numerous physiologic functions in the body including maintaining bowel function, providing bulk, delaying gastric emptying time by making contents more viscous, binding bile acids and hormones, and altering the environment of the colon. Some of the effects of fiber are the result of the presence of fiber in the GI tract. Others are the result of fermentation of the fiber by colonic bacteria . When fermented by colonic bacteria, fiber is broken down to short chain fatty acids and gases . The various types of fiber differ in their physiologic effects and in the extent to which they are fermented. The table on the following page summarizes types of fiber, their physiologic actions, sources and conditions on which they may have an effect.

Research has shown that specific types of fiber may be beneficial in treating constipation, diarrhea, diverticular disease, diabetes, obesity, and cardiovascular disease, and in preventing cancer. By providing bulk, fiber may increase satiety. Bulk in the colon will increase stool weight and volume, promoting comfortable laxation and diluting other lumenal contents. By slowing gastric emptying, fiber may aid in weight and glucose control. Although the mechanism is not entirely clear, some sources of dietary fiber have been shown to lower serum cholesterol. Short chain fatty acids provide fuel to colonic epithelium, are a source of calories, and may decrease the pH in the lumen of the colon. Dietary fiber may protect against colon cancer through the combined effects of dilution of contents, binding bile acids, increasing transit time, and lowering colonic pH. Fiber also appears to protect against breast cancer . When short chain fatty acids are absorbed, water and sodium are also absorbed, which may be helpful in some cases of diarrhea.

On the other hand, excessive dietary fiber has been shown to decrease the availability or increase the losses of zinc, calcium, iron, copper, magnesium, riboflavin, niacin, and B6 as well as various drugs.

Children consuming the recommended number of servings from the Food Guide Pyramid in the appropriate amounts for age will consume approximately 5 - 8 grams dietary fiber for preschoolers, 10 - 15 grams dietary fiber for school-aged children and 12 - 18 grams dietary fiber for adolescents. Levels of fiber intake in excess of 14 grams of dietary fiber per day have been associated with increased fecal loss of zinc, calcium, iron, copper, and magnesium in young children. Also, the caloric density of high-fiber foods is low and can lead to ingestion of too few calories for adequate growth. For these reasons, arbitrary use of the High Fiber Diet in children is NOT recommended. The minimal amount of dietary fiber recommended for children three years and older is equivalent to age plus 5 gm/day. A safe range of fiber intake is between age plus 5 and age plus 10 gm/day.

HIGH-FIBER DIET

Description

Emphasis is placed on modifying the normal diet by increasing intake of whole grains, legumes, fruits, and vegetables. Refined carbohydrates are replaced by unrefined foods. The calorie level of the diet is essentially unchanged. Emphasis is placed on modifying the existing diet rather than on eating a specific amount of fiber. There is no established Recommended Dietary Allowance (RDA) for dietary fiber. Recommendations range from 20 to 50 grams per day for adults, and 15-25 grams for children. The National Cancer Institute recommends a goal of doubling an individual's present intake. A gradual increase of fiber in the diet is recommended. A High-Fiber Diet initially may result in flatulence and bloating in some individuals.

One popular way to consider different types of dietary fiber is by their solubility in water, so that fibers are referred to as insoluble or soluble. Insoluble fibers are thought to aid in relieving constipation by adding bulk and by holding water . Soluble fibers are more fermentable and increase bulk by increasing the bacterial mass in the colon. The division is not clear-cut, however. Most sources of fiber contain both soluble and insoluble fibers, and insoluble fibers can be fermented, so they provide some of the advantages of soluble fibers.

It is not possible to predict which fiber source or even what precise amount of fiber will achieve the desired result of the high fiber diet in an individual; therefore, a variety of fiber sources are encouraged. However, if the diet is being used as therapy for hypercholesterolemia or diabetes, soluble fibers should be emphasized. Oatmeal, legumes, fruits, and most vegetables are good sources of soluble fiber. If the diet is prescribed for constipation or diverticular disease, insoluble fibers are more important. Insoluble fibers are found in wheat bran, wheat germ, other whole grains, and corn.

The purpose of the High-Fiber Diet is to

- Increase the volume and weight of the stool that reaches the distal colon
- Increase gastrointestinal motility
- Decrease the intraluminal colonic pressure

Indications for use

- Constipation and encopresis
- Whenever increased stool volume is desired
- Irritable bowel syndrome

Adequacy

This diet is nutritionally adequate, according to the Recommended Dietary Allowances of the National Research Council. It may potentially have the undesirable effect of impairing the absorption of calcium, iron, zinc, copper, and possibly other trace minerals. For this reason, the High Fiber Diet should be used only in those children for whom a diagnosis requiring this type of intervention has been established. A multivitamin preparation with minerals is recommended.

Professional references

1.   American Academy of Pediatric Committee on Nutrition. Plant Fiber Intake in the Pediatric Diet. Pediatrics 1981; 67(4):572-575

2.   Slavin JL. Dietary fiber. Dietetic Currents 1983; 10(6):27-32.

3.   Back to fiber. Minneapolis: General Mills, 1986.

4.   Modified fiber diet: terms related to fiber. In: American Dietetic Association. Handbook of clinical dietetics. New Haven and London: Yale University Press, 1981:B9-B21.

5.   Anderson JW, Clark JT. Soluble dietary fiber: metabolic and physiologic considerations. Contemporary Nutrition 1986; 11(9).

6.   Achord JL. Irritable bowel syndrome and dietary fiber. J Am Dietetic Assoc 1979; 75:452-3.

7.   Fiber and residue control. In: Pemberton CM, Gastineau CF, eds. Mayo Clinic diet manual--a handbook of dietary practice. Philadelphia: W.B. Saunders, 1981:138-44.

8.   Slavin JL. Dietary fiber: classification, chemical analysis, and food sources. J Am Dietetic Assoc 1987; 87(9):1164-71.

9.   Marotta R. Practical methods of increasing fiber intake. In: Floch MH, ed. Clinical value of dietary fiber (proceedings of a symposium sponsored by the Department of Medicine, Norwalk Hospital, Yale University School of Medicine). Norwalk, Conn.: Purdue Frederick, 1982:35-41.

10. Lanza E, Ritva A. A critical review of food fiber analysis and data. J Am Diet Assoc 1986; 86:732.

11. Emerson AP. Foods high in fiber and phytobezoar formation. J Am Diet Assoc 1987; 87(12):1675-77.

12. Position of the American Dietetic Association. Health implications of dietary fiber. J Am Diet Assoc 1988; 88(2):216.

13. Gorman MA, Bowman MS. Position of the American Dietetic Association. Health implications of dietary fiber: technical support paper. J Am Diet Assoc 1988; 88(2):217-21..

14. Slavin JL. The Availability of Minerals in Fibre Diets In: The Clinical Role of Fibre. (Proceedings of a symposium held in Toronto, Canada). Ontario, Canada: Medical Education Services (Canada) Inc., 1985: 43-49.

15. Owens-Stively J, McCain D, Wynne E. Childhood Constipation and Soilng. Minneapolis: Minneapolis Children's Medical Center, 1986.

16. VanOss-Tymchuck EM. Update on Dietary Fiber. "Notes from the Nutritionist". Med-Diet Labs, Inc., Newsletter, 1989.

17. Williams CL, Bollella M, Wynder EL. A New Recommendation for Dietary Fiber in Childhood. Pediatrics 1995; Vol 96, Number 5: 985-988.

HIGH-FIBER DIET
FIBER CONTENT OF SELECTED FOODS

This list groups foods according to approximate grams of dietary fiber per serving size as indicated.

You should consume a total of _____ grams of fiber each day.

CEREALS

Approximately 8 grams of fiber per serving

100% Bran®	1/2 cup
All Bran®	1/3 cup
Bran Buds®	1/3 cup
Fiber One®	1/3 cup

Approximately 4 grams of fiber per serving

Cracklin' Oat Bran®	1/3 cup
Fruit and Fibre®	3/4 cup
Raisin Bran® (or similar)	1 cup
Shredded Wheat 'n Bran®	3/4 cup
Raisin Squares®	3/4 cup
Bran Muffin Crisp®	3/4 cup

Approximately 3 grams of fiber per serving

Bran Chex®	1/2 cup
Corn Bran®	1/2 cup
Corn Chex®	3/4 cup
40% Bran® (or similar)	2/3 cup
Grape Nuts®	2/3 cup
Grape-Nuts® Flakes	2/3 cup
Grits	1/4 cup
Honey Bran®	7/8 cup
Most®	2/3 cup
Oatmeal, cooked	3/4 cup
Post Toasties®	1 cup
Puffed Wheat®	1-1/4 cups
Ralston®, cooked	1/2 cup
Shredded Wheat®	1 large biscuit
Total®	3/4 cup
Wheat germ	1/4 cup

Approximately 2 grams of fiber per serving

Cheerios®	1 cup
Nutri-Grain® (barley, corn, rye, or wheat)	3/4 cup
Wheat Chex®	3/4 cup
Wheaties®	1 cup
Grape-Nuts®	1/4 cup
Ralston®	2/3 cup

Approximately 1 gram of fiber per serving

100% Natural® cereal, plain	3/4 cup
Corn flakes	3/4 cup
Crispy Wheat 'n Raisins®	3/4 cup
Frosted Mini-Wheats®	4 biscuits
Heartland® Natural cereal, plain	1/4 cup
Rice Krispies®	3/4 cup
Special K®	1 cup

BREADS

Approximately 2 grams of fiber per serving

Bran muffin	1 small
Graham crackers	2
Rye crackers	3
Whole wheat bread	1 slice
Whole wheat crackers	6
Whole wheat rolls	1
Cornbread	1 square (2")

Approximately 1 gram of fiber per serving

Cracked wheat bread	1 slice
Mixed grain bread	1 slice
Oatmeal bread	2 slices
Raisin bread	1 slice
Pumpernickel bread	1 slice
Rye bread	1 slice
White Enriched Bread	1 slice

Less than 1 gram of fiber per serving

Bagel	1
French bread	1 slice
Italian bread	1 slice
Pita bread	1 piece
Saltines	6

GRAINS, FLOUR, AND PASTA

More than 5 grams of fiber per serving

Unprocessed bran (Miller's)	1/2 cup*
Whole meal flour	1/2 cup**

*   13 grams of dietary fiber
**   6 grams of dietary fiber

Approximately 2 grams of fiber per serving

Barley grits, cooked	1/3 cup
Barley, raw	1/2 cup
Brown rice	1/2 cup
Buckwheat	1/2 cup
Bulgur	1/3 cup
Cracked wheat	1/4 cup
Ground millet	3/4 cup
Rolled oats	4 cups
White flour	1/2 cup
Whole wheat pasta	1/2 cup
Wild rice	1/2 cup

LEGUMES

Approximately 6 grams of fiber per serving (cooked)

Baked beans	1/2 cup
Kidney beans	1/3 cup
Lentils	3/4 cup
Lima beans	1/2-2/3 cup
Navy beans	1/2 cup
Pinto beans	2/3 cup
White beans	1/2 cup

NUTS, SEEDS, AND COCONUT

Approximately 3 grams of fiber per serving

Almonds	2 tbsp.
Brazil nuts	1/4 cup
Coconut, shredded	3 tbsp.
Filberts	30 nuts
Olives	15 medium
Peanut butter	3 tbsp.
Peanuts	1/4 cup
Popcorn	1 cup
Pumpkin seeds	2 tbsp.
Sesame seeds	2 tbsp.
Soy nuts	2 tbsp.
Sunflower seeds	2 tbsp.
Walnuts	3 tbsp.

FRESH FRUIT

Approximately 4 grams of fiber per serving

Blackberries	3/4 cup
Blueberries	1 cup
Pear	1 medium

Approximately 3 grams of fiber per serving

Nectarine	1 medium
Raspberries	1 cup
Strawberries	1 cup
Apple	1 medium

Approximately 2 grams of fiber per serving

Apricots	2 medium
Banana	1 small
Cantaloupe	1/4 cup
Grapes	1 cup
Mango	1
Orange	1 medium
Papaya	1
Peach	1 medium
Tangerine	1 medium

Approximately 1 gram of fiber per serving

Cherries	10 large
Grapefruit	1/2
Pineapple	1/2 cup
Plums	2-3 medium
Rhubarb, raw	1/2 cup
Watermelon	3 cups

FRUIT JUICES

Approximately 0.5 grams of fiber per serving

Apple juice	1/2 cup
Grape juice	1/2 cup
Grapefruit juice	1/2 cup
Orange juice	1/2 cup
Papaya juice	1/2 cup

DRIED FRUIT

Approximately 3.5 grams of fiber per serving

Dates	5
Prunes	3
Raisins	6 tbsp.
Apricots	4

CANNED FRUIT

Approximately 0.5 grams of fiber per serving

Applesauce	1/2 cup
Apricots	3 halves
Cherries	1/2 cup
Grapefruit	1/2 cup
Mandarin oranges	1/2 cup
Pears	1/4 cup
Pineapple	1/4 cup
Plums	3

VEGETABLES

Approximately 4 grams of fiber per serving

Baked potato with skin	1 medium
Parsnips, raw	1/2 large
Peas (frozen), cooked	1/2 cup
Sweet potato	1 medium

Approximately 3 grams of fiber per serving

Broccoli tops	1/2 cup
Carrots, cooked	1/2 cup, or 1 medium
Corn	1/2 cup

Approximately 2 grams of fiber per serving

Avocado	1/2 medium
Beets	1/2 cup
Brussels sprouts	4 or 1/2 cup
Cabbage, boiled or raw	1/2 cup
Eggplant	1/2 cup
Green beans	1/2 cup
Onions, cooked	3/4 cup
Onions, raw	1/2 cup
Spinach	1 cup
String beans, raw	1/2 cup
Turnips, raw	2/3 cup
Zucchini, raw	1/2 cup

Approximately 1 gram of fiber per serving

Asparagus	1/2 cup
Bean sprouts, raw	1/2 cup
Cauliflower, raw	1/2 cup
Dill pickle	1 medium
French fried potatoes	10 medium
Mushrooms, raw	1/2 cup
Potatoes, mashed	1/2 cup
Tomato, fresh	1 medium

Less than 1 gram of dietary fiber per serving

Celery, raw	1 stalk
Cucumber, raw	6 slices
Green pepper, raw	2 rings
Cooked	1/2 cup
Lettuce, raw	1/2 cup

Brand names mentioned are for the purpose of providing examples only, and do not constitute an endorsement or recommendation for any particular product. It is best to check actual product labeling for a more accurate value for grams of dietary fiber.

Values provided are averages compiled from the following sources. Tables vary in values, so an average estimate had to be made for some foods.

Professional references

1. Slavin J. Fiber in the diet. Food, Science, and Nutrition fact sheet. St. Paul: University of Minnesota Agricultural Extension Service, 1982:35.
2. Fiber content of foods. In: Back to fiber. Minneapolis: General Mills, 1986.
3. What are some good sources of fiber? In: Dietary fiber to lower cancer risk. Washington, D.C.: American Institute for Cancer Research, 1985.
4. American Dietetic Association. Handbook of clinical dietetics. New Haven and London: Yale University Press, 1981:B11-12.
5. Lanza E, Butrum RR. A critical review of food fiber analysis and data. J Am Dietetic Assoc 1986; 86(6):732-40.
6. Park Nicollet Medical Foundation and the International Diabetes Center. 1st ed., rev. 1987. Adding fiber to your diet. Minneapolis: Diabetes Center, Inc., 1982.

GUIDELINES FOR INCREASING FIBER IN THE DIET

Some guidelines that may be helpful while increasing the fiber content of the diet follow:

1. Include a variety of fiber sources. Do not rely on a single source.

2. Increase fiber intake slowly. A gradual increase is best. Too rapid of an increase may result in flatulence and bloating.

3. Replace refined grains with whole grains, and incorporate other fiber sources. The goal is to change the types of food eaten, not to supplement your present diet with high-fiber foods.

4. Include additional fruits and vegetables each day.

5. Increase fluid intake when increasing dietary fiber intake. An additional 4 cups of fluid per day is recommended for younger children and an additional 6 to 8 cups for the older child and adolescent (not including cola and other caffeine containing soft drinks. Inadequate fluid consumption may result in constipation.

6. Start by gradually replacing the following items in the diet:

Eat more of these foods	Eat less of these foods
Whole grain breads	White bread
High-fiber bran cereals	Low-fiber, refined cereals
Whole wheat flour	White flour
Brown or wild rice	White rice
Fresh fruit	Canned fruit

7. For 1 cup white flour, you may use one of the following substitutions:

    1 cup whole wheat flour minus 2 tbsp.
    1/2 cup white flour plus 1/2 cup whole wheat flour
    3/4 cup white flour and 1/4 cup wheat germ or 1/4 cup 100% Bran®

HIGH-FIBER DIET
SAMPLE MENU
APPROXIMATELY 15 GRAMS OF DIETARY FIBER
FOR USE WITH PRESCHOOL CHILDREN

	Approximate grams of Dietary Fiber
Breakfast	
1/2 small banana	1
1/2 cup Cheerios®	1
1 slice whole wheat bread	2
Margarine	0
1/2-3/4 cup milk	0
Morning Snack	
1/2-1 cup Juice	0.5
3 whole wheat crackers	1
Lunch	
1-2 oz. sliced turkey	0
1 slice whole wheat bread	2
1/2 medium orange	1
1/2-3/4 cup milk	0
Afternoon Snack	
1/2 medium apple	1.5
Evening Meal	
1-2 oz. broiled fish	0
1/2 cup mashed potato	1
1/2 whole wheat roll	1
Margarine	0
1/4 cup green beans	1
1/2-3/4 cup milk	0
Evening Snack	
2 Graham Crackers	2
1/2-3/4 cup milk	0

* The above menu is provided as a sample; your daily meal plans will vary. Combination foods may count as full or partial servings from various food groups. Fats, desserts, and sweets may be added to the meal plan after the requirements for essential nutrients are met.

HIGH-FIBER DIET
SAMPLE MENU
APPROXIMATELY 20 GRAMS OF DIETARY FIBER
FOR USE WITH SCHOOL-AGED CHILDREN

	Approximate grams of Dietary Fiber
Breakfast	
1/2 small banana	1
1/2 cup Cheerios®	1
1 slice whole wheat bread	2
Margarine	0
1 cup milk	0
Lunch	
1-2 oz. sliced turkey	0
2 slices whole wheat bread	4
1 lettuce leaf	-
1 medium orange	2
1 cup milk	0
Afternoon Snack	
1 medium apple	3
Evening Meal	
2-3 oz. broiled fish	0
1/2 mashed potato	1
1 whole wheat roll	2
Margarine	0
1/2 cup green beans	2
1 cup milk	0
Evening Snack	
2 Graham Crackers	2
1 cup milk	0

* The above menu is provided as a sample; your daily meal plans will vary. Combination foods may count as full or partial servings from various food groups. Fats, desserts, and sweets may be added to the meal plan after the requirements for essential nutrients are met.

HIGH-FIBER DIET
SAMPLE MENU
APPROXIMATELY 25 GRAMS OF DIETARY FIBER
FOR USE WITH ADOLESCENTS

	Approximate grams of Dietary Fiber
Breakfast	
1/2 small banana	1
1 cup Cheerios®	2
1 poached egg	0
2 slices whole wheat bread	4
Margarine	0
1 cup milk	0
Lunch	
2-3 oz. sliced turkey	0
2 slices whole wheat bread	4
1 lettuce leaf	-
1 medium orange	2
1 cup milk	0
Afternoon Snack	
1 medium apple	3
Evening Meal	
3-4 oz. broiled fish	0
1 cup mashed potatoes	2
1 whole wheat roll	2
Margarine	0
1/2 cup green beans	2
1 cup lettuce and tomato salad	1
2 tbsp. salad dressing	0
1 cup milk	0
Evening Snack	
2 Graham Crackers	2
1 cup milk	0

* The above menu is provided as a sample; your daily meal plans will vary. Combination foods may count as full or partial servings from various food groups. Fats, desserts, and sweets may be added to the meal plan after the requirements for essential nutrients are met.

FIBER- AND RESIDUE-CONTROLLED DIETS

The terms *fiber* and *residue* are not equivalent. Residue refers to the total solids in feces made up of undigested or unabsorbed dietary constituents in addition to sloughed cells from the gastrointestinal tract, intestinal bacteria, and some metabolic products of bacteria.

The term residue has often been referred to with a dual meaning:

(a) The indigestible content of food, as in dietary fiber
(b) The increase in fecal output regardless of whether any portion of the food being referred to remains in the colon after digestion

For example, prune juice does not yield a residue after digestion; however, it is considered a high-residue food because it contains a natural laxative, diphenyllisatin, which results indirectly in an increased stool volume. Milk also contributes to stool volume, even though it is not a high-fiber food. It has been proposed that the term *residue* should no longer be used because of its dual meaning.[1]

The meaning of residue in this text shall be (b) as listed above.

Fiber has been defined earlier in this section.

Professional references

1. American Dietetic Association. Handbook of clinical dietetics. New Haven, Conn.: Yale University Press, 1982:B9-B21.

2. Pemberton CM, Gastineau CF, eds. Mayo clinic diet manual--a handbook of dietary practices. Philadelphia: W.B. Saunders, 1988:140-48.

3. Krause MV, Mahan LK. Food, nutrition and diet therapy. 7th ed. Philadelphia: W.B. Saunders, 1984:438-51.

LOW-FIBER OR FIBER-CONTROLLED DIET

Description

A Low-Fiber or Fiber-Controlled Diet contains a minimal amount of fiber and connective tissue. The diet results in reduced stool weight and bulk and in a delayed intestinal transit time. The goal of this diet is to prevent the formation of a bolus of high-fiber foods that may act as an obstruction in individuals who have narrowed intestinal or esophageal lumens, therefore preventing distention and further aggravation of inflamed tissue. The diet averages approximately 10 grams of dietary fiber.

The diet should be individualized to meet the patient's needs depending on the type of surgery, illness, or patient tolerance.

Indications for Use

The Low-Fiber or Fiber-Controlled Diet may be used:

- As a transitional diet between a liquid and a Regular Diet following surgery, trauma, or other illness.
- During an acute phase of diverticulosis, ulcerative colitis, or infectious enterocolitis.
- In the management of some of the gastrointestinal complications of radiation therapy.
- When distention would result in pain, as in stenosis of intestinal or esophageal lumen resulting from inflammatory changes, or in the case of esophageal varices.

Adequacy

This diet is nutritionally adequate, according to the Recommended Dietary Allowances of the National Research Council.

Professional references

1. American Dietetic Association. Handbook of clinical dietetics. New Haven, Conn.: Yale University Press, 1982:B9-B21.

2. Pemberton CM, Gastineau CF, eds. Mayo clinic diet manual--a handbook of dietary practices. Philadelphia: W.B. Saunders, 1988:140-48.

3. Krause MV, Mahan LK. Food, nutrition and diet therapy. 7th ed. Philadelphia: W.B. Saunders, 1984:438-51.

LOW-RESIDUE DIET

A Low-Residue Diet allows those foods that are low in fiber. In addition, it restricts those foods that are low in fiber, but may affect stool volume, such as connective tissue, milk, prunes, and prune juice. The avoidance of these foods is based more on tradition and common practice rather than on confirmed scientific evidence.

The purpose of the diet is to limit or minimize fecal volume.

A Low-Residue Diet may be achieved by altering the Fiber-Controlled Diet in the following manner:

1. Restricting milk to 2 cups per day.
2. Eliminating prunes and prune juice.

Indications for Use

The Low-Residue Diet may be used in acute stages of ulcerative colitis and Crohn's disease.

Adequacy

The Low-Residue diet may be low in calcium, according to the Recommended Dietary Allowances of the National Research Council.

Professional references

1. American Dietetic Association. Handbook of clinical dietetics. New Haven, Conn.: Yale University Press, 1982:B9-B21.

2. Pemberton CM, Gastineau CF, eds. Mayo clinic diet manual--a handbook of dietary practices. Philadelphia: W.B. Saunders, 1988 140-48.

3. Krause MV, Mahan LK. Food, nutrition and diet therapy. 7th ed. Philadelphia: W.B. Saunders, 1984:438-51.

MINIMUM-RESIDUE DIET

Description

The Minimum-Residue Diet allows only those foods with no or very little crude fiber. Foods that increase stool volume, such as prunes, prune juice, and milk, are also omitted. It may be low in nutrients and only short-term use is recommended.

Indications for Use

The Minimum-Residue Diet may be used:

- As a transitional diet between Full Liquids and a Soft Diet.
- Before or after surgery.
- Temporarily in disorders such as partial bowel obstruction affecting the lower portion of the small or large bowel.
- In some cases of radiation colitis.

Adequacy

The Minimum-Residue Diet is low in calcium and several other nutrients, according to the Recommended Dietary Allowances of the National Research Council. If long-term use is required, an appropriate low-residue supplement should be used.

Professional references

1. American Dietetic Association. Handbook of clinical dietetics. New Haven, Conn.: Yale University Press, 1982:B9-B21.

2. Pemberton CM, Gastineau CF, eds. Mayo clinic diet manual--a handbook of dietary practices. Philadelphia: W.B. Saunders, 1988:140-48.

3. Krause MV, Mahan LK. Food, nutrition and diet therapy. 7th ed. Philadelphia: W.B. Saunders, 1984:438-51.

LOW-FIBER OR FIBER-CONTROLLED DIET

Special notes

The Low-Fiber Diet is prescribed in the treatment of colitis, diarrhea, or other gastrointestinal disturbances; or before and/or after abdominal surgery.

FOOD GROUP	ALLOWED/RECOMMENDED	AVOID/USE SPARINGLY
BREADS/STARCHES *6-11 servings or more**	Bread or rolls: white, fine rye, graham. Plain sweet rolls, doughnuts, waffles, pancakes, French toast, bagels. Plain sweet breads, baking powder biscuits, matzoth.	Bread, rolls, or crackers made made with whole wheat, bran, seeds, nuts, or coconut.
Crackers:	Soda, saltine, or graham crackers. Pretzels, rusks, melba toast, zwieback.	See above.
Cereals:	Cooked cereals: cornmeal, farina, cream of wheat, cream of rice, Malt-O-Meal®, Coco Wheats®. Well-cooked oatmeal or pettijohns. Dry cereals: corn, rice, oat, and refined wheat cereals.	Cereals with whole grain or bran. Dry, coarse wheat cereals. Granola, "High fiber" cereals.
Potatoes/Pasta/Rice:	Mashed, baked (without skin), and creamed potatoes. Macaroni, spaghetti, noodles, refined-flour pasta, refined rice, hominy.	Potato skins. Whole-grain pasta, wild or brown rice. Popcorn.
VEGETABLES *3 servings or more*	Strained tomato and vegetable juices. Fresh: tender lettuce	All other vegetables, cooked or raw.
FRUIT *2 servings or more*	All fruit juices except prune juice. Cooked or canned: applesauce, apricots, cherries, cranberry sauce, grapefruit, grapes, melons, mandarin oranges, grapefruit, nectarines, peaches, plums, pears, pineapple, raspberries	All other fruits: fresh, cooked or canned.

FOOD GROUP	ALLOWED/RECOMMENDED	AVOID/USE SPARINGLY
MEAT & **SUBSTITUTES** *2 servings or more*	Ground or well-cooked, tender beef, ham, veal, lamb, pork, or poultry. Tender steaks or chops. Eggs and plain cheese. Fish, oysters, shrimp, lobster, clams, liver.	Tough, fibrous meats with gristle. Peanut butter, smooth or chunky. Cheese with seeds or nuts. Nuts and seeds; dried peas, beans and lentils.
MILK *2-3 cups or equivalent*	All except those listed to avoid. Plain yogurt.	Yogurt that contains nuts or seeds.
SOUPS & COMBINATION FOODS	Bouillon, broth, or cream soups made from allowed foods. Any strained soup.	Soups or mixed dishes that are not allowed.
DESSERTS & **SWEETS**	Plain cakes and cookies; gelatin; fruit ice; sherbet; ice cream or ice milk; popsicles. Pudding or custard; cream pie; pie made with allowed fruits. Plain hard candy, honey, jelly, molasses, syrup, sugar, chocolate syrup, gum drops, marshmallows.	Desserts or candy that contains nuts, coconut, or dried fruits. Jam, preserves, or marmalade.
FATS & OILS *in moderation*	Margarine, butter, cream, mayonnaise, salad oils, plain salad dressings made from allowed foods, plain gravy, crisp bacon.	Seeds, nuts, olives. Avocados.
BEVERAGES	All, except those listed to avoid.	Beverages made from fruits and vegetables not allowed, or from other foods not allowed.

FOOD GROUP	ALLOWED/RECOMMENDED	AVOID/USE SPARINGLY
CONDIMENTS/ MISCELLANEOUS	Catsup, horseradish, prepared mustard, cream sauce, vinegar, cocoa powder. Cornstarch and the following spices in moderation: allspice, basil, bay leaves, celery powder or leaves, cinnamon, cumin powder, ginger, mace, marjoram, onion powder, oregano, paprika, parsley flakes, pepper (black, ground fine), rosemary, sage, savory, tarragon, thyme, turmeric.	Coconut, pickles; any other food not on the allowed list.

LOW-FIBER DIET
SAMPLE MENU

* The amounts noted on the food listing indicate the **minimum** number of servings needed from the basic food groups to provide a variety of nutrients essential to good health. A maximum amount (limit) is indicated when amounts of certain foods must be controlled. Combination foods may count as full or partial servings from the food groups. Dark green, leafy or orange vegetables are recommended 3 or 4 times weekly to provide vitamin A. A good source of vitamin C is recommended daily. Potatoes may be included as a serving of vegetables. The menu below is provided as a sample; your daily menus will vary.

SAMPLE MENU

Breakfast	Noon Meal	Evening Meal
1/2 cup orange juice	1/2 cup chicken noodle soup	3 oz. baked chicken breast
1 egg	2 oz. sliced roast beef	1/2 cup mashed potato
1 slice white toast	White bread	1/2 cup cooked green beans
Margarine	Mayonnaise or margarine	White dinner roll
3/4 cup corn flakes	1/2 cup apple juice	Margarine
1 cup milk	1 small banana	1/2 cup canned
peaches or		
	1 cup milk	1/2 cup fruit ice
		1 cup milk

MINIMUM-RESIDUE DIET

Special notes

The Minimum-Residue Diet may be used, as prescribed, in the short-term treatment of certain surgeries, bowel obstruction, or acute phase of Inflammatory Bowel Disease.

FOOD GROUP	ALLOWED/RECOMMENDED	AVOID/USE SPARINGLY
BREADS/STARCHES *4 servings or more**	Bread or rolls: white, plain. Plain sweet rolls, doughnuts, waffles, pancakes, French toast, bagels. Plain sweet breads, baking powder biscuits, matzoth.	Any others, including whole grain bread items.
Crackers:	Soda, saltine, or graham crackers. Pretzels, rusks, melba toast, zwieback.	Any others, including whole grain crackers.
Cereals:	Cooked cereals: fine cornmeal, farina, cream of wheat, cream of rice, Malt-O-Meal®, Coco Wheats®. Dry cereals: corn, rice, oat, and refined wheat cereals.	Any others.
Potatoes/Pasta/Rice:	Macaroni, spaghetti, noodles, refined rice.	Potatoes, hominy, Whole-grain pasta, wild or brown rice.
VEGETABLES *2 servings or more*	Strained tomato and vegetable juices.	Any other canned, fresh, or frozen vegetables.
FRUIT *2 servings or more*	Strained fruit juice, including one serving of strained citrus juice or vitamin C-fortified juice daily.	Any others, including prune juice. Any canned fresh, or dried fruits.
MEAT & SUBSTITUTES *2 servings or more (4 to 6 oz. total per day)*	Ground or well-cooked, tender beef, ham, veal, lamb, pork, poultry, or fish (roasted, broiled, or tough meats). Eggs cooked any way but fried.	Any others. Cottage cheese, cheese. Fried eggs.

FOOD GROUP	ALLOWED/RECOMMENDED	AVOID/USE SPARINGLY
MILK	No milk is allowed.	Milk in any form.
SOUPS & **COMBINATION** **FOODS**	Bouillon, broth, or soups made from allowed foods. Casseroles or mixed dishes made with allowed foods.	Any others, including cream soups.
DESSERTS & **SWEETS** *in moderation*	Plain cake and cookies; gelatin; fruit ice; sherbet; angel food and sponge cake. Arrowroot cookies. Clear pudding made with strained fruit juice or water. Plain hard candy, honey, clear jelly, molasses, syrup, sugar, chocolate syrup, marshmallows, gum drops.	Any others. Ice cream, pudding, pie, custard, candy, marmalade. with fruit or nuts,
FATS & OILS *in moderation*	Margarine, butter, heavy cream, mayonnaise, salad oils, whipped cream, cream cheese.	Any others, including salad dressing.
BEVERAGES	All, except those listed to avoid.	Malt.
CONDIMENTS Olives, pickles.	Iodized salt, flavoring.	Any others.

*   These amounts indicate the **minimum** number of servings needed from the basic food groups to provide a variety of nutrients essential to good health. A maximum amount (limit) is indicated when amounts of certain foods must be controlled. Combination foods may count as full or partial servings from the food groups. Dark green, leafy or orange vegetables are recommended 3 or 4 times weekly to provide vitamin A. A good source of vitamin C is recommended daily. Potatoes may be included as a serving of vegetables. The menu below is provided as a sample; your daily menus will vary.

Note: This diet cannot provide all the basic nutrients needed for good health, and should not be continued for more than 2-3 days without the guidance of your physician or dietitian.

SAMPLE MENU

Breakfast
1/2 cup strained orange juice

1 soft-cooked egg (optional)
1 slice white toast

Margarine
1/2 cup cream of wheat

Noon Meal
2 oz. sliced roast beef

White bread
Mayonnaise

1/2 cup strained apple juice
1/2 cup apple cider

Evening Meal
3 oz. baked chicken
breast
1/2 cup noodles
1/2 cup strained
vegetable juice
Plain, white dinner roll
Margarine
water or 1/2 c
strained fruit juice

MEDICAL NUTRITION THERAPY
FOR TYPE 1 DIABETES IN THE PEDIATRIC POPULATION

DESCRIPTION

Type 1 diabetes is the third most common chronic illness in children and adolescents under 18 years of age. The risk of developing type 1 diabetes is higher than most other chronic diseases of childhood. The prevalence of type 1 diabetes in people younger than 20 years is 1.7 cases per 1000.

Therapy includes an individualized food plan matched by an appropriate insulin regimen, combined with daily self-blood glucose monitoring, and routine medical evaluation and diabetes education, and is aimed at correcting the acute complications (hypoglycemia and hyperglycemia), and preventing intermediate complications (failure to grow and develop optimally) and long-term complications (microvascular and macrovascular) associated with insulin dependent diabetes mellitus.

The overall goals of medical nutrition therapy are:

1.   Achievement of glucose levels as close to normal as possible with age-appropriate target ranges taken into account, and:

      a.   prevention of hypoglycemia and diabetic ketoacidosis (DKA)
      b.   elimination of symptoms of hyperglycemia
      c.   quality of life factors considered

Blood glucose goals must be realistic for the pediatric population and are dependent on many factors, including comfort level of the patient and caregivers. It is generally recommended that blood glucose target ranges for children less than 5 years be between 100 - 200 mg/dl because of risk of hypoglycemia/hypoglycemia unawareness. Target blood glucose goals may be tightened as the child gets older and as determined by their physician and parents.

Results of the Diabetes Control and Complications Trial (DCCT) and associated intensified diabetes management are not applicable in children less than 13 years. Tight control of diabetes in contraindicated in children less than 2 years old. The American Diabetes Association recommends "extreme caution" when employing intensive management in children ages 2 to 7 years old because of the possible risk of hypoglycemia associated with abnormal brain growth and development.

It should be noted that the phrase "intensive management" is a relative one, and can apply to any child/adolescent/family utilizing a team of health professionals and who is involved in a diabetes management plan designed to improve blood glucose by any increment, since any decrease in glycosylated hemoglobin is associated with a lower risk of complications.

If intensified diabetes management is employed in the pediatric population, an experienced team including a physician specializing in pediatric diabetes, diabetes nurse specialist, diabetes nutrition specialist, and licensed psychologist should be consulted.

2. Normalization or maintenance of acceptable serum lipid levels.*

National Cholesterol Education Program (NCEP) Treatment Guidelines

Ages 2 - 19 years

	Total Cholesterol (mg/dl)	LDL Cholesterol (mg/dl)
Desirable	<170	<110
Borderline high	170 - 199	110 - 129
High	>200	>130

*Adapted from the Report of the Expert Panel on Blood Cholesterol Levels in Children and Adolescents, National Cholesterol Education Program, National Institutes of Health, US Department of Health and Human Services, 1991

"The NCEP Expert Panel on Blood Cholesterol Levels in Children and Adolescents and the American Academy of Pediatrics (AAP) have recommended selective screening of children and adolescents who have a family history of premature CVD or at least one parent with high cholesterol (NCEP Expert Panel, 1991, and AAP statement, 1992). If additional risk factors such as smoking, hypertension, obesity, and IDDM are present, it is recommended that physicians screen at their own discretion." Fasting lipid profiles (total cholesterol, triglycerides, HDL cholesterol, LDL cholesterol, and triglycerides) should be obtained at baseline, and done annually to assess lipid status. It should be noted that metabolic control of blood glucose levels is strongly related to lipid levels, and achievement of relatively tighter blood glucose control should be a first step in lipid improvement. In addition, nutritional guidelines as recommended in the Step I diet (less than 300 mg cholesterol daily, 30% or less of total calories from fat, less than 10% from saturated fat, up to 10% from polyunsaturated fat, and the remainder from monounsaturated fat) are appropriate for children and adolescents. If achievement of acceptable lipid levels is not obtained after achievement of acceptable metabolic control and incorporation of Step I diet guidelines, then advancement to Step II diet guidelines, and possibly drug intervention can be initiated." (National Cholesterol Education Program Report of the Expert Panel on Blood Cholesterol Levels in Children and Adolescents, 1991)

3. Provision of adequate calories for normal growth and development rates and energy needs for children and adolescents.

It is estimated that approximately 5 - 10% of all children with diabetes will not grow optimally; poor control of blood glucose levels is related to suboptimal growth. Growth and weight changes should be assessed at each visit (ideally every 3 - 4 months), and plotted on percentile growth charts developed by the National Center for Health Statistics (NCHS). Deceleration in growth (i.e.; a child "falling off" of their normal curve) may be an indicator of poor glycemic control. It is important to monitor both height and weight changes since a decline may indicate very poor diabetes control, an endocrine disorder or another disease.

Assessment of height and/or weight deviations should include:
- replotting of height and weight changes for accuracy
- diet history and assessment of under/over- nutrition
- referral to physician for further evaluation if not food/lifestyle-related

Additionally, an excessive acceleration of weight may be an indicator of other factors or the need to decrease current caloric/increase energy output level in children and adolescents.

Determination of Caloric Requirements for the Pediatric Population
A variety of methods are available to use as guidelines for calculations of energy needs in the pediatric population. Probably the best determination of energy needs is to ascertain usual intake from a diet assessment to devise a food plan, and use guidelines for comparison purposes. Energy requirements vary with age, weight, and activity level. The following are guidelines for assistance in determining/evaluating energy requirements for the pediatric population:

1. National Academy of Science/Recommended Daily Allowances Guidelines
    (please refer to page 2 for complete listing of RDAs)
    General guidelines:
    - infants   98 - 108 calories/kg/day
    - children, 1 - 3 years   100 calories/kg/day
    - children, 4 - 10 years   70 - 90 calories/kg/day

2. General Guidelines*
    - 1000 kcals for the 1st year
    - add 100 kcals for each additional year until 10 - 12 years
        - boys 11 - 15 years: add 200 kcals per year
        - girls 11 - 15 years: may need less depending on activity level
    - after age 15, calculate as an adult

3. General Guidelines*
    - 1000 kcals for the 1st year
        - add:
        - 125 kcals x age for boys
        - 100 kcals x age for girls
    - up to 20% more kcals for activity

    - for toddlers between 1 - 3 years, 40 kcals per inch length

*Adapted from Joslin Diabetes Center: Joslin Diabetes Center Management of the Pediatric and Adolescent Patient Education Program Policies and Procedures, Boston, MA, 1990

It should be emphasized that these methods are estimates only of energy needs in the pediatric population. Consideration of usual food intake and activity level should be strongly weighed.

Nutritional assessment and revision of food plans should be done every 3 - 6 months in this population. Factors such as growth and weight change and change in activity levels should be assessed at each visit.

The food plan should never be restricted to control blood sugar levels, and this fact should be emphasized to parents and caregivers. It is rarely necessary to restrict calories in pediatric patients with type 1 diabetes.

4.   Inclusion of basic nutrition principles as summarized in the US Dietary Guidelines for Americans and the Food Guide Pyramid.

- Eat a variety of foods

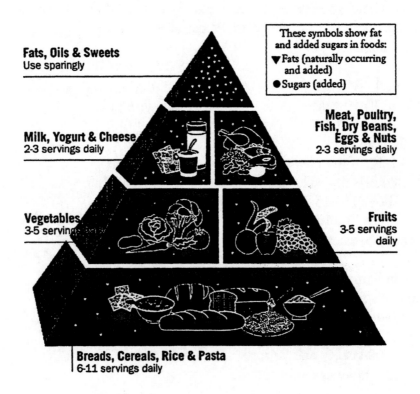

- Balance the food you eat with physical activity-maintain or improve your weight or for children, to promote growth and development and prevent overweight
- Choose a diet with plenty of grain products, vegetables, and fruits
- Choose a diet low in fat, saturated fat, and cholesterol (fat restrictions should not be applied to infants and toddlers below the age of 2 years; after that, children should gradually develop a dietary intake that contains no more than 30 percent of calories from fat by age 5 years)
- Choose a diet moderate in sugars
- Choose a diet moderate in salt and sodium

Nutrition assessments by a Registered Dietitian should include complete evaluation of caloric and nutrient intake with the Recommended Daily Allowances for pediatric patients used for comparison purposes **(refer to the appendix for RDA's in the pediatric population).**

MEDICAL NUTRITION THERAPY
FOR TYPE 1 DIABETES IN THE PEDIATRIC POPULATION

INDICATIONS
Type 1 diabetes in the pediatric population 18 years and younger.

All pediatric patients with diabetes should be managed by a team of health professionals with expertise in diabetes in the pediatric population.

It should be noted that infants and toddlers less than 5 years of age with type 1 diabetes pose a unique set of concerns and needs requiring medical support and education from a team of diabetes specialists with expertise in this area. Education, support, therapy, management, follow-up and day to day care should be undertaken with the special needs of this population taken into consideration. Recommendations in this section should be used in conjunction with referral to such a team.

PROFESSIONAL REFERENCES/EDUCATIONAL TOOLS
Professional references and selected educational tools are summarized at the end of this topic.

MEDICAL NUTRITION THERAPY CONSIDERATIONS AND TYPE 1 DIABETES IN THE PEDIATRIC POPULATION
General Information:
A child's or adolescent's usual food intake and activity schedule should be used to determine a food plan which in turn should be used as a basis for establishing an insulin regimen. Once the diabetes management plan is determined based on usual habits and activities, individuals using insulin should then try to be consistent with that particular plan to maintain optimal glucose control. The food plan should be devised to incorporate consistency in intake for blood glucose control and sound nutrition principles for growth and development.

Nutrition assessment and education of children and their families should be done by a Registered Dietitian who has experience in working with diabetes in the pediatric population.

To contact a registered dietitian, call:
*The American Dietetic Association/National Center for Nutrition and Dietetics Hot Line (800)366-1655
or
*The American Association of Diabetes Educators, (312)644-4411

NUTRIENT COMPOSITION OF THE DIET
Carbohydrate
It has been widely accepted by most health professionals that elimination of "simple" sugars is the ultimate goal of the diet for people with type 1 diabetes. Additionally, it has been recommended that complex carbohydrates be substituted for these sugars. This

recommendation, however, was based on theoretical reasoning that simple sugars entered the bloodstream much quicker than complex ones. Little scientific evidence was used to support this information. Some foods produce lower glycemic responses than others, but from a clinical standpoint, it is recommended that first priority be given to the amount of carbohydrate rather than to the type.

Many studies support the fact that sucrose affects blood glucose levels similarly to other types of carbohydrates, and can be incorporated into diets of people with type 1 diabetes (methods for doing so will be discussed in "Meal Planning Approaches" section). This does not suggest that people with diabetes should consume foods high in sugar, but rather, that recommendations should be given to people that allow them to properly substitute these foods into their meal plans without disrupting blood glucose control. It should be emphasized that foods containing high amounts of sugar offer little nutritional value to the diet, and are also typically void of vitamins and minerals, and high in calories and fat. Addition of high sugar foods must be limited, especially in children, to allow for adequate ingestion of more nutritionally valuable food items.

The most recently published recommendations (1997) for IDDM diets suggests variance of carbohydrate percentage in the diet based on the person's usual eating habits and glucose and lipid levels. No set range is recommended. Once carbohydrate intake at meals and snacks is determined, the diabetes team should match an appropriate insulin regimen to the food plan.

Protein
There is currently not enough evidence to suggest restriction of dietary protein for all persons with IDDM. A mixture of animal and vegetable sources should be incorporated to provide approximately 10 - 20% of the calories from protein. If nephropathy is present, a restriction of not less than the US RDA for protein of 0.8 grams protein/kg body weight per day is recommended. Any restriction of protein in a child's meal plan for diabetes should be done by a registered dietitian.

There is currently no evidence to support the notion that 50 to 60 percent of protein consumed changes into blood glucose, and in fact, current research available suggests that protein has little or no effect on blood glucose levels. It should be noted that protein does require insulin to be metabolized and can delay digestion, and therefore may theoretically affect blood glucose levels if consumed in large quantities.

Traditional recommendations for people with diabetes to consume protein with snacks to "hold them over" is not based on scientific evidence, and should be made with caution especially in children and adolescents who are overweight.

Further research on the effects of protein consumed by people with diabetes is warranted.

153

**Fat
(See previous section on NCEP guidelines, page 148)**

It is theorized that 10 percent of the fat one eats changes into blood glucose, however, no studies verifying this have been done. Dietary fat requires insulin to be metabolized and can alter digestion of foods eaten, and may change the way in which carbohydrate affects blood glucose levels.

Because people with diabetes are at an increased risk for heart disease and the other health-related risks associated with an excessive intake of dietary fat, it is important to teach children and adolescents to gradually incorporate low fat guidelines into their everyday eating patterns.

Fiber
The American Academy of Pediatrics, Committee on Nutrition recommends that fiber should be eaten to ensure normal laxation in children. It is recommended that a level of 0.5 grams dietary fiber/kg body weight (not to exceed 35 grams per day) be consumed.

In general, whole grain breads, cereals and crackers are the best sources of fiber. Fruits and vegetables have varying amounts of fiber in them.

No evidence is available that demonstrates a lowering of blood glucose levels in persons consuming soluble fiber.

Care must be taken in adding fiber to the diets of children and adolescents to prevent gastrointestinal problems associated with an increased fiber diet. It is recommended that additional fiber be added slowly, and increased amounts of water be consumed to help prevent GI disturbances.

Sodium
Recommended levels of 2400 - 3000 mg per day are acceptable in the pediatric population.

Micronutrients (vitamins and minerals)
No current evidence suggests a need for micronutrient replacement in persons with diabetes who are consuming an adequate diet. In persons with a known deficiency (i.e.; chromium, magnesium), supplementation may be required.

Recommendations for vitamin and mineral supplementation should not exceed 100% of the RDA for children and adolescents.

MEDICAL NUTRITION THERAPY
FOR TYPE 1 DIABETES IN THE PEDIATRIC POPULATION

MEAL PLANNING APPROACHES
General Factors to Consider

- The child's/adolescent's usual food pattern should be considered first when devising a meal plan. A complete nutrition assessment and food history should be obtained prior to devising a food plan (a sample nutrition assessment and food record log are included in this section). The food plan should then be tailored to incorporate favorite foods, and meals and snacks should be planned around routine daily activities and schedules, and instruction should be included to address schedule changes, special occasions, and changes in everyday activity.

- Consideration to the type of insulin and regimen should be given to match usual habits and food intake:
  - Planned snacks should be considered if insulins are peaking at particular times.
  - Bedtime snacks should be included in children on overnight long-acting insulin.
  - Morning and afternoon snacks should be deleted or limited (no more than 30 grams carbohydrate) in children or adolescents using Humalog insulin.

- Active times (i.e.; gym, sports practices, birthday parties, etc.) should be considered, and appropriate food and/or insulin adjustments should be suggested to prevent low blood sugars.

- Instruction should be focused on a balance of achieving optimal blood glucose control through consistency in intake and sound nutritional principles for growth and development in children and adolescents.

- Families should be instructed not to vary food plan based on blood glucose levels (i.e.; do not omit food for high blood glucoses), but rather add only if less than target blood glucose range or if active.

- Physicians and health care teams should make usual eating patterns and activities the top priority when devising an insulin regimen to make the least (if any) changes in a child's/adolescent's daily routine.

Exchange Lists for Meal Planning

The Exchange Lists for Meal Planning from the American Diabetes Association can be used to teach children and adolescents meal planning. The Exchange Lists systematically categorize foods into groups: the carbohydrate-containing groups including starch, fruit, milk, other, and vegetable; the meat and meat substitute group; and the fat group. The portions on each list are roughly similar in carbohydrate, protein, fat and calorie content, and can thus be "exchanged" for one another.

An advantage to using the Exchange Lists is that, if followed, this method can provide nutritional adequacy. However, the Exchange Lists are also rigid, and offer little variety in food choices if followed strictly. The following chart demonstrates the nutrient composition of each of the groups:

Group/Lists	Carbohydrate (grams)	Protein (grams)	Fat (grams)	Calories (grams)
Carbohydrate Group				
Starch	15	3	1 or less	80
Fruit	15	-	-	60
Milk				
Skim	12	8	0-3	90
Low-fat	12	8	5	120
Whole	12	8	8	150
Other carbohydrates	15	varies	varies	varies
Vegetables	5	2	-	25
Meat and Meat Substitute Group				
Very lean	-	7	0 - 1	35
Lean	-	7	3	55
Medium-fat	-	7	5	75
High-fat	-	7	8	100
Fat Group	-	-	5	45

"The following Exchange Lists are the basis of a meal planning system designed by a committee of the American Diabetes Association and The American Dietetic Association. While designed primarily for people with diabetes and others who must follow special diets, the Exchange Lists are based on principles of good nutrition that apply to everyone. ©1995 American Diabetes Association, Inc., The American Dietetic Association."

Exchange Lists

Starch Exchanges

One starch exchange equals 15 grams carbohydrate, 3 grams protein, 0-1 grams fat, and 80 calories

Bread		**Cereals and Grains**	
Bagel	½ (1 oz)	Bran cereals	½ cup
Bread, reduced-calorie	2 slices (1½ oz)	Bulgur	½ cup
Bread, white, whole-wheat, pumpernickel, rye	1 slice (1 oz)	Cereals	½ cup
		Cereals, unsweetened, ready-to-eat	¾ cup
Bread sticks, crisp, 4 in. long x ½ in.	2 (2/3 oz)	Cornmeal (dry)	3 Tbsp
English muffin	½	Couscous	1/3 cup
Hot dog or hamburger bun	½ (1 oz)	Flour (dry)	3 Tbsp
Pita, 6 in. across	½	Granola, low-fat	¼ cup

Starch Exchanges, continued

One starch exchange equals 15 grams carbohydrate, 3 grams protein, 0-1 grams fat, and 80 calories

Bread

Raisin bread, unfrosted	1 slice (1 oz)
Roll, plain, small	1 (1 oz)
Tortilla, corn, 6 in. across	1
Tortilla, flour, 7-8 in. across	1
Waffle, 4½ in. square, reduced-fat	1

Starchy Vegetables

Baked beans	1/3 cup
Corn	½ cup
Corn on cob, medium	1 (5 oz)
Mixed vegetables with corn, peas or pasta	1 cup
Peas, green	½ cup
Plantain	½ cup
Potato, baked or boiled	1 small (3 oz)
Potato, mashed	½ cup
Squash, winter (acorn, butternut)	1 cup
Yam, sweet potato, plain	½ cup

Beans, Peas, and Lentils

Beans and peas (garbanzo, pinto, kidney, white, split, black-eyed)	½ cup
Lima beans	2/3 cup
Lentils	½ cup
Miso*	3 Tbsp

Starchy Foods Prepared With Fat

(Count as 1 starch exchange, plus 1 fat exchange.)

Biscuit, 2½ in. across	1
Chow mein noodles	½ cup
Corn bread, 2 in. cube	1 (2 oz)
Crackers, round butter type	6
Croutons	1 cup
French-fried potatoes	16-25 (3 oz)
Granola	¼ cup
Muffin, small	1 (1½ oz)
Pancake, 4 in. across	2
Popcorn, microwave	3 cups
Sandwich crackers, cheese or peanut butter filling	3
Stuffing, bread (prepared)	1/3 cup
Taco shell, 6 in. across	2
Waffle, 4½ in. square	1
Whole-wheat crackers, fat added	4-6 (1 oz)

Cereals and Grains

Grape-Nuts®	¼ cup
Grits	½ cup
Kasha	½ cup
Millett	¼ cup
Muesli	¼ cup
Oats	½ cup
Pasta	½ cup
Puffed cereal	1 ½ cups
Rice milk	½ cups
Rice, white or brown	1/3 cup
Shredded Wheat®	½ cup
Sugar-frosted cereal	½ cup
Wheat germ	3 Tbsp

Crackers and Snacks

Animal crackers	8
Graham crackers, 2 ½ in. square	3
Matzoh	¾ oz
Melba toast	4 slices
Oyster crackers	24
Popcorn (popped, no fat added or low-fat microwave)	3 cups
Pretzels	¾ oz
Rice cakes, 4 in. across	2
Saltine-type crackers	6
Snack chips, fat-free (tortilla, potato)	15-20 (3/4 oz)
Whole-wheat crackers, no fat added	2-5 (3/4 oz)

* =400 mg or more sodium per exchange

Fruit Exchanges
15 grams carbohydrate and 60 calories. The weight includes skin, core, seeds, and rind.

Fruit

Apple, unpeeled, small	1 (4 oz)	Papaya	½ fruit (8 oz) or 1 cup cubes
Applesauce, unsweetened	½ cup	Peach, medium, fresh	1 (6 oz)
Apples, dried	4 rings	Peaches, canned	½ cup
Apricots, fresh	4 whole (5½ oz)	Pear, large, fresh	½ (4 oz)
Apricots, dried	8 halves	Pears, canned	½ cup
Apricots, canned	½ cup	Pineapple, fresh	¾ cup
Banana, small	1 (4 oz)	Pineapple, canned	½ cup
Blackberries	¾ cup	Plums, small	2 (5 oz)
Blueberries	¾ cup	Plums, canned	½ cup
Cantaloupe, small	1/3 melon (11 oz) or 1 cup cubes	Prunes, dried	3
		Raisins	2 Tbsp
Cherries, sweet, fresh	12 (3 oz)	Raspberries	1 cup
Cherries, sweet, canned	½ cup	Strawberries	1¼ cup whole berries
Dates	3	Tangerines, small	2 (8 oz)
Figs, fresh	1½ large or 2 medium (3½ oz)	Watermelon	1 slice (13½ oz) or 1¼ cup cubes
Figs, dried	1½		
Fruit cocktail	½ cup	### Fruit Juice	
Grapefruit, large	½ (11 oz)	Apple juice/cider	½ cup
Grapefruit sections, canned	¾ cup	Cranberry juice cocktail	1/3 cup
Grapes, small	17 (3 oz)	Cranberry juice cocktail, reduced-calorie	1 cup
Honeydew melon	1 slice (10 oz) or 1 cup cubes	Fruit juice blends, 100% juice	1/3 cup
Kiwi	1 (3½ oz)	Grape juice	1/3 cup
Mandarin oranges, canned	¾ cup	Grapefruit juice	½ cup
Mango, small	½ fruit (5½ oz) or ½ cup	Orange juice	½ cup
		Pineapple juice	½ cup
Nectarine, small	1 (5 oz)	Prune juice	1/3 cup
Orange, small	1 (6½ oz)		

Milk Exchanges
One milk exchange equals 12 grams carbohydrate and 8 grams protein.

Skim and Very Low-fat Milk
(0-3 grams fat per serving)

Skim Milk	1 cup	**Low-fat** (5 grams fat per serving	
½% milk	1 cup	2% milk	1 cup
1% milk	1 cup	Plain low-fat yogurt	¾ cup
Nonfat or low-fat buttermilk	1 cup	Sweet acidophilus milk	1 cup
Evaporated skim milk	½ cup		
Nonfat dry milk	1/3 cup dry	**Whole Milk** (8 grams fat per serving)	
Plain nonfat yogurt	¾ cup	Whole milk	1 cup
Nonfat or low-fat fruit-flavored yogurt sweetened with aspartame or with a nonnutritive sweetener	1 cup	Evaporated whole milk	½ cup
		Goat's Milk	1 cup
		Kefir	1 cup

Other Carbohydrates List
One exchange equals 15 grams carbohydrate, or 1 starch, or 1 fruit, or 1 milk.

Food	Serving Size	Exchanges per Serving
Angel food cake, unfrosted	1/12th cake	2 carbohydrates
Brownie, small, unfrosted	2 in. square	1 carbohydrate, 1 fat
Cake, unfrosted	2 in. square	1 carbohydrate, 1 fat
Cake, frosted	2 in. square	2 carbohydrates, 1 fat
Cookie, fat-free	2 small	1 carbohydrate
Cookie or sandwich cookie with crème filling	2 small	1 carbohydrate, 1 fat
Cranberry sauce, jellied	¼ cup	1½ carbohydrates
Cupcake, frosted	1 small	2 carbohydrates, 1 fat
Doughnut, plain cake	1 medium (1½ oz)	1½ carbohydrates, 2 fats
Doughnut, glazed	3 ¾ in. across (2 oz)	2 carbohydrates, 2 fats
Fruit juice bars, frozen, 100% juice	1 bar (3 oz)	1 carbohydrate
Fruit snacks, chewy (pureed fruit concentrate)	1 roll (3/4 oz)	1 carbohydrate
Fruit spreads, 100% fruit	1 Tbsp	1 carbohydrate
Gelatin, regular	½ cup	1 carbohydrate
Gingersnaps	3	1 carbohydrate
Granola bar	1 bar	1 carbohydrate, 1 fat
Granola bar, fat-free	1 bar	2 carbohydrates
Hummus	1/3 cup	1 carbohydrate, 1 fat
Ice cream	½ cup	1 carbohydrate, 2 fats
Ice cream, light	½ cup	1 carbohydrate, 1 fat
Ice cream, fat-free, no sugar added	½ cup	1 carbohydrate
Jam or jelly, regular	1 Tbsp	1 carbohydrate
Milk, chocolate, whole	1 cup	2 carbohydrates, 1 fat
Pie, fruit, 2 crusts	1/6 pie	3 carbohydrates, 2 fats
Pie, pumpkin or custard	1/8 pie	1 carbohydrate, 2 fats
Potato chips	12-18 (1 oz)	1 carbohydrate, 2 fats
Pudding, regular (made with low-fat milk)	½ cup	2 carbohydrates
Pudding, sugar-free (made with low-fat milk)	½ cup	1 carbohydrate
Salad dressing, fat-free*	¼ cup	1 carbohydrate
Sherbet, sorbet	½ cup	2 carbohydrates
Spaghetti or pasta sauce, canned*	½ cup	1 carbohydrate, 1 fat
Sweet roll or Danish	1 (2½ oz)	2½ carbohydrates, 2 fats
Syrup, light	2 Tbsp	1 carbohydrate
Syrup, regular	1 Tbsp	1 carbohydrate
Syrup, regular	¼ cup	4 carbohydrates
Tortilla chips	6-12 (1 oz)	1 carbohydrate, 2 fats
Vanilla wafers	5	1 carbohydrate, 1 fat
Yogurt, frozen, low-fat, fat-free	1/3 cup	1 carbohydrate, 0-1 fat
Yogurt, frozen, fat-free, no sugar added	½ cup	1 carbohydrate
Yogurt, low-fat with fruit	1 cup	3 carbohydrates, 0-1 fat

* =400 mg or more sodium per exchange

Vegetable Exchanges

One vegetable exchange equals 5 grams carbohydrate, 2 grams protein, 0 grams fat, and 25 calories.
In general, one vegetable exchange is:
1/2 cup of cooked vegetables or vegetable juice, or 1 cup of raw vegetables

Artichoke
Artichoke hearts
Asparagus
Beans (green, wax, Italian)
Bean sprouts
Beets
Broccoli
Brussels sprouts
Cabbage
Carrots
Cauliflower
Celery
Cucumber
Eggplant
Green onions or scallions
Greens (collard, kale, mustard, turnip)
Kohlrabi
Leeks
Mixed vegetables (without corn, peas, or pasta)

Mushrooms
Okra
Onions
Pea pods
Peppers (all varieties)
Radishes
Salad greens (endive, escarole, lettuce, romaine, spina
Sauerkraut*
Spinach
Summer squash
Tomato
Tomatoes, canned
Tomato sauce*
Tomato/vegetable juice*
Turnips
Water chestnuts
Watercress
Zucchini

* = 400 mg or more sodium per exchange

Meat and Meat Substitutes

Meat and meat substitutes that contain both protein and fat are on this list. In general, one meat exchange is:

    1 oz meat, fish, poultry, or cheese
    ½ cup beans, peas, and lentils

Once ounce (one exchange) of meat includes:

	Carbohydrate (grams)	Protein (grams)	Fat (grams)	Calories
Very Lean	0	7	0-1	35
Lean	0	7	3	55
Medium-fat	0	7	5	75
High-fat	0	7	8	100

Very Lean Meat and Substitutes List
One exchange equals 0 grams carbohydrate, 7 grams protein, 0-1 grams fat, and 35 calories.

One very lean meat exchange is equal to any one of the following items:**

Poultry: Chicken or turkey (white meat, no skin), Cornish hen (no skin)	1 oz
Fish: Fresh or frozen cod, flounder, haddock, halibut, trout; tuna fresh or canned in water	1 oz
Shellfish: Clams, crab, lobster, scallops, shrimp, imitation shellfish	1 oz
Game: Duck or pheasant (no skin), venison buffalo, ostrich	1 oz
Cheese with 1 gram or less fat per ounce:	¼ cup
Nonfat or low-fat cottage cheese	
Fat-free cheese	1 oz

Lean Meat and Substitutes List
One exchange equals 0 grams carbohydrate, 7 grams protein, 3 grams fat, and 55 calories.

One lean meat exchange is equal to any one of the following items**

Beef: USDA Select or Choice grades of lean beef trimmed of fat, such as round, sirloin, and flank steak; tenderloin; roast (rib, chuck, rump); steak (T-bone, porterhouse, cubed), ground round	1 oz
Pork Lean pork, such as fresh ham; canned, cured, or boiled ham; Canadian bacon*; tenderloin, center loin chop	1 oz
Lamb: Roast, chop, leg	1 oz
Veal: Lean chop, roast	1 oz
Poultry: Chicken, turkey (dark meat, no skin), chicken (white meat, with skin), domestic duck or goose (well-drained of fat, no skin)	1 oz

Very Lean Meat and Substitutes List
One exchange equals 0 grams carbohydrate, 7 grams protein, 0-1 grams fat, and 35 calories.

Other:

Processed sandwich meats with 1 gram or less fat per ounce, such as deli thin, shaved meats, chipped beef*, turkey ham	1 oz
Egg whites	2
Egg substitutes, plain	¼ cup
Hot dogs with 1 gram or less fat per ounce*	1 oz
Kidney (high in cholesterol)	1 oz
Sausage with 1 gram or less fat per ounce	1 oz

** Count as one very lean meat and one starch exchange.

Beans, peas, lentils (cooked)	½ cup

* = 400 mg or more sodium per exchange

Lean Meat and Substitutes List
One exchange equals 0 grams carbohydrate, 7 grams protein, 3 grams fat, and 55 calories.

Fish:

Herring (uncreamed or smoked)	■
Oysters	6 medi■
Salmon (fresh or canned), catfish	■
Sardines (canned)	2 medi■
Tuna (canned in oil, drained)	■

Game: Goose (no skin), rabbit ■

Cheese:

4.5%-fat cottage cheese	¼ ■
Grated Parmesan	2 T■
Cheeses with 3 grams or less fat per ounce	■

Other:

Hot dogs with 3 grams or less fat per ounce*	1½■
Processed sandwich meat with 3 grams or less fat per ounce, such as turkey pastrami or kielbasa	■
Liver, heart (high in cholesterol)	■

162

Medium-Fat Meat and Substitutes List
One exchange equals 0 grams carbohydrate, 7 grams protein, 5 grams fat, and 75 calories

One medium-fat meat exchange is equal to any one of the following items.**

Beef: Most beef products fall into this category (ground beef, meatloaf, corned beef, short ribs, Prime grades of meat trimmed of fat, such as prime rib)	1 oz
Pork: Top loin, chop, Boston butt, cutlet	1 oz
Lamb: Rib roast, ground	1 oz
Veal: Cutlet (ground or cubed, unbreaded)	1 oz
Poultry: Chicken (dark meat, with skin), ground turkey or ground chicken, fried chicken (with skin)	1 oz
Fish: Any fried fish product	1 oz
Cheese: With 5 grams or less fat per ounce	1 oz
Feta	1 oz
Mozzarella	¼ cup (2 oz)
Ricotta	
Other:	
Egg (high in cholesterol, limit to 3 per week)	1
Sausage with 5 grams or less fat per ounce	1 oz
Soy milk	1 cup
Tempeh	¼ cup
Tofu	4 oz or ½ cup

High-Fat Meat and Substitutes List
One exchange equals 0 grams carbohydrate, 7 grams protein, 8 grams fat, and 100 calories

One high-fat meat exchange is equal to any one of the following items.**

Pork: Spareribs, ground pork, pork sausage	1 oz
Cheese: All regular cheeses, such as American*, cheddar, Monterey Jack, Swiss	1 oz
Other: Processed sandwich meats with 8 Grams or less fat per ounce, such as bologna, pimento loaf, salami	1 oz
Sausage, such as bratwurst, Italian knockwurst, Polish, smoked	1 oz
Hot dog (turkey or chicken)*	1 (10/lb)
Bacon	3 slices (20 slices/lb)

** Count as one very lean meat and one starch exchange.

Hot dog (beef, pork, or combination)*	1 (1/10 lb)
Peanut butter (contains unsaturated fat)	2 Tbsp

*   = 400 mg or more sodium per exchange

Fat List

Monounsaturated Fats List
One fat exchange equals 5 grams fat and 45 calories

Avocado, medium	1/8 (1 oz)
Oil (canola, olive, peanut)	1 tsp
Olives: ripe (black)	8 large
Green, stuffed*	10 large
Nuts	
Almonds, cashews	6 nuts
Mixed (50% peanuts)	6 nuts
Peanuts	10 nuts
Pecans	4 halves
Peanut butter, smooth or crunchy	2 tsp
Sesame seeds	1 Tbsp
Tahini paste	2 tsp

Polyunsaturated Fats List
One fat exchange equals 5 grams fat and 45 calories

Margarine: stick, tub, or squeeze	1 tsp
Lower-fat (30% to 50% vegetable oil)	1 Tbsp
Mayonnaise: regular	1 tsp
reduced-fat	1 Tbsp
Nuts, walnuts, English	4 halves
Oil (corn, safflower, soybean)	1 tsp
Salad dressing: regular*	1 Tbsp
reduced-fat	2 Tbsp
Miracle Whip Salad Dressing®	
regular	2 tsp
reduced-fat	1 Tbsp
Seeds: pumpkin, sunflower	1 Tbsp

* = 400 mg or more sodium per exchange

Saturated Fats List*
One fat exchange equals 5 grams of fat and 45 cal[...]

Bacon, cooked	1 slic[...]
	slice
Bacon, grease	
Butter: stick	
whipped	
Reduced-fat	1 [...]
Chitterlings, boiled	2 Tbsp (½ [...]
Coconut, sweetened, shredded	2 [...]
Cream, half and half	2 [...]
Cream cheese: regular	1 Tbsp (½ [...]
Reduced-fat	2 Tbsp ([...]
Fatback or salt pork, see below**	
Shortening or lard	
Sour cream: regular	2 [...]
Reduced-fat	3 [...]

* Saturated fats can raise blood cholesterol levels.

** Use a piece 1 in. x 1 in. x ¼ in. if you
Plan to eat the fatback cooked with
½ in. when eating only the
vegetables with the fatback
removed.

Free Foods List

Free foods are foods or drinks that contain less than 20 calories or less than 5 grams of carbohydrate per serving. Foods with a serving size listed should be limited to three servings per day spread out throughout the day. Foods listed without a serving size can be eaten as often as you like.

Fat-free or Reduced-fat Foods

Cream cheese, fat-free	1 Tbsp
Creamers, nondairy, liquid	1 Tbsp
Creamers, nondairy, powdered	2 tsp
Mayonnaise, fat-free	1 Tbsp
Mayonnaise, reduced-fat	1 tsp
Margarine, fat-free	4 Tbsp
Margarine, reduced-fat	1 tsp
Miracle Whip®, nonfat	1 Tbsp
Miracle Whip®, reduced-fat	1 tsp
Nonstick cooking spray	
Salad dressing, fat-free	1 Tbsp
Salad dressing, fat-free, Italian	2 Tbsp
Salsa	¼ cup
Sour cream, fat-free, reduced-fat	1 Tbsp
Whipped topping, regular or light	2 Tbsp

Drinks

Bouillon, broth, consommé*	
Bouillon or broth, low-sodium	
Carbonated or mineral water	
Club soda	
Cocoa powder, unsweetened	1 Tbsp
Coffee	
Diet soft drinks, sugar-free	
Drink mixes, sugar-free	
Tea	
Tonic water, sugar-free	

Condiments

Catsup	1 Tbps
Horseradish	
Lemon juice	
Lime juice	
Mustard	
Pickles, dill*	1½ large
Soy sauce, regular or light*	
Taco sauce	
Vinegar	1 Tbsp

Sugar-free or Low-sugar Foods

Candy, hard, sugar-free	1 candy
Gelatin dessert, sugar-free	
Gelatin, unflavored	
Gum, sugar-free	
Jam or jelly, low-sugar or light	2 tsp
Sugar substitutes*	
Syrup, sugar-free	2 Tbsp

* Sugar substitutes, alternatives, or replacements that are approved by the Food and Drug Administration (FDA) are safe to use. Common brand names include:

> Equal® (aspartame)
> Sprinkle Sweet® (saccharin)
> Sweet One® (acesulfame K)
> Sweet-10® (saccharin)
> Sugar Twin® (saccharin)
> Sweet 'n Low® (saccharin)

Seasonings

Be careful with seasonings that contain sodium or are salts, Such as garlic or celery salt, and lemon pepper.

Flavoring extracts
Garlic
Herbs, fresh or dried
Pimento
Spices
Tabasco® or hot pepper sauce
Wine, used in cooking
Wine, used in cooking
Worcestershire sauce

* = 400 mg or more of sodium per exchange

Combination Foods List

These combination foods do not fit into any one exchange list. This is a list of exchanges for some typical combination foods.

Food	Serving Size	Exchanges Per Serving
Entrees		
Tuna noodle casserole, lasagna, spaghetti with meatballs, chili with beans, macaroni and cheese*	1 cup (8 oz)	2 carbohydrates, 2 medium-fat meat
Chow mein (without noodles or rice)*	2 cups (16 oz)	1 carbohydrate, 2 lean meats
Pizza, cheese, thin crust*	¼ of 10 in. (5 oz)	2 carbohydrates, 2 medium-fat meats, 1 fat
Pizza, meat topping, thin crust*	¼ of 10 in. (5 oz)	2 carbohydrates, 2 medium-fat meats, 2 fats
Pot pie*	1 (7 oz)	2 carbohydrates, 1 medium-fat meat, 4 fats
Frozen entrees		
Salisbury steak with gravy, mashed potato*	1 (11 oz)	2 carbohydrates, 3 medium-fat meats, 3-4 fats
Turkey and gravy, mashed potato, dressing*	1 (11 oz)	2 carbohydrates, 2 medium-fat meats, 2 fat
Entrée with less than 300 calories*	1 (8 oz)	2 carbohydrates, 3 lean meats
Soups		
Bean*	1 cup	1 carbohydrate, 1 very lean mea
Cream (made with water)*	1 cup (8 oz)	1 carbohydrate, 1 fat
Split pea (made with water)*	½ cup (4 oz)	1 carbohydrate
Tomato (made with water)*	1 cup (8 oz)	1 carbohydrate
Vegetable beef, chicken noodle, or other broth-type*	1 cup (8 oz)	1 carbohydrate

* = 400 or more sodium per exchange.

Fast Foods**

Food	Serving Size	Exchanges per Serving
Burritos with beef*	2	4 carbohydrates, 2 medium-fat meats, 2 fats
Chicken nuggets*	6	1 carbohydrate, 2 medium-fat meats, 1 fa
Chicken breast and wing, breaded and fried*	1 each	1 carbohydrate, 4 medium-fat meats, 2 fats
Fish sandwich/tartar sauce*	1	3 carbohydrates, 1 medium-fat meat, 3 fat
French fries, thin*	20-25	2 carbohydrates, 2 fat
Hamburger, regular	1	2 carbohydrates, 2 medium-fat meats
Hamburger, large*	1	2 carbohydrates, 3 medium-fat meats, 1 fa
Hot dog with bun*	1	1 carbohydrate, 1 high-fat meat, 1 fa
Individual pan pizza*	1	5 carbohydrates, 3 medium-fat meats, 3 fats
Soft-serve cone	1 medium	2 carbohydrates, 1 fa
Submarine sandwich*	1 sub (6 in.)	3 carbohydrates, 1 vegetable, 2 medium-fat meats, 1 fa
Taco, hard shell*	1 (6 oz)	2 carbohydrates, 2 medium-fat meats, 2 fats
Taco, soft shell	1 (3 oz)	1 carbohydrate, 1 medium-fat meat, 1 fa

* = 400 or more sodium per exchange.

** Ask at your fast-food restaurant for nutrition information about your favorite fast foods.

How to use Exchange Lists

A description of how to use Exchange Lists for meal planning follows:

(See sample calculation form, page 168)

1. Complete nutrition assessment **(sample form provided on page 173).**
2. Record usual intake from diet history on calculation form according to exchange groups (i.e.; if usual intake is 1 cup cereal, 1 cup milk, 1 cup orange juice, and 2 slices of toast with margarine, then mark 3 - 4 starches, 0 - 2 meat, 1 - 2 fruits, 0 - 1 milks, and 0 - 2 fats). A diet history is used as the basis for an initial meal plan. A range of intake for each of the groups should be given (see Sample Meal Plan, page 170).
3. Total the number of servings from each of the exchange groups for the day, and write this number under the "Total for Day" column for each group.
4. Fill in the gram composition of exchanges (carbohydrate, protein, and fat) by multiplying "Total for Day" by gram content (located in lower left corner of each box). Use a combination of very lean, lean, medium-fat and high-fat meat nutrient contents for determination of fat content in meat according to usual intake.
5. Total the grams of carbohydrate, protein, and fat and write these numbers in "Total" box under each nutrient.
6. Determine caloric level from each nutrient by multiplying each "Total Grams" by corresponding number of calories per gram (located in lower left corner of each box below "Total" box).
7. Determine "Total Calories" by adding total calories from carbohydrate, protein, and fat, and write figure in corresponding box.
8. Determine the percentage of carbohydrate, protein, and fat by using the following formulas:

$$\frac{\text{Total calories carbohydrate}}{\text{Total calories}} \quad \times \quad 100 \quad = \quad \text{\%carbohydrate}$$

$$\frac{\text{Total calories protein}}{\text{Total calories}} \quad \times \quad 100 \quad = \quad \text{\%protein}$$

$$\frac{\text{Total calories fat}}{\text{Total calories}} \quad \times \quad 100 \quad = \quad \text{\%fat}$$

SAMPLE CALCULATION FORM

Time	Bkfst 7:00 a.m.	Snack 9:30	Lunch 12:00	Snack 3:00	Dinner 6:30	Snack 8:30 pm	Total serving /day	CHO (g)	Protein (g)	Fat	Calories
Starch	1-2	1	2-3	1-2	2-3	1	9-10	15 / 142.5	3 / 28.5	t / 9.5	80 / 760
Fruit	0-1	0-1	1-2	1-2	1	1	5	15 / 75	-	-	60 / 300
Milk	1-2		1		1		4-5	12 / 54	8 / 36	1 / 4.5	90 / 405
Veg.	-	0-1	0-1		0-1		1-2	5 / 7.5	2 / 3	-	25 / 37.5
Meat/ Sub	0-2		2-3		3		6-7	-	7 / 45.5	5(3) / 32.5	75(55) / 487.5
Fat	1-2	0-1	1-2	0-1	1-2	0-1	6			5 / 30	45 / 270
Other				diet pop							
Total g								279	113	76.5	Total = 2257
Calories								1116 x4	452 x4	689 x9	
Percent calories								49%	20%	31%	

Source: International Diabetes Center, 1997, used with permission

168

SAMPLE CALCULATION FORM

	Bkft	Snack	Lunch	Snack	Dinner	Snack	Total serving /day	CHO (g)	Protein (g)	Fat	Calories
Time											
Starch								15	3	1	80
Fruit								15			60
Milk								12	8	1	90
Veg.								5	2		25
Meat/ Sub									7	5(3)	75(55)
Fat										5	45
Other											
Total g											
Calories								x4	x4	x9	Total =
Percent calories											

Source: International Diabetes Center, 1997, used with permission

Meal Plan

| Meal Plan for: | Johnny Doe | Date: | 7-27-97 |
| Dietitian: | Nancy Miller | Phone: | 555-1000 |

Carbohydrate	Grams	Percent
Carbohydrate	289 g	49%
Protein	113	20%
Fat	76.5	31%
Calories	2200-2300	

Time	Number of Exchanges/Choices	Menu Ideas	Menu Ideas
7:00 a.m.	3-4 Carbohydrate group 0-1 Starch 1-2 Fruit _____ Milk _skim_ 0-2 Meat group 1-2 Fat group	1½ cups dry cereal 1 cup skim milk ½ banana - sliced	2 eggs scrambled 2 slice wheat toast w/ 2 tsp margarine ½ cup orange juice 1 cup milk
9:30 a.m.	1-2 Carbohydrate Choices	1 package fruit snacks raw vegetables	small juice box 2 caramel rice cakes
12:00 noon	4-5 Carbohydrate group 2-3 Starch 1-2 Fruit 1 Milk ✓ Vegetables 2-3 Meat group 1-2 Fat group	sandwich with meat/cheese small bag chips 1 piece fruit 8 oz. milk	McDonalds hamburger small fries lowfat milk
3:00 p.m.	2-3 Carbohydrate Choices	2 small tortillas with melted mozzarella cheese	½ sandwich - pbanj small glass milk
6:30 p.m.	4-5 Carbohydrate group 2-3 Starch 1 Fruit ✓ Milk ✓ Vegetables 3 Meat group 1-2 Fat group	Chicken breast small baked potato with margarine dinner roll fruit cocktail - ½ cup 1 cup milk broccoli	1 cup noodle casserole with lettuce salad with light dressing small piece of dessert 1 cup milk
8:30 p.m.	1-2 Carbohydrate Choices	1 bag light microwave popcorn	1 cup cereal 1 cup milk

170

ONE DAY FOOD RECORD

NAME_____

HEIGHT_____   WEIGHT_____

(INSTRUCTIONS ON REVERSE SIDE)

INDICATE ACTUAL TIME FOOD IS EATEN	AMOUNT	FOOD & BEVERAGE	METHOD OF PREPARATION	DO NOT WRITE IN THIS SPACE
When you get up				
Breakfast				
Middle of the morning snack				
Lunch				
Middle of the afternoon snack				
Supper				
Evening snack				

What has your doctor told you about eating?

171

INTERNATIONAL DIABETES CENTER
3800 Park Nicollet Boulevard
Minneapolis, MN 55416

ONE DAY FOOD RECORD

Instructions for food diary:

1. Write down everything that you eat and drink for one day, on the reverse side of this page.

2. Show the amount actually eaten, not how much was put on the dish.

3. Specify type of food used, i.e. 1 cup skim milk or 2% or whole.

4. Count "how much" as cups or part of cups.

5. For food that does not fit into a cup or spoon, write down size. For meat or fish, record cooked ounces. For poultry, describe piece.

6. Note what is in mixed dishes and amount eaten in cups.

7. Describe the preparation method used.

8. Remember to record butter, margarine, sauces or salad dressing added to food.

9. Include alcoholic beverages.

NUTRITION ASSESSMENT

Date _____
Dietitian _____
Chart # _____
Physician _____

Name _____ Age _____

Diagnosis of Diabetes _____ Present Diabetes Treatment _____
Medical History _____ Other Medications _____
_____

Lab Data

HbA1c _____ BG _____
Cholesterol _____ HDL-C _____ Triglycerides _____ LDL-C _____
BP _____ Microalbumin _____ Other _____

Target Goals

Target BG's _____ mg/dl to _____ mg/dl
Target HbA1c _____ %

SMBG: Frequency _____ Times of day _____ Method _____

Medical clearance for exercise: Y / N   Exercise limitations _____

Time	Bkft	Snack	Lunch	Snack	Dinner	Snack	Total serving /day	CHO (g)	Protein (g)	Fat	Calories
Starch								15	3	1 .	80
Fruit								15			60
Milk								12	8	1	90
Veg.								5	2		25
Meat/ Sub									7	5(3)	75(55)
Fat										5	45
Other							Total g				
							Calories	x4	x4	x9	Total =
							Percent calories				

Ht _____ (_____ %) Wt History _____
Wt _____ (_____ %) Reasonable Wt _____
Estimated calorie expenditure + Activity factor = Total calorie needs _____

History

Occupation _____   Hours worked _____
Lives with _____   Meal preparation _____
Hypoglycemia _____   Eating out _____
Alcohol use _____   Travel _____
Schedule changes/Weekends/School schedule _____
Exercise: Type/Frequency _____
Appetite/GI problems/Allergies/Intolerances _____
Vitamin & mineral supplements _____
Psychosocial/Economic _____
Assessment

_____
_____
_____
_____

Goals (Nutrition/Exercise/SMBG)

_____
_____
_____

©1996 International Diabetes Center. Institute for Research and Education HealthSystem Minnesota   IDC 0003 (10/95)

Carbohydrate Counting

Carbohydrate counting is a method of food planning for people with diabetes that considers only the carbohydrate content of foods for consistency. It is based on the premise that carbohydrate is the nutrient that affects blood sugar levels first and the most. Research shows that most sugars, whether "simple" or "complex", basically affect blood glucose levels the same as long as same amounts are eaten. For instance, 15 grams of carbohydrate from chocolate cake will likely affect blood sugar levels the same as 15 grams of carbohydrate from a piece of bread.

It is especially important that families are taught nutrition principles combined with carbohydrate counting to prevent excessive weight gain and poor nutritional choices when using carbohydrate counting.

The common unit in teaching carbohydrate counting is a "carbohydrate choice" which is equal to 15 grams of carbohydrate. When a person is given a meal plan using carbohydrate counting, they will be told to eat a specific range of carbohydrate choices or carbohydrate grams at each meal and snack. Additionally, they will receive guidelines for amounts of meat, vegetables, and fat to eat throughout the day.

The Exchange Lists for Meal Planning have been revised to incorporate carbohydrate counting principles. The groups of foods in the Exchange Lists that contain carbohydrate are the starch, fruit, milk, and other carbohydrate lists. Each of the portions listed in these groups contains approximately 15 grams of carbohydrate and can be counted as one carbohydrate choice. Although vegetables contain carbohydrate, the amount is so minimal that it is commonly recommended that people using carbohydrate counting do not need to include them as choices. Additionally, the carbohydrate content of many vegetables is dietary fiber which is not totally digested and will not affect blood glucoses significantly.

A sample of a meal plan using carbohydrate counting is shown below:

Name: Jane Doe	Calories: 1800 - 1900	Date: 6/1/97
Carbohydrate: 216 grams Cals from Carb: 864 (46%)	Protein: 103 grams Cals from Protein: 412 (22%)	Fat: 67 grams Cals from Fat: 604 (32%)

Breakfast
Carbohydrate Choices 3 - 4
(45 - 60 grams)
   Starch 2
   Fruit 0-1
   Milk 1
Meat 0 - 2
Fat 0 - 2
	Lunch
	Carbohydrate Choices 4 - 5
	(60 - 75 grams)
	   Starch 2
	   Fruit 1 - 2
	   Milk 1
	Meat 2 - 3
	Vegetable 1 - 2
	Fat 1 - 2
		Evening Meal
		Carbohydrate Choices 5 - 6
		(75 - 90 grams)
		   Starch. 2 - 3
		   Fruit 0 - 1
		   Milk 2
		Meat 3 - 4
		Vegetable 1 - 2
		Fat 1 - 2

Morning Snack Carbohydrate Choices 2 - 3 (30 - 45 grams)	Afternoon Snack Carbohydrate Choices 1 - 2 (15 - 30 grams)	Evening Snack Carbohydrate Choices 1 - 2 (15 - 30 grams)

The meal plan card shown gives total carbohydrate choices for each meal and snack, and also shows guidelines for amounts of each of the carbohydrate-containing groups (i.e.; starch, fruit, milk) to consume to maintain variety of food choices.

Flexibility in intake using carbohydrate counting can be demonstrated in the following example:
If a family was having pizza at their evening meal, then the child could use all of their carbohydrate choices for consumption of pizza rather than having the proposed fruit and milk exchanges that usually are eaten. In this instance, the patient is given freedom to choose according to occasion and flexibility is offered additionally.

It is again important to recognize that examples such as the above should be included in the instruction to families, however, **emphasis should be placed on inclusion of basic nutrition principles and food variety.**

Ranges of intake for carbohydrate choices, as well as, meat, vegetables, and fat are given to guide the patient in making all food choices at any meal or snack. It is important that general guidelines are given for sugar and fat intake also, since good nutrition may be neglected if people only concentrate on consistency with carbohydrate. Also, especially with children and adolescents, excessive intakes of high-sugar/high-fat foods can cause more nutritious foods to be deleted, excessive weight gain, and poor eating habits in the future. Guidelines for sucrose intake will be discussed in more detail later in this section.

The table below can help when determining the number of carbohydrate choices that corresponds to grams of carbohydrate:

Carbohydrate Grams	Carbohydrate Choices
0 - 5	0
6 - 10	1/2
11 - 20	1
21 - 25	1 1/2
26 - 35	2
36 - 40	2 1/2
41 - 50	3
51 - 55	3 1/2
56 - 65	4
66 - 70	4 1/2
71 - 80	5

References for Teaching Carbohydrate Counting
- Tools for teaching carbohydrate counting can be found at the end of this section

USING FOOD LABELS IN DIABETES MEAL PLANNING

In January 1993, the US Government created new rules governing food labels. These were meant to end the confusion surrounding labeling, provide accurate and useable information to the consumer, and provide a consistent format for comparison between similar foods.

An example of a food label is shown below with explanations of some of its features:

Nutrition Facts

Serving Size 1 cup (248g)
Servings Per Container 4

Amount Per Serving

Calories 150   Calories from Fat 35

	% Daily Value*
Total Fat 4g	**6%**
Saturated Fat 2.5g	**12%**
Cholesterol 20mg	**7%**
Sodium 170mg	**7%**
Total Carbohydrate 17g	**6%**
Dietary Fiber 0g	**0%**
Sugars 17g	
Protein 13g	

Vitamin A 4%	•	Vitamin C 6%
Calcium 40%	•	Iron 0%

* Percent Daily Values are based on a 2,000 calorie diet. Your daily values may be higher or lower depending on your calorie needs:

	Calories:	2,000	2,500
Total Fat	Less than	65g	80g
Sat Fat	Less than	20g	25g
Cholesterol	Less than	300mg	300mg
Sodium	Less than	2,400mg	2,400mg
Total Carbohydrate		300g	375g
Dietary Fiber		25g	30g

Calories per gram:

Fat 9   •   Carbohydrate 4   •   Protein 4

- Nutrition Facts - the heading for the new food label
- Serving Size - listed in similar amounts for similar foods for comparison. Based on realistic servings.
- Vitamins and Minerals - vitamins A & C, and iron and calcium are required. Others are voluntary.
- % Daily Value - based on a 2000 calorie diet. Used to compare like foods for nutrient content.
- Daily Value Footnote - reference values for a 2000 and 2500 calorie diet.
- Calories Per Gram Footnote - tell calories per gram of carbohydrate, protein, and fat.

USING LABELS WITH CARBOHYDRATE COUNTING

The Nutrition Facts Panel can be used to determine how to use various convenience and packaged foods for persons using carbohydrate counting. Families should be instructed to use the lines entitled **serving size** and **total carbohydrate** to determine how to incorporate foods into a child's or adolescent's food plan. Additionally, the serving size listed should be noted since the total carbohydrate in grams corresponds to that specific portion. If one consumes twice that portion, then the total carbohydrate must subsequently be multiplied by two.

One carbohydrate choice is equal to 15 grams of carbohydrate. If a convenience food contains 34 grams of carbohydrate per 1 cup serving, then it is counted as two carbohydrate choices. Two cups of the same food would be equal to 68 grams of carbohydrate or roughly 4 1/2 carbohydrate choices (**see carbohydrate choices page 175).**

On the nutrition facts panel, the sugar and dietary fiber are already calculated as part of the total carbohydrate, and therefore do not need to be considered separately. However, since dietary fiber is not digested and will not affect blood glucose levels, patients should be instructed to subtract grams of dietary fiber from the total carbohydrate amount if dietary fiber equal 5 grams or more per serving.

Additional instruction related to nutritious food choices, fat, sodium and calories should be included for children and adolescents consuming convenience and packaged foods on a regular basis.

Patients should be instructed that the term "sugar-free" on a label does not necessarily mean carbohydrate-free, and that these foods must sometimes be substituted into the food plan using carbohydrate counting.

Food manufacturers are still required to list ingredients in foods from most to least with respect to weight. Under new labeling regulations, certain terms now have a specific definition from food to food. The following is a list of regulated labeling terms and their definitions:

- Calories
    - calorie-free - less than 5 calories per serving
    - low calorie - 40 calories or less per serving
    - reduced calorie - at least 25% fewer calories per serving when compared with a similar food
    - light, lite - one third fewer calories or 50% less fat per serving; if more than half the calories are from fat, fat content must be reduced by 50% or more
- Sugar
    - sugar-free - less than 1/2 gram sugars per serving
    - low sugar - may not be used as a claim
    reduced sugar - at least 25% less sugar per serving when compared with a similar food

- no added sugars, without added sugar, no sugar added - no amount of sugars or any other ingredient that contains sugars that functionally substitute for contains no ingredients that contain added sugars, such as jam, jelly, or concentrated fruit juice; the product it resembles and substitutes for normally contains added sugars; and the label declares that the food is not "low calorie" or "calorie reduced" as appropriate
- Fat
    - fat-free - less that 1/2 gram fat per serving
    - 100% fat free - meets requirements for fat free
    - low fat - 3 grams or less fat per serving
    - ___% fat free - meets requirements for low fat; the percentage is based on the amount of fat (by weight) in 100 grams of the food.
    - reduced fat - at least 25% less fat when compared with a similar food
    - saturated fat free - less than 1/2 gram saturated fat per serving
    - low saturated fat - 1 gram or less saturated fat per serving and no more than 15% of calories from saturated fat
    - reduced saturated fat - at least 25% less saturated fat per serving when compared with a similar food
- Cholesterol
    - cholesterol-free - less than 2 milligrams cholesterol per serving and 2 grams or less saturated fat per serving
    - low cholesterol - 20 milligrams or less cholesterol per serving and 2 grams or less saturated fat per serving
    - reduced cholesterol - at least 25% less cholesterol when compared with a similar food, and 2 grams or less saturated fat per serving
- Sodium
    - sodium-free - less than 5 milligrams sodium per serving
    - salt free - meets requirements for sodium free
    - very low sodium - 35 milligrams or less sodium per serving
    - low sodium - 140 milligrams or less sodium per serving
    - reduced sodium - at least 25% less sodium when compared with a similar food
    - light in sodium - 50% less sodium per serving; restricted to foods with more than 40 calories per serving or more than 3 grams of fat per serving
    - unsalted, without added salt, no salt added - no salt is added during processing; the product it resembles and substitutes for is normally processed with salt; and the label bears the statement "not a sodium-free food" or "not for control of sodium in the diet" if the food is not sodium free

NUTRITIVE AND NON-NUTRITIVE SWEETENERS

Nutritive Sweeteners

Nutritive sweeteners are so named because they contribute calories to a person's diet when consumed.

- **Sucrose**

Many studies show that incorporating sucrose into the diets of people with diabetes has no adverse effects on overall blood glucose control. Sucrose does not cause a higher increase in blood glucose compared to equivalent amounts of other carbohydrates. It is important to remember that added sugars are found in such foods as soft drinks, candy, heavy syrups, jams, jellies and desserts, all of which contain too many calories and too few nutrients, and therefore should be added less often and after inclusion of more nutritious foods that will contribute to optimal growth and development in children and adolescents.

Other nutritive sweeteners such as corn syrup, fruit juice concentrate, lactose, hydrogenated starch hydrolysates, fructose, molasses, honey, dextrose, maltose, all contain carbohydrate and will affect blood glucoses similarly to sucrose, and therefore must be substituted into the meal plan of people with diabetes.

Sugar alcohols and other polyols are included in the total carbohydrate listed on the nutrition label. Because they only contribute half the calories (on average) per gram compared to other carbohydrates, families should be taught to subtract half the grams from sugar alcohols if the amount listed is more than 5 grams.

Guidelines for sucrose intake:
- Inclusion of sucrose into the diet for diabetes is not meant to encourage its use.
- Foods that contain sucrose must be properly substituted into the diet in place of another carbohydrate-containing food. Portions of these foods are often small since the carbohydrate content is typically more concentrated.
- Foods that contain sucrose are often high in fat, and so must be limited to keep the fat content of the diet minimal.
- Labels appearing on snack foods should be used to calculate a food's use (i.e., 15 grams of carbohydrate equals a carbohydrate choice).

Non-Nutritive Sweeteners

Non-nutritive sweeteners add no or very few additional calories to a person's diet when consumed in products or alone. They are particularly sweet in very small amounts. The Food and Drug Administration (FDA) sets acceptable daily intakes (ADI) for all artificial sweeteners which is the amount determined to be safe for humans to consume daily over their lifetime with a safety factor. The amount is based on the kilogram weight of a person. For a child weighing fifty pounds (23 kilograms), the limit would be approximately equal to seven cans of a soft drink containing an artificial sweetener each day.

Non-nutritive sweeteners will have no effect on blood glucose levels, and their consumption should be determined based on ADI, family preferences and the nutritional content of a child's or adolescent's usual intake. Foods containing artificial sweeteners that have limited or no nutritional value (soft drinks, frozen desserts, etc.) should not replace more nutritious beverages and foods in the diets of persons with diabetes.

The non-nutritive sweeteners currently available in the United States include saccharin (Sweet n Low), Aspartame (Nutrasweet, Equal) and acesulfame-K (Sunette, SweetOne, Swiss Sweet).

DIABETES AND SNACKS

Children and adolescents often have snacks as part of their food plan, and should be instructed on how to work a variety of snacks into their food plan and to include choices that offer sound nutrition without excessive amounts of calories, fat and salt. Families should be given guidelines for working "treats" and sweets into the food plan, if desired, but the emphasis should be placed on encouraging healthful eating while snacking.

The following tips can be used when instructing families:
- Try to include whole grain crackers and snacks, and fresh fruits and vegetables
- Limit the fat in snacks by choosing ones that contain 3 grams or less per serving
- Use labels to work convenience and packaged snacks into food plans (15 grams of carbohydrate equals one carbohydrate choice)
- Beware of "sugar-free" and "fat-free" - these terms do not mean "calorie-free", and foods described this way often need to be worked into the food plan
- Families need to determine the frequency of sweets and "treats" according to family rules and nutritional balance of their child's food intake
- If families inquire regarding the use of candy or candy bars, they should be instructed that it is okay to use the label to determine how to work the correct amount in as a snack, but caution families regarding the poor nutritional value of such items

Below is a generic and limited snack list that contains various choices for children and adolescents. The carbohydrate choices and fat grams have been listed for the portion listed:

	carbohydrate choices	fat grams*
Animal crackers, 8	1	2
Breakfast bar, 1	2 - 3	3 - 6
Crackers, 5 - 6	1	0 - 8
Caramel corn, 1/2 cup	2	2.5
Cheese puffs, 25	1	11
Cookie, 3" diameter	1	5
Corn chips, 34 (1 oz)	1	9
Fresh fruit, 1 medium piece	1	0
Frozen yogurt, lowfat, 1/2 cup	1 - 1 1/2	0 - 3
Fruit bars, 1	1	0
Fruit juice, 1/2 cup	1 - 1 1/2	0
Fruit snacks, 1 pouch	1 - 1 1/2	0
Gelatin snack cup, 1	1	0
Gelatin, sugar free, 1 cup	0	0
Granola bar, 1	1 1/2 - 2	0 - 3
Ice cream, 1/2 cup	1	8
Popcorn, 3 cups popped	1	0 - 10
Potato chips, 12 - 18 chips	1	10
Pretzels, 65 sticks or 4 large twists	1	0 - 1
Pudding snacks, 1 cup	1 1/2 - 2	3 - 5

	carbohydrate choices	fat grams*
Rice cakes, 2	1	0
Toaster pastry, 1	2 - 3	3 - 8
Tortilla chips, 15 - 18 chips	1	6
Trail mix, 1/4 cup	1	8
Yogurt, artificially sweetened, 1 cup	1	0 - 3
Yogurt, fruit on bottom, 1 cup	2 - 3	3

*The fat content of items will vary. It is best to look at the label for actual carbohydrate and fat content of snacks consumed.

DIABETES IN THE SCHOOL AND DAYCARE FACILITIES

Children and adolescents with diabetes often spend a large part of their day outside of the home and in the care and presence of non-family members. In order to fully ensure the well-being and proper management of a young person with diabetes, it is important that families work closely with outside providers including school and daycare personnel to develop a diabetes care plan that outlines all aspects of the child's care. Conferences between school and daycare personnel should occur and a written plan be devised that addresses all topics related to diabetes.

Factors to consider when devising a care plan for children with diabetes include:
- hours of school/daycare
- meal and snack times
- gym, recess, sports practice times
- blood glucose monitoring times and place
- guidelines for action by school personnel/caregivers (i.e.; treatment of hypoglycemia, checking for ketones, when to call parents)
- guidelines for illnesses
- insulin injection times, place (if applicable)

The information below can be used when teaching school personnel or daycare providers:

- **Hypoglycemia**

If people on insulin receive too much insulin, too little food, or are very active, their blood sugar level might go too low (usually less than 70 or 80 mg/dl). If this happens, children may exhibit certain **symptoms** such as:

paleness	**hunger**	**dizziness**
sweatiness	**blurred vision**	**shakiness**
confusion	**inattentiveness**	**irritability**
drowsiness		

It is important that these symptoms be recognized by someone so that proper treatment can be initiated. Some children/adolescents will not display any symptoms of a low blood sugar. If treatment is not initiated, the student may experience unconsciousness or convulsions. **If you notice any difference in a student's behavior, they may need to test their blood sugar or initiate treatment.**

Treatment is aimed at raising the blood sugar to normal levels. This is done by administering some form of carbohydrate (15 grams) to the child. Examples of this are:

1/2 cup juice	**1/2 cup regular pop**	**fruit snacks**
6 - 7 lifesavers	**3 Glucose Tablets**	**4 -5 sugar cubes**
piece of fruit	**small tube frosting**	**5 - 6 crackers**

People with diabetes are advised to carry something on them at all times in case of a reaction. However, it is important to have something in the classroom or on hand should a child be unprepared.

After treatment, you should notice improvement in 10 - 15 minutes. If not, then treatment should be repeated. If improvement still does not occur, the child's parents should be contacted for instructions. If initial treatment is successful, the child should be given 15 grams of carbohydrate more if it is one hour or more until the next snack or meal.

- **Meal Plan**

People on insulin are asked to follow a consistent pattern of eating based on assessment by a dietitian. New nutrition recommendations allow for foods that have been traditionally deleted to be worked into the meal plan in place of other foods. School lunch personnel should be instructed to make sure to observe the student only in relation to them eating their entire meal rather than for what they choose to eat.

Teachers should allow students to eat foods brought for special occasions. Parents can teach students how to work these foods into the meal plan.

Most children with diabetes will require a midmorning and afternoon snack to prevent hypoglycemia at these times. Teachers or caregivers may be asked to remind them to take these snacks. Please be sure to allow ample time for these snacks to be consumed by the child with diabetes. Snacks are often necessary before, during or right after gym class.

Families should be advised that typical school lunches include:
> 2 - 4 starches
> 0 - 2 fruits
> 1 milk
> 2 meat
> 0 - 2 vegetables
> 3 - 4 fat
> (total of 4 - 6 carbohydrate choices or approximately 60 - 90 grams of carbohydrate)

- **Blood glucose monitoring**

Students with diabetes will need to monitor their blood sugars. This is usually done with a device called a meter. Schools differ on the location in which this process should occur. Parents should clarify this with school personnel prior to the first day of classes. Blood glucose monitoring should be done before each meal and anytime the student feels "funny" such as during hypoglycemia.

- **Other information**

It is important that there is good communication between families of students with diabetes and all school personnel. A meeting should be held with families to determine expectations of students and school personnel, and for emergency contact information.

EXERCISE AND DIABETES IN CHILDREN AND ADOLESCENTS

Research in persons with type 1 diabetes has shown that glycemic control is not always affected positively neither short nor long term as exercise is added to the overall management plan. This is mainly because of the difficulty in this group of making accurate food and/or insulin adjustments to prevent blood glucose excursions resulting from exercise. Regardless of this fact, exercise continues to be a recommended addition to the management plans of all persons with type 1 diabetes.

Children and adolescents should be encouraged to participate in physical activity on a regular basis to promote health, prevent disease later in life, and provide socialization.

It is recommended that children/adolescents work closely with their diabetes team for guidance in making insulin and/or food changes to accommodate increases in physical activity associated with sports, camping trips, field trips or other such activities. Schedules of practices, games, etc. must be considered to provide the best recommendations to families regarding changes in insulin amounts or regimens and food plans to prevent problems with blood glucose responses.

Additionally, athletes should be given guidelines for fluid replacement with endurance activities. It is recommended that these individuals work closely with a diabetes team for insulin/carbohydrate adjustments.

Various insulin types/regimens are more beneficial based on the time and duration of exercise. Additionally, insulin administration devices can provide convenience to children and adolescents who must transport insulin during extracurricular activities.

Risks associated with an increase in physical activity, whether planned or unplanned, include: hypoglycemia, hyperglycemia/ketosis, and possible exacerbation of associated diabetes complications (if present in children and adolescents). Appropriate education should be given to clients and families to avoid these possible risks.

The following general recommendations can be used when educating regarding exercise in children and adolescents:

- **Hypoglycemia with Exercise**

Hypoglycemia (low blood glucose) can occur during or up to 30 hours after physical activity (post-exercise hypoglycemia) depending on the duration and intensity of the exercise session. People with diabetes should be given guidelines for either adding food and/or decreasing insulin to prevent hypoglycemia with exercise.

Adding Carbohydrate to Prevent Hypoglycemia with Exercise

A general rule of thumb for adding carbohydrate to prevent hypoglycemia with exercise is to add 15 grams of carbohydrate for every 60 minutes of extra activity. For example, if a child was going to go out and play hard or ride his bicycle for one hour, adding a medium piece of fruit or 5 to 6 crackers should provide the carbohydrate necessary to prevent hypoglycemia. Children and adolescents may need more or less depending on a variety of factors including type and intensity of activity, overall blood glucose control, when the last meal or snack was eaten, current blood glucose level, and fitness level.

Another set of guidelines to follow for adding carbohydrate to prevent hypoglycemia is by assessing the type of activity to be performed and the current blood glucose level. The table below gives guidelines for using this method:

Making Food Adjustments for Exercise:

General Guidelines

Type of Exercise and Examples	If Blood Glucose Is:	Increase Food Intake By:	Suggestions of Food to Use:
Exercise of short duration and of low to moderate intensity (walking a half mile or leisurely bicycling for less than 30 minutes)	less than 100 mg/dl	10 to 15 gms of carbohydrate per hour	1 fruit or 1 starch/bread exchange
	100 mg/dl or above	not necessary to increase food	
Exercise of moderate intensity (one hour of tennis, swimming, jogging, leisurely bicycling, golfing, etc)	less than 100 mg/dl	25 to 50 gms of carbohydrate before exercise, then 10 to 15 gms per hour of exercise	1/2 meat sandwich with a milk or fruit exchange
	100 to 180 mg/dl	10 to 15 gms of carbohdrate	1 fruit or 1 starch/bread exchange
	180 to 300 mg/dl	not necessrry to increase	
	300 mg/dl or above	don't begin exercise until blood glucose is under better control	
Strenuous activity or exercise (about one to two hours of football, hockey, recquetball, or basketball; strenuous bicycling or swimming; shoveling heavy snow)	less than 100 mg/dl	50 gms of carbohydrate, monitor blood glucose carefully	1 meat sandwch (2 slices of bread) with a milk and fruit exchange
	100 to 180 mg/dl	25 to 50 gms of carbohydrate depending on intensity and duration	1/2 meat sandwich with a milk or fruit exchange
	180 to 300 mg/dl	10 to 15 gms of carbohydrate	1 fruit or 1 starch/bread exchange
	300 mg/dl or above	don't begin exercise until blood glucose is under better control	

Reprinted, with permission, from Diabetes Actively Staying Healthy (DASH): Your Game Plan for Diabetes and Exercise, *by Marion J. Franz, MS, RD and Jane Norstrom, MA. Minneapolis: International Diabetes Center, 1990.*

To prevent post-exercise hypoglycemia, patients should be advised to consume the additional carbohydrate either during or directly after exercise.

Adjusting insulin to prevent hypoglycemia
When adjusting insulin to prevent hypoglycemia during exercise, the following general guidelines can be employed:
1. Determine insulin that is working the hardest during physical activity
2. Decrease that insulin by 1 - 2 units (1/2 unit increments may be required in younger children less than 10 years old)

Sample of insulin adjustment to prevent hypoglycemia:
A 7 year old child is on an insulin regimen of 4 units Regular/6 units NPH in the morning before breakfast, 2 units of Regular at lunch, and 3 units Regular/4 units NPH at evening meal. The child will be going to gymnastics practice in the afternoon from 3:00 p.m. to 4:00 p.m.
Answer:
Since the Regular insulin at lunch will be working the hardest during the gymnastics practice, it would be appropriate for this family to decrease that dose by
1/2 to 1 unit to prevent hypoglycemia. The family would also be advised to have the child eat their afternoon snack and take extra carbohydrate to treat a hypoglycemic reaction if one occurs.

For activity of long duration (more than one hour), the following guidelines can be used:
1. Determine insulin that is working the hardest during physical activity
2. Calculate total daily dose of insulin (all types)
3. Multiply total daily dose by 10%
4. Decrease insulin working while active by 10% total daily dose

To prevent post-exercise hypoglycemia, it may be useful to adjust insulin(s) taken subsequent to activity by 1 - 2 units.

General Guidelines and Information for Exercisers:
- Adding carbohydrate to prevent hypoglycemia is more predictable than adjusting insulin doses.
- Adjusting short acting insulins is more predictable than adjusting longer acting insulins.
- Persons using Regular or Humalog insulin can ask their physician for active Vs inactive doses of insulin based on blood glucose results.
- Patients should be instructed to:
    - test their blood glucoses before, during (if longer than one hour) and after exercise (up to 10 hours) to see the effects on blood glucose.
    - always wear medical ID
    - carry a carbohydrate source to treat hypoglycemia.
    - carry their blood glucose meter with them during exercise (if possible).
    - not inject insulin into an area of the body that will be exercising within one hour

It should be noted that the previous sections on adding carbohydrate or decreasing insulin to prevent hypoglycemia during physical activity are only guidelines. It is recommended that families work closely with a team of diabetes experts for consultation in making adjustments that are individualized to their particular child's needs.

- **Hyperglycemia with Exercise**
Hyperglycemia after exercise can occur for two reasons:

- Poor glycemic control and lack of adequate insulin
It is important to note that exercise can only assist in lowering blood glucose levels if adequate insulin is available. Insulin is required for exercising muscle tissues to utilize glucose for energy. In other words, if a person is in poor diabetes control, exercise will not lower blood glucose levels. In this case, if exercise is begun, the active muscle will send a message to the liver to produce glucose (glycogenolysis) for energy to accommodate increased needs during exercise. Without adequate insulin (i.e.; poor glycemic control), the additional glucose from the liver will increase blood glucose levels even further.
Recommendations for exercise:
    - If a person has been experiencing high blood sugars (> 240 mg/dl) and metabolic control is questionable, have them check for ketones
    - If ketones are present (greater than trace to small or > 40 mg/dl), it is necessary to consult with the diabetes care team before exercising for assistance in problem solving and obtaining better diabetes control; exercising in this situation will worsen metabolic control

- Intensive exercise
Hyperglycemia can also occur in individuals who exercise intensively or beyond their body's normal capacity. This happens because the body's normal hormonal response to heavy exercise is to produce extra glucose from the liver to accommodate extra physical activity. Sometimes this response is excessive causing a rise in blood glucose levels subsequent to particularly heavy exercise.

Patients should be instructed that this increase is often transient, and if metabolic control is good (i.e.; adequate insulin is available), then blood glucoses will likely continue to decrease over the next few hours.

- **Diabetes Complications and Exercise**
If a child or adolescent has any complications (retinopathy, neuropathy, nephropathy, high blood pressure) associated with diabetes, it is important that exercises that could exacerbate problems be avoided. Consultation with a diabetes professional prior to beginning a program would be advised in this situation.

DIABETES AND MANAGEMENT OF ILLNESS

It is typical for the body to respond to illness (stress) with an increase in blood glucose levels. An increase in blood glucose levels is usually the first sign to a person with diabetes that an illness or infection is present. To prevent progression to diabetic ketoacidosis (DKA), certain guidelines must be followed by the person with diabetes.

The following are guidelines for management during brief (less than 24 hours) illness:

- **Check for ketones**
  During illness insulin needs may increase to accommodate high glucose levels related to stress hormone production. When the body's insulin is deficient, fat will be metabolized by the body for energy in place of glucose. Fat is generally an inefficient fuel for the body to use as an initial energy source, and is incompletely broken down, and will produce ketones in the blood and urine. Ketones are an acidic substance in the body and can be fatal. Ketones will cause a person to feel nauseated and have severe abdominal pain.

  When a person with diabetes is ill, they must check for ketones. If the level of ketones is moderate to large (>40 mg/dl), the patient should be instructed to contact their physician.

  Patients should be instructed to check for ketones anytime they are ill or if blood glucose readings are > 240 mg/dl two times in a row.

- **Continue to take insulin**
  People with diabetes typically have high blood glucoses during illness or infection and need to continue taking their insulin doses. This is usually true even if a person is unable to eat their usual food plan. If a person is unable to eat their food plan or vomiting, they should be instructed to contact their physician for further recommendations. General guidelines for substituting carbohydrate-containing foods are provided later in this section.

  Physicians will often give patients guidelines for adding extra short-acting insulin during illness if ketones are present.

- **Continue to test blood glucoses**
  It is important to continue to test blood glucose levels during illness to track progression of treatment measures. It may be necessary to check blood glucoses more often during illness. Blood glucoses should be provided to physicians to assist in managing the patient and instruct regarding insulin adjustments during illness

- **Continue to eat usual food plan, if tolerated**
  If able, the patient should be instructed to continue following their usual food plan consistently. This is especially true if additional insulin has been added to clear ketones.

If unable to eat the usual food plan, it is recommended that patients try to consume 50 grams of carbohydrate every 3 - 4 hours to replace meals and snacks. Samples of foods (in 15 gram portions) that could be used for carbohydrate replacement during illness are:

- 1/2 cup of regular soft drink (not diet)
- 1/2 twin popsicle
- 1/4 cup sweetened gelatin
- 6 - 7 lifesavers
- 1/2 cup frozen dessert
- 1/2 cup fruit juice
- 1 slice dry toast
- 1 cup artificially sweetened yogurt
- 8 oz Gatorade

If blood glucose levels are >200 mg/dl, consuming carbohydrate-containing foods may not be necessary, however, families should be instructed to have their child eat if able, and continue to monitor blood glucose levels.

If a patient has ketones or is vomiting or has diarrhea, it is particularly important to maintain a steady intake of fluids via plain water, bouillon, popsicles or any other appropriate source.

- **Contact your physician, if needed**
  It is important that families are given guidance as to who to contact at any time should they require assistance in dealing with an illness in their child. DKA and dehydration can develop rapidly during illness, especially in children.

It should be noted that the previous sections are only guidelines for management of diabetes during brief illnesses. Complete guidelines for illness should be received from the child's physician and/or diabetes team.

DIABETES AND SPECIAL OCCASIONS AND SCHEDULE CHANGES

Families should be given instruction related to recommendations for handling special occasions such as birthday parties, holidays, sleepovers, school trips, family outings, and other such events. Emphasis should be placed on giving guidelines for adjusting insulin regimens or doses and how to alter the food plan to accommodate various types of foods and timing of meals and snacks.

Adjustments in food/insulin for schedule changes:
It is generally recommended that timing of insulin/meals/snacks occur within 1 - 1 1/2 hours variance day to day ideally so as not to upset diabetes management plan. If meal times are going to occur outside of 2 hours from the usual time, the following general recommendations can be made:

Possible adjustments in insulin regimen and carbohydrate spacing for schedule changes:

Usual schedule:		**Brunch schedule**	
7:00 am	test	7:00 am	test
	insulin (R and NPH)		insulin (NPH only)
7:30 am	breakfast		snack
	4 - 5 carbohydrate choices		1 - 2 carbohydrate choices
10:00 am	1 - 2 carbohydrate choices	10:30 am	test
11:55 am	test		insulin (R only)
12:00	lunch	11:00 am	lunch
	4 - 5 carbohydrate choices		7 - 8 carbohydrate choices
3:00 pm	2 - 3 carbohydrate choices	3:00 pm	2 - 3 carbohydrate choices
5:30 pm	test	5:30 pm	test
	insulin (R and NPH)		insulin (R and NPH)
6:00 pm	evening meal	6:00 pm	evening meal
	4 - 5 carbohydrate choices		4 - 5 carbohydrate choices
9:00 pm	test	9:00 pm	test
	bedtime snack		bedtime snack
	1 - 2 carbohydrate choices		1 - 2 carbohydrate choices

Late Afternoon Meal		**Late Evening Meal**	
7:00 am	test	7:00 am	test
	insulin (R and NPH)		insulin (R and NPH)
7:30 am	breakfast	7:30 am	breakfast
	4 - 5 carbohydrate choices		4 - 5 carbohydrate choices
10:00 am	morning snack	10:00 am	morning snack
	1 - 2 carbohydrate choices		1 - 2 carbohydrate choices
11:55 am	test	11:55 am	test
12:00	2 - 3 carbohydrate choices	12:00	4 - 5 carbohydrate choices
2:30 pm	insulin (evening meal R only)	3:00 pm	2 - 3 carbohydrate choices
3:00 pm	meal	5:30 pm	test
	7 - 8 carbohydrate choices		insulin (NPH only)
5:30 pm	test		1 - 2 carbohydrate choices
	insulin (NPH only)	7:30 pm	insulin (R only)
	snack (if BG <80 - 100)	8:00 pm	evening meal
	1 - 2 carbohydrate choices		4 - 5 carbohydrate choices
9:00 pm	test	9:00 pm	test
	bedtime snack		snack (if BG < 100)
	1 - 2 carbohydrate choices		1 - 2 carbohydrate choices

It is important to teach families that short-acting insulin (regular or Humalog) should be given to cover meals, and thus shifted to before the main meal times. Additionally, carbohydrate choices will be spaced differently throughout the day to accommodate various eating times during holidays or other special occasions. It may be necessary to add extra short-acting insulin to cover larger meals during special occasions. Families can be instructed to add approximately 1 unit of short-acting insulin for each additional carbohydrate choice to be eaten at meal time. It should be noted that if extra activity is also occurring, the extra food may be used to prevent hypoglycemia. It is important to look at all factors and determine adjustments in food and insulin during special occasions.

Again, it is important for families to work closely with their diabetes team to determine a schedule of insulin and carbohydrate choices that is appropriate for them during special occasions.

DIABETES AND PSYCHOSOCIAL CONCERNS IN CHILDREN AND ADOLESCENTS

An important person of the diabetes team is a psychologist or family counselor. Since diabetes is a chronic disease that affects many aspects of a child's life, it is important that families are given the opportunity to visit and receive assessment by a behavioral specialist familiar with chronic illness.

Family counselors are particularly important for families who are dealing with stressors in addition to diabetes, or who need assistance in working diabetes into their everyday life.

As children and adolescents go through life stages and have new experiences, it is helpful to offer families referral sources for psychologists or counselors who have expertise in offering support and guidance with diabetes issues. Additionally, peer support groups, diabetes camps and similar such meetings are extremely valuable for both children and adolescents who are faced with feelings of not belonging or frustrations related to general difficulties associated with managing a chronic illness.

Bibliography

American Academy of Pediatrics: (1993). <u>Pediatric Nutrition Handbook</u>, AAP, Elk Grove Village, IL.

American Diabetes Association: (1997): "Clinical practice recommendations, 1997." <u>Diabetes Care</u>, 20:Supp 1.

American Diabetes Association: (1996). <u>Diabetes 1996: Vital Statistics</u>, American Diabetes Association, Inc., Alexandria, VA.

Boland, EA, & Grey, M: (1997). "Coping strategies of school-age children with diabetes mellitus". <u>The Diabetes Educator</u>, 22:6, 592-597.

Connell, JE, Thomas-Dobersen, D: (1991). "Nutritional management of children and adolescents with insulin-dependent diabetes mellitus: a review by the diabetes care and education practice group". <u>Journal of the American Dietetic Association</u>, 91, 1556-1564.

Franz, MJ, Horton, ES, Bantle, JP et al: (1994). "Nutrition principles for the management of diabetes and related complications (technical review)". <u>Diabetes Care</u>, 17, 490-518.

Franz, MJ (1993). "Avoiding sugar: does research support traditional beliefs?". <u>The Diabetes Educator</u>, 19:2, 144-150.

Kushion, W, Salisbury, PJ, Seitz, KW, Wilson, BE: (1991). "Issues in the care of infants and toddlers with insulin-dependent diabetes mellitus". <u>The Diabetes Educator</u>, 17:3, 107-110.

National Research Council: (1989). <u>Recommended Dietary Allowances, 10th edition</u>, National Academy Press, Washington, DC.

Pond, JS, Peters, ML, Pannell, DL, Rogers, CS: (1995). "Psychosocial challenges for children with insulin-dependent diabetes mellitus". <u>The Diabetes Educator</u>, 21:4, 297-299.

Thomas-Dobersen, D et al: (1993). "Selected aspects of diabetes nutrition-prevention and management in infants and children". <u>On the Cutting Edge</u> (a newsletter of the Diabetes Care and Education Practice Group, American Dietetic Association), 14:3.

US Department of Health and Human Services (1995). <u>Nutrition and Your Health - Dietary Guidelines for Americans</u>. Home and Garden Bulletin No. 232.

US Department of Health and Human Services (1991). <u>National Cholesterol Education Program - Report of the Expert Panel on Blood Cholesterol Levels in Children and Adolescents</u>, NIH Publication No. 91-2732.

Wheeler, ML, Franz, MJ, Barrier, P, Holler, H, Cronmiller, N, Delahanty, L: (1996). "Macronutrient and energy database for the 1995 exchange lists for meal planning: a rationale for clinical practice decisions". <u>Journal of the American Dietetic Association</u>, 96:11, 1167-1171.

Wise, JE, Kolb, EL, Sauder, SE: (1992). "Effect of glycemic control on growth velocity in children with IDDM". <u>Diabetes Care</u>, 15:7, 826-830.

Selected Resources for Teaching Pediatric Patients about Diabetes:

American Diabetes Association: (1996). Children with Diabetes-Information for Teachers and Child-Care Providers, American Diabetes Association, Alexandria, VA.

American Diabetes Association/American Dietetic Association: (1995). Exchange Lists for Meal Planning, American Diabetes Association, Inc. and American Dietetic Association.

American Diabetes Association: (1994). The Fitness Book for People with Diabetes, American Diabetes Association, Alexandria, VA.

American Diabetes Association/American Dietetic Association: (1995). Single Topic Diabetes Resources, American Diabetes Association/American Dietetic Association.

Barry, B & Castle, G: (1994). Carbohydrate Counting - Adding Flexibility to Your Food Choices, IDC Publishing, Minneapolis, MN.

Betschart, J: (1991). It's Time to Learn About Diabetes (workbook and video tape), Chronimed Publishing, Minneapolis, MN.

Betschart, J & Thom, S: (1995). In Control: A Guide for Teens with Diabetes, Chronimed Publishing, Minneapolis, MN.

Daly, A, Barry, B, Gillespie, S, Kulkarni, K, Richardson, M: (1995). Carbohydrate Counting-Getting Started, American Diabetes Association/American Dietetic Association.

Eli Lilly and Company: (1995). Nutrition in the Fast Lane, Franklin Publishing Inc, Indianapolis, IN.

Elliott, J: (1990). If Your Child Has Diabetes, Putnam Publishing Group, New York, NY.

Franz, MJ: (1997). Exchange for All Occasions, IDC Publishing, Minneapolis, MN.

Hess, MA: (1995). The Art of Cooking for the Diabetic, Contemporary Books, Inc, Chicago, IL.

International Diabetes Center: (1996). My Food Plan, IDC Publishing, Minneapolis, MN.

Moynihan, PM, Balik, B, Eliason, S: (1988). Diabetes Youth Curriculum-A Toolbox for Educators, Chronimed Publishing, Minneapolis, MN.

To order educational materials:

- American Diabetes Association   1-800-232-3472

- American Dietetic Association   1-800-877-1600

- International Diabetes Center   1-612-993-3393

- Chronimed Publishing   1-800-848-2793

- American Association of Diabetes Educators   1-800-338-3633

WEIGHT MANAGEMENT FOR CHILDREN

Description

Evidence from recent studies has shown that the prevalence of obesity among children and adolescents is increasing. These studies indicate that healthy children, over two years of age who exhibit a discernible increase in body fat should be monitored by parents and health professionals, and early interventions planned as necessary. As obesity is associated with an increased risk of diabetes mellitus, hypertension and coronary artery disease, the overweight child should be seen by a Registered Dietitian and other health professionals as needed in an effort to assess and control obesity before adulthood.

Philosophy of Treatment

Treatment of obesity in children should be based on the following recommendations:

- Children should not be placed on restricted calories diets. Instead, efforts should be made to encourage the child to be physically active, to eat a well-balanced diet, and to return to internal control of eating.
- Interventions to treat obesity in children should not interfere with normal growth or promote the development of eating disorders.
- The feeding relationship between the caregiver and the child should be evaluated and normalized if needed.
- Positive behavioral management techniques should be included and self-esteem, attitudes, or body image improved.

Weight management for children needs to focus on normalizing eating behaviors and finding a balance of calories intake and energy expenditure to achieve a healthy weight goal range. A healthy weight goal range should be identified first. This goal will depend on the age, degree of overweight, sex, and height of the child, and whether they have reached puberty. For very young children an appropriate goal is to gain weight at a slower rate, or to maintain their current weight until their height and development can catch-up to their weight. Some weight loss at a slow rate may be appropriate for adolescents, older children, or severely obese younger children. Appropriate weight range goals can be identified using standard nutritional assessment techniques.

Weight management diets for children should not be based on severe caloric restriction. It is most appropriate to work with current eating behaviors and food choices to identify modifications which will lead to lower caloric intakes. Sample eating guides used for educational purposes should not be viewed as restrictive, but should represent normal diets for children and adolescents according to their growth and developmental requirements. These guides may be used as models or goals for eating patterns. It is most appropriate, however, to gradually modify a child's current eating patterns based on their lifestyle and needs.

Overweight children who have appropriate eating patterns, make nutritious food choices, are physically active, and have a normal parent-child feeding relations may not need intervention. Some children may be overweight by medical standards, but may be normal for their genetic predisposition. These children and their families may need guidance in accepting the child's body size and shape, and then allowing the child to grow in the pattern that is normal for them. These children should be monitored for sudden changes in weight, gain or loss, and for support in maintaining good habits and self image.

Assessment

A child's weight for stature should be evaluated to determine the degree of over weight. For prepubescent children, moderate obesity is defined by a weight for height in the 75th to 89th percentiles is defined as the 90th percentile or greater. Prepubescent children who show a pattern of increasing weight for stature over a period of six months or more should also be monitored.

For pubescent children, that is, females whose height is greater than 137 cm and males with a height greater than 145 cm, moderate obesity is defined by a weight greater than the 75th to 90th percentiles of weight for height for age. It is inappropriate to evaluate only the weight for height in pubescent children because of the varied growth patterns of puberty. Pubescent children who are greater than the 75th percentile of weight for height for age should be evaluated further using triceps skinfold measurements to determine obesity, using standard assessment techniques, and information on adolescent nutrition.

Further assessment of the overweight child is necessary to determine the appropriate interventions. In addition, eating patterns, the parent-child relationship, and physical activity levels should be evaluated.

Nutritional Adequacy

Dietary intakes below 1200 calories are generally not recommended for children and will be inadequate in energy, as well as other nutrients, such as iron and calcium, which are required to meet the needs for growth and development. The nutritional adequacy of dietary intakes over 1200 calories will vary depending on the age the child. Reduced caloric intakes for children should be evaluated for each individual according to nutrient needs for the child's age, sex, height, weight, and activity level. Intakes which contain a variety of nutrient dense foods should be adequate for most children. However, without careful food selection, iron and calcium may be low or of marginal levels.

Children under two years of age should not be placed on a reduced calorie or reduced fat diet. Low caloric or low fat diets are nutritionally inadequate and may be harmful to their growth and development.

Other Considerations

Although food intake modification is an important part of weight management for children, equally important are behavior modifications and exercise. All three components are essential for maintaining a healthy weight range over the long term.

Behavior Modification

Behavior modifications, especially for young children, need to include the family. It should focus on normalization of the feeding relationship and may be related to the parent-child relationship. This is often complex and is different for each child. It may require the special skills of other health professionals, such as social workers, family therapists, parenting or family education specialists.

Physical Activity

Physical activity is an essential component of effective long term weight control, and can help children achieve and maintain a healthy weight, and has many other long term health and social benefits. To maintain an activity program, it is important to choose activities that are enjoyable and accessible. If the exercise is fun and easy to do it is more likely to be continued. Children are naturally active and need only a safe, developmentally appropriate environment, suggestions and encouragement.

The best physical activity plans are those that fit the family's life-style. Assist families in identifying ways that more activity can be incorporated into daily life and leisure activities. Families may need to identify times of the day for physical activity, a safe place for the activity, and age appropriate activities. Some regular ways to encourage more daily actuate might include:

- Ask children to help with active chores, such as walking pets, taking out the trash, vacuuming.
- Encourage children, and family members, to walk or bike, when possible.
- Limit time spent watching TV and playing video games.

If all family members make an effort to be more active everyday, children will also be more active. Involving others as role models and for support and encouragement is also helpful. Assistance in developing an exercise program for children may be available from physical therapists, physical education teachers, occupational therapists or recreation leaders at local community centers or organizations such as the YMCA or YWCA.

How to Evaluate Weight-Loss Programs/Diets

Obesity is a significant health problem in our society today and is associated with many chronic diseases. Americans spend millions of dollars in attempts to lose weight, often without much success. Most people who lose weight by diet alone regain the weight lost. (Robison, 1993).

It can be difficult to determine which of the approximately 30,000 weight-loss programs available is effective and safe. The following criteria are designed to help you evaluate weight-loss regimens to determine if they are nutritionally sound, safe, effective, and appropriate for children.

Weight management programs should:
1. Include no fewer than 1,200 calories per day for children and adolescents.
2. Have an individual meal plan including sufficient calories and nutrients for individual growth.
3. Include a variety of foods from all of the basic food groups (meat, milk, grain, fruit, and vegetables.)
4. Include foods that are affordable, culturally acceptable, and easy to obtain and prepare.
5. Promote a gradual rate of weight loss of 1/2 pound per week, or no more that two pounds per month for children and adolescents during the growing years. Some children, especially the very young, should try to maintain their current weight or gain weight at a slower rate until they grow into their weight range.
6. Include behavior modification techniques to identify and change problem eating behaviors.
7. Include planned, continuous physical activity three or more times per week for 30 minutes or more each time.
8. Promote healthy eating behavior and exercise habits that can be followed throughout life.
9. Include a family assessment component and improve or normalize the feeding relationship between the child and the parents/caregivers, if necessary.
10. Be medically sound and approved by a Registered Dietitian and a physician.
11. Include cultivation of self, that is, self-image, self-confidence, and sound body image.
12. Discuss stress management as appropriate for the age of the child.
13. Acknowledge that the process of making lifetime changes takes time and patience and may involve the whole family.
14. Include a system of support and encouragement.

Professional References:

1. American Dietetic Association. Position of the American Dietetic Association: Optimal weight as a health promotion strategy. J Am Dietetic Assoc 1989; 89(12):1814.
2. Blaak, EE, KR Westerterp, O Bar-Or, LJM Marchitelli, and JA Vogel. Total energy expenditure and spontaneous activity in relation to training in obese boys. Am J Clin Nutr 1992; 55:777-782.
3. Epstein, LH, A Valiski, RR Wing, J McCurley. Ten-year follow-up of behavioral, family-based treatment of obese children. J Am Medical Assoc 1990; 264:2519-2523.
4. Kosharek, SM. If Your Child Is Overweight. American Dietetic Association, 1993.
5. Mahan, LK and JM Rees. Nutrition in Adolescence. Times Mirror/Mosby Company 1984.
6. Mellin, L. To: President Clinton re: Combating childhood obesity. J Am Dietetic Assoc 1993; 93(3)265-266.
7. Minnesota Department of Health WIC Program. Growing Healthy: Promoting Healthy Body Weight for Overweight Children One to Five. Minnesota Department of Health WIC Program, 1991.
8. Peck, EB and HD Ullrich. Children and Weight: A Changing Perspective. Nutrition Communications Associates, Berkeley, CA, 1992.
9. Pipes, PL and CM Trahms. Nutrition in Infancy and Childhood, 5th ed. Mosby-Year Book, Inc, 1992.
10. Quality Assurance Committee, Dietitians in Pediatric Practice. Quality Assurance Criteria for Pediatric Nutrition Conditions: A Model, Section XVII. Weight Management. American Dietetic Association, 1988.
11. Robison, J, SL Hoerr, J Strandmark and B. Mavis. Obesity, weight loss, and health. J. Am Dietetic Assoc 1993: 93:445-449.
12. Satter, E. How to Get Your Kid to Eat...But Not Too Much. Bull Publishing Co, 1987.
13. Serdula, MK, D. Ivery, RJ Coates, DS Freedman, DF Williamson, and T Byers. Do obese children become obese Adults? A review of the literature. Preventive Med 1993; 22:167-177.

Calorie-Controlled Meal Plans and Information

1,200 CALORIE DAILY MEAL PLAN

Food Group	Total Number of Servings/Day
Milk, skim*	2 cups
Vegetables, cooked	2
Vegetables, raw	as desired
Fruit or juice	3
Breads or Starches	4
Meat or substitute	4 oz.
Fats	3

Sample Menu:
Servings/Exchanges

Breakfast

1 fruit or juice — 1/2 cup unsweetened canned fruit or juice; OR
1 piece fresh fruit

1 bread or starch — 1/2 cup hot cereal; OR
3/4 cup unsweetened dry cereal; OR
1 slice toast; OR ½ English muffin; OR 1/2 bagel

1 fat — 1 tsp. margarine; OR 1 strip bacon

1 milk, skim — 1 cup skim milk or plain, nonfat yogurt

Noon Meal

1-2 oz. meat or substitute — 2 oz. lean beef, pork, poultry, or fish; OR
2 oz. cheese; OR 1/2 cup low-fat cottage cheese; OR 1/2 cup
water-packed tuna

2 breads or starches — 2 slices bread; OR 1 cup potatoes or pasta; OR
2/3 cup rice; OR 1 bagel

1 fat — 1 tsp. margarine or mayonnaise; OR
1 tbsp. salad dressing

1 vegetable, cooked — 1/2 cup unbuttered, cooked vegetables

Free raw vegetables — lettuce salad; OR vegetable sticks

1 fruit or juice — 1/2 cup unsweetened, canned fruit or juice; OR
1 piece fresh fruit

1/2 milk, skim — 1/2 cup skim milk or plain, nonfat yogurt

Evening Meal

2-3 oz. meat or substitute	2 oz. lean beef, pork, poultry, or fish; OR 2 oz. cheese or 1/2 cup low-fat cottage cheese; OR 1/2 cup water-packed tuna
1 bread or starch	1 slice bread; OR 1/2 cup potatoes or pasta OR 1/3 cup rice; OR 1/2 bagel
1 fat	1 tsp. margarine or mayonnaise; OR 1 tbsp. salad dressing
1 vegetable, cooked	1/2 cup unbuttered, cooked vegetables
Free raw vegetables	lettuce salad or vegetable sticks
1 fruit or juice	1/2 cup unsweetened, canned fruit or juice; OR 1 piece fresh fruit
1/2 milk, skim	1/2 cup skim or plain, nonfat yogurt

*If you do not drink milk or are intolerant to it, you may substitute 1 oz. cheddar cheese or 8 oz. plain nonfat yogurt for 1 cup skim milk (to provide equivalent calcium value).

1,500 Calorie Daily Meal Plan

Food Group   **Total Number of Servings/Day**

Food Group	Total Number of Servings/Day
Milk, skim*	2 cups
Vegetables, cooked	2
Vegetables, raw	as desired
Fruit or juice	4
Breads or Starches	6
Meat or substitute	5 oz.
Fats	4

Sample Menu:

Servings/Exchanges

Breakfast

1 fruit or juice	1/2 cup unsweetened canned fruit or juice; OR 1 piece fresh fruit
2 breads or starches	1/2 cup hot cereal; OR 3/4 cup unsweetened dry cereal; OR 1 slice toast; OR 1 English muffin; OR 1 bagel
1 fat	1 tsp. margarine; OR 1 strip bacon
1 milk, skim	1 cup skim milk or plain, nonfat yogurt

Noon Meal

2 oz. meat or substitute	2 oz. lean beef, pork, poultry, or fish; OR 2 oz. cheese; OR 1/2 cup low-fat cottage cheese; OR 1/2 cup water-packed tuna
2 breads or starches	2 slices bread; OR 1 cup potatoes or pasta; OR 2/3 cup rice; OR 1 bagel; OR 1 English muffin
1 fat	1 tsp. margarine or mayonnaise; OR 1 tbsp. salad dressing
1 vegetable, cooked	1/2 cup unbuttered, cooked vegetables
Free raw vegetables	lettuce salad or vegetable sticks
1 fruit or juice	1/2 cup unsweetened, canned fruit or juice; OR 1 piece fresh fruit
1/2 milk, skim	1/2 cup skim milk or plain, nonfat yogurt

Snack

1 fruit or juice

1/2 cup unsweetened, canned fruit or juice; OR
1 piece fresh fruit

Evening Meal

3 oz. meat or substitute

3 oz. lean beef, pork, poultry, or fish; OR
3 oz. cheese; OR 3/4 cup low-fat cottage cheese; OR
3/4 cup water-packed tuna

1 bread or starch

1 slice bread; OR 1/2 cup potatoes or pasta; OR
OR 1/3 cup rice

2 fats

2 tsp. margarine or mayonnaise; OR
2 tbsp. salad dressing

1 vegetable, cooked

1/2 cup unbuttered, cooked vegetables

Free raw vegetables

lettuce salad or vegetable sticks

1 fruit or juice

1/2 cup unsweetened, canned fruit or juice; OR
1 piece fresh fruit

1/2 milk, skim

1/2 cup skim or plain, nonfat yogurt

Snack

1 bread or starch

3 cups unbuttered popcorn; OR
3 graham cracker squares

*If you do not drink milk or are intolerant to it, you may substitute 1 oz. cheddar cheese or 8 oz. plain, nonfat yogurt for 1 cup skim milk (to provide equivalent calcium value).

1,800 Calorie Daily Meal Plan

Food Group	Total Number of Servings/Day
Milk, skim*	3 cups
Vegetables, cooked	4
Vegetables, raw	as desired
Fruit or juice	4
Breads or Starches	8
Meat or substitute	6 oz.
Fats	5

Sample Menu:

Servings/Exchanges

Breakfast

1 fruit or juice	1/2 cup unsweetened canned fruit or juice; OR 1 piece fresh fruit
2 breads or starches	1/2 cup hot cereal; OR 3/4 cup unsweetened dry cereal; OR 1 slice toast; OR 1 bagel; OR 1 English muffin
1 fat	1 tsp. margarine; OR 1 strip bacon
1 milk, skim	1 cup skim milk or plain, nonfat yogurt

Noon Meal

2 oz. meat or substitute	2 oz. lean beef, pork, poultry, or fish; OR 2 oz. cheese; OR 1/2 cup low-fat cottage cheese; OR 1/2 cup water-packed tuna
2 breads or starches	2 slices bread; OR 1 cup potatoes or pasta; OR 2/3 cup rice OR 1 bagel
2 fats	2 tsp. margarine or mayonnaise; OR 2 tbsp. salad dressing
2 vegetables, cooked	1/2 cup unbuttered, cooked vegetables
Free raw vegetables	lettuce salad or vegetable sticks
1 fruit or juice	1/2 cup unsweetened, canned fruit or juice, OR 1 piece fresh fruit
1 milk, skim	1 cup skim milk or plain, nonfat yogurt

Snack

1 fruit or juice	1/2 cup unsweetened, canned fruit or juice, OR 1 piece fresh fruit

Evening Meal

4 oz. meat or substitute	4 oz. lean beef, pork, poultry, or fish; OR 4 oz. cheese or 1 cup low-fat cottage cheese; OR 1 cup water-packed tuna
3 breads or starches	3 slices bread; OR 1-1/2 cup potatoes or pasta; OR 1 cup rice
2 fats	2 tsp. margarine or mayonnaise; OR 2 tbsp. salad dressing
1 vegetable, cooked	1/2 cup unbuttered, cooked vegetables
Free raw vegetables	lettuce salad or vegetable sticks
1 fruit or juice	1/2 cup unsweetened, canned fruit or juice; OR 1 piece fresh fruit
1 milk, skim	1 cup skim or plain, nonfat yogurt

Snack

1 bread or starch	3 cups unbuttered popcorn; OR 3 graham cracker squares

*If you do not drink milk or are intolerant to it, you may substitute 1 oz. cheddar cheese or 8 oz. plain, nonfat yogurt for 1 cup skim milk (to provide equivalent calcium value).

2,000 CALORIE DAILY MEAL PLAN

Food Group	Total Number of Servings/Day
Milk, skim*	3 cups
Vegetables, cooked	4
Vegetables, raw	as desired
Fruit or juice	4
Breads or Starches	10
Meat or substitute	6 oz.
Fats	6

Sample Menu:

Servings/Exchanges

Breakfast

1 fruit or juice	1/2 cup unsweetened canned fruit or juice; OR 1 piece fresh fruit
2 breads or starches	1/2 cup hot cereal; OR 3/4 cup unsweetened dry cereal; OR 1 slice toast
2 fats	2 tsp. margarine; OR 2 strips bacon
1 milk, skim	1 cup skim milk or plain, nonfat yogurt

Noon Meal

2 oz. meat or substitute	2 oz. lean beef, pork, poultry, or fish; OR 2 oz. cheese; OR 1/2 cup low-fat cottage cheese; OR 1/2 cup water-packed tuna
3 breads or starches	2 slices bread and 1/2 cup potatoes or pasta; OR 1 cup rice
2 fats	2 tsp. margarine or mayonnaise; OR 2 tbsp. salad dressing
2 vegetables, cooked	1/2 cup unbuttered, cooked vegetables
Free raw vegetables	lettuce salad or vegetable sticks
1 fruit or juice	1/2 cup unsweetened, canned fruit or juice; OR 1 piece fresh fruit
1 milk, skim	1 cup skim milk or plain, nonfat yogurt

Snack

1 fruit or juice	1/2 cup unsweetened, canned fruit or juice; OR 1 piece fresh fruit

Evening Meal

4 oz. meat or substitute	4 oz. lean beef, pork, poultry, or fish; OR 4 oz. cheese; OR 1 cup low-fat cottage cheese; OR 1 cup water-packed tuna
3 breads or starches	3 slices bread; OR 1-1/2 cup potatoes or pasta; OR OR 1 cup rice
2 fats	2 tsp. margarine or mayonnaise; OR 2 tbsp. salad dressing
1 vegetable, cooked	1/2 cup unbuttered, cooked vegetables
Free raw vegetables	lettuce salad OR vegetable sticks
1 fruit or juice	1/2 cup unsweetened, canned fruit or juice; OR 1 piece fresh fruit
1 milk, skim	1 cup skim or plain, nonfat yogurt

Snack

2 breads or starches	6 cups unbuttered popcorn; OR 6 graham cracker squares

*If you do not drink milk or are intolerant to it, you may substitute 1 oz. cheddar cheese or 8 oz. plain, nonfat yogurt for 1 cup skim milk (to provide equivalent calcium value).

2,200 Calorie Daily Meal Plan

Food Group	Total Number of Servings/Day
Milk, skim*	4 cups
Vegetables, raw and cooked	4 or more, as desired
Fruit or juice	5
Breads or Starches	10
Meat or substitute	6 oz.
Fats	7

Sample Menu:

Servings/Exchanges

Breakfast

2 fruit or juice	1 cup unsweetened canned fruit or juice; OR 1 small piece fresh fruit PLUS 1/2 cup unsweetened juice
2 breads or starches	2 slices toast; OR 1/2 cup hot cereal PLUS 1 slice toast
2 fats	2 tsp. margarine
1 milk, skim	1 cup skim milk or plain, nonfat yogurt

Snack

1 bread	2 bread sticks

Noon Meal

2 oz. meat or substitute	2 oz. lean beef, pork, poultry, or fish; OR 2 oz. cheese; OR 1/2 cup low-fat cottage cheese; OR 1/2 cup water-packed tuna
2 breads or starches	2 slices whole wheat bread
2 fats	2 tbsp. reduced-calorie mayonnaise; OR 2 tsp. salad dressing
2 vegetables, cooked	1 cup unbuttered, cooked vegetables
Free raw vegetables	lettuce salad or vegetable sticks
1 fruit or juice	1 piece fresh fruit
1 milk, skim	1 cup skim milk

Snack

1 bread or starch	3 cups popcorn
1 fat	1 tsp. margarine

Evening Meal

4 oz. meat or substitute	4 oz. lean beef, pork, poultry, or fish
2 breads or starches	2 slices bread; OR 1 cup potatoes or pasta; OR 2/3 cup rice
2 fats	2 tsp. margarine or mayonnaise; OR 2 tbsp. salad dressing
2 vegetable, cooked	1/2 cup unbuttered, cooked vegetables
Free raw vegetables	salad greens or vegetable sticks
1 fruit or juice	1/2 cup unsweetened, canned fruit or juice; OR 1 piece fresh fruit
1 milk, skim	1 cup skim or plain, nonfat yogurt

Snack

1 fruit or juice	1/2 cup unsweetened fruit or juice; OR 1 piece fresh fruit
2 breads or starches	6 graham cracker squares
1 cup milk, skim	1 cup skim milk

*If you do not drink milk or are intolerant to it, you may substitute 1 oz. low-fat cheese or 8 oz. plain, nonfat yogurt for 1 cup skim milk (to provide equivalent calcium value).

2,400 CALORIE DAILY MEAL PLAN

Food Group	Total Number of Servings/Day
Milk, skim*	4 cups
Vegetables, raw and cooked	5 or more, as desired
Fruit or juice	5
Breads or Starches	12
Meat or substitute	6 oz.
Fats	7

Sample Menu:

Servings/Exchanges

Breakfast

2 fruit or juice	1 cup unsweetened canned fruit or juice; OR 1 piece fresh fruit PLUS 1/2 cup unsweetened juice
3 breads or starches	2 slices toast PLUS 1/2 cup hot cereal
2 fats	2 tsp. margarine
1 milk, skim	1 cup skim milk

Snack

1 milk, skim	1 cup nonfat yogurt
1 fruit or juice	1 piece fresh fruit
1 bread or starch	1/2 bagel

Noon Meal

2 oz. meat or substitute	2 oz. lean beef, pork, poultry, or fish; OR 2 oz. cheese; OR 1/2 cup low-fat cottage cheese; OR 1/2 cup water-packed tuna
2 breads or starches	2 slices whole wheat bread
2 fats	1 tbsp. reduced-calorie mayonnaise PLUS 1 tsp. salad dressing
2 vegetables, cooked	1 cup unbuttered, cooked vegetables
Free raw vegetables	salad greens or vegetable sticks
1 fruit or juice	1 piece fresh fruit
1 milk, skim	1 cup skim milk

Snack

1 bread or starch	3 cups popcorn
1 fat	1 tsp. margarine
1 raw vegetables	10 vegetable sticks

Evening Meal

4 oz. meat or substitute	4 oz. lean beef, pork, poultry, or fish
3 breads or starches	3 slices bread, 1-1/2 cup potatoes or pasta; OR 1 cup rice
2 fats	1 tsp. margarine or mayonnaise PLUS 1 tbsp. salad dressing
2 vegetable, cooked	1 cup unbuttered, cooked vegetables
Free raw vegetables	salad greens or vegetable sticks
1 fruit or juice	1/2 cup unsweetened, canned fruit or juice; OR 1 piece fresh fruit

Snack

2 breads or starches	6 graham cracker squares
1 cup milk, skim	1 cup skim milk

*If you do not drink milk or are intolerant to it, you may substitute 1 oz. low-fat cheese or 8 oz. plain, nonfat yogurt for 1 cup skim milk (to provide equivalent calcium value).

2,800 CALORIE DAILY MEAL PLAN

Food Group	Total Number of Servings/Day
Milk, skim*	4 cups
Vegetables, raw and cooked	5
Fruit or juice	6
Breads or Starches	15
Meat or substitute	7 oz.
Fats	8

Sample Menu:

Servings/Exchanges

Breakfast

2 fruit or juice	1 cup unsweetened canned fruit or juice; OR 1 piece fresh fruit PLUS 1/2 cup unsweetened juice
3 breads or starches	2 slices toast PLUS 1/2 cup hot cereal
2 fats	2 tsp. margarine
1 meat**	1 tbsp. peanut butter; OR 1 egg (no added fat)
1 milk, skim	1 cup skim milk

Snack

1 fruit or juice	1 piece fresh fruit
1 bread or starch	1 whole bagel

Noon Meal

2 oz. meat or substitute	2 oz. lean beef, pork, poultry, or fish; OR 2 oz. cheese or 1/2 cup low-fat cottage cheese; OR 1/2 cup water-packed tuna
3 breads or starches	2 slices whole wheat bread PLUS 2 graham cracker squares
2 fats	2 tbsp. reduced-calorie mayonnaise; OR 2 tsp. salad dressing; OR 2 tsp. margarine
2 vegetables, cooked	1 cup unbuttered, cooked vegetables
Free raw vegetables	salad greens or vegetable sticks

Noon Meal, continued

1 fruit or juice	1 piece fresh fruit
1 milk, skim	1 cup skim milk

Snack

1 bread or starch	3 cups popcorn, plain
2 fats	2 tsp. margarine or vegetable oil

Evening Meal

4 oz. meat or substitute	4 oz. lean beef, pork, poultry, or fish
5 breads or starches	1-1/2 cups potatoes or pasta PLUS 2 slices bread
2 fats	2 tsp. margarine or mayonnaise; OR 2 tbsp. salad dressing
2 vegetables, cooked	1 cup unbuttered, cooked vegetables
Free raw vegetables	salad greens or vegetable sticks
1 fruit or juice	1/2 cup unsweetened, canned fruit or juice; OR 1 piece fresh fruit
1 milk, skim	1 cup skim milk

Snack

2 bread or starch	6 graham cracker squares
1 cup milk, skim	1 cup skim milk
1 fruit or juice	1 piece fresh fruit

*If you do not drink milk or are intolerant to it, you may substitute 1 oz. cheese or 8 oz. plain, nonfat yogurt for 1 cup skim milk (to provide equivalent calcium value).
**If you do not choose to have a Meat or Substitute at breakfast, you may add 1 oz. Meat or Substitute to the noon or the evening meal. A maximum of 3 egg yolks per week is recommended.

Dining Out Guidelines for Healthy Eating

The following are guidelines to help you select foods that are lower in sodium, cholesterol, fat, and calories when dining out. Making wise menu choices will help you control weight and will promote better health.

Food Group	Wise Choices	Avoid/Use Sparingly
Appetizers	Fruit juices, fruit cup, fresh vegetables such as radishes, celery, carrot sticks	Vegetable juices, soups, including broth, consommé, or cream soups. Pickles, olives, cheese & crackers, potato chips & dips. Assorted snack crackers. Shrimp cocktail, pickled herring, chopped liver, pate.
Salads	Vegetable salads without added dressings or fat. Ask for lemon wedges, oil, and vinegar, French, Italian, or low-calorie dressings "on the side." Fresh fruit salads or tomatoes.	Prepared salads with dressing, such as coleslaw or potato salad. Pickled vegetables, bacon bits, croutons, cheese, anchovies. Nuts, seeds, guacamole, avocado, or gelatins.
Breads/Starches	Any kind of plain bread or dinner rolls. All cereals, except granola or sugar-coated cereals. (Be sure to limit your pre-dinner eating to one dinner roll.)	Biscuits, croutons, garlic toast, croissants, muffins, corn bread, sweet rolls, coffee cake, salted crackers, bread sticks, popcorn, bread stuffing, pancakes, waffles.
Potatoes/Rice	Baked, mashed, steamed, or boiled potatoes. Rice without added salt or fat. Try a dash of Parmesan cheese, lemon juice, pepper, or plain yogurt for potato topping.	Creamed, fried, hash browned, scalloped, or au gratin potatoes. Chow mien noodles. Pasta or rice in cream, cheese, or butter sauce.
Vegetables	Plain, cooked vegetables (without sauces or fat). Try lemon juice, pepper, or vinegar for flavor. (See "salads.")	Creamed, buttered, scalloped, or au gratin vegetables. V-8 juice, sauerkraut, stewed tomatoes, French fried foods, pickled vegetables.
Fruit	Fruit juices, fruit cup, fresh salads, mix with orange concentrate or dip pieces of fruit into lemon yogurt. (See "appetizers.")	Fruit salads with dressing, sour cream, or sugar added. Canned fruit that contains sugar or syrup.

Food Group	Wise Choices	Avoid/Use Sparingly
Meat & Substitutes	Roasted, baked, broiled, or grilled lean meat, fish, or poultry without added salt or fat. Low-fat cottage cheese or cheese. Lean meat examples: Beef: filet mignon, sirloin or rump roast, lean ground beef, kabobs. Pork: loin chop or roast. Veal: all cuts except breast. Poultry: chicken, turkey, or pheasant (remove skin). Fish: all varieties, except batter-dipped or fried. Eggs: poached, cooked, or scrambled (not more than one). Substitute 2 egg whites for 1 egg.	Deep fried, pan fried, or breaded meats. Meats or fish in gravies, cream cheese, or barbecue sauce. Stews, casseroles, rich pastas, and pizza. Smoked or cured meat; e.g. wieners, bacon, sausage. Prime rib, New York strip, other high-fat meats. Sardines, pickled herring, caviar. Creamed, scalloped or fried eggs. Omelets with cheese, smoked meat, or cured meat. Eggs Benedict.
Milk	Skim milk or 1%.	Whole, 2% milk. Milk shakes or malts; buttermilk; chocolate milk.
Desserts and Sweets	Fruit (dried, cooked or fresh); fruit ice (nonfat yogurt, sherbet, sorbet). Angel food cake, sponge cake, fig bars, ginger snaps, vanilla wafers, fat-free desserts.	Pastries, puddings, pies, cakes, doughnuts, cheesecake, custard, ice cream, chocolate sundaes.
Fats & Oils	Margarine (first ingredient vegetable oil). Oil (and vinegar). Ask for these "on the side." Use less than 20 calories of low-calorie salad dressing or use your Fat servings for regular salad dressing.	Butter, cream, cream cheese, cream substitute, sour cream, mayonnaise, cream sauces. Salad dressings, gravy, bacon, tartar sauce, cheese sauces. Deep-fried foods.
Beverages	Coffee (regular or decaffeinated), tea, herbal tea, sugar-free pop or fruit juice. Mineral water, club soda.	Lemonade, hot cocoa, sweetened carbonated beverages or sweetened fruit drinks. Alcohol (unless approved by physician).
Condiments/ Miscellaneous	Lemon juice, pepper, vinegar. Jam or jelly fruit spread. Catsup, mustard, horseradish, Worcestershire sauce (limit to 1 tbsp. of each). Artificial sweeteners and diet syrup.	Pickles, pickle relish, soy sauce, meat sauce, chili sauce, salt, seasoned salt, meat tenderizers, meat marinades, barbecue sauce.

General Food Information Hints

Here are steps you can take to lower the fat and calories in the foods you cook:

1. Begin by measuring all foods (for one or two weeks) in order to be aware of correct portion sizes. Then occasionally spot check portion sizes.
2. Remove fat from soups, stews, and gravies by chilling them first; then skim off the fat.
3. Use plain yogurt instead of sour cream or mayonnaise in salad dressings, vegetable dips, or potato toppings. Experiment with your own seasoning combinations. Try fat free dairy products.
4. To reheat leftovers, use a microwave, a rack, or a vegetable steamer in a frying pan. Add water, then cover, and steam the leftovers for a few minutes.
5. Reduce sugar by 1/3 to 1/2 in recipes.
6. Reduce fat by 1/4 to 1/2 in recipes.
7. Remove all visible fat from meat (and skin from poultry) before cooking.
8. Use a rack or grill when roasting to allow the fat to drip out of the meat.
9. Select low-fat cuts of meat (tenderize them by pounding or roasting at a low temperature for a longer period of time).
10. Broil fish or chicken slowly. Brush it with lemon juice or low calorie salad dressings and/or herbs and paprika.
11. Poach fish fillets in a heavy aluminum foil packet. Pour lemon juice or white wine over fish, adding onion, chives, parsley and/or seasonings on top. Fold the top ends securely, and bake for 30 minutes at 350°.
12. Fry eggs in a nonstick pan, using 1/2 teaspoon fat melted or brushed around the pan. Fry eggs slowly, then add a few drops of water to the pan. Cover the pan and let eggs steam for a "basted" or "over easy" look. Nonstick spray is also a good option.
13. Stir-fry sliced, diced or chopped vegetables in a Chinese wok or a frying pan with a minimum amount of oil (1 to 2 tsp.) or in broth.
14 Instead of butter or margarine, use herbs such as dill weed, thyme, oregano, basil or marjoram to season vegetables. Lemon or lime juice or salad vinegars are also good additions.
15. Use butter flavors, available in extract, powder, or liquid form on vegetables.
16. Sprinkle Parmesan cheese on potatoes, vegetables, or salads to add zest without adding many calories.
17. Base meals around grain products (noodles, rice, potatoes, etc.) instead of focusing largely on the meat item.
18. Prepare occasional meatless meals by using high fiber, low-fat legumes (dried peas and beans).
19. Substitute oatmeal or whole wheat flour for part of white flour in recipes.
20. Select breads, cereals, and crackers which list whole wheat, rye, oats, or corn as first ingredient.

Experiment with a variety of grains, such as barley, brown rice, bulgur, cornmeal, or buckwheat.
(Can be prepared without fat in low sodium bouillon. When cooking brown rice, do not add salt if necessary until after cooked as it tends to harden the kernels.)

Trimming Fat and Calories

Instead of These:	Choose These:
sour cream	lowfat or nonfat yogurt or mix together in a blender 2 tbsp. skim milk, 1 tbsp. lemon juice and 1 cup lowfat or nonfat cottage cheese
creamed cottage cheese (4% fat)	lowfat cottage cheese (1% fat), pot cheese, or farmer's cheese
ricotta cheese	part-skim ricotta cheese
heavy cream	evaporated skim or lowfat milk
whole milk	1%, skim milk, or buttermilk
butter	margarine made with vegetable oil, tub or liquid margarine
luncheon meats, sausage, bacon, spare ribs	turkey and chicken breast, fish, lean beef, lamb, pork, or veal
tuna packed in oil	tuna packed in water
self-basting turkey	baste your own turkey
hard cheeses — cheddar, Swiss	part skim mozzarella varieties
1 cup solid shortening	2/3 cup vegetable oil
1 whole egg	2 egg whites or 1/4 cup egg substitute
1 ounce unsweetened baking chocolate	3 tbsp. cocoa
meat	legumes
fats when sautéing foods	chicken or beef broth
fats when frying foods	low-calorie cooking spray
fats for seasoning foods	herbs and spices to season foods
butter on vegetables	use butter flavors, available in extract, powder, or liquid
cream cheese	Neufchatel cheese
1/2 cup oil in baking	1/2 cup applesauce or 1/4 cup oil + 1/4 cup nonfat milk

Instead of These:	Choose These:
ice cream	sorbet, sherbet, ice milk, lowfat frozen yogurt, nonfat yogurt
baked goods	angel food cake, lowfat cookies, canned fruit in its own juice
canned creamed soups	white sauce thickened with cornstarch, add mushrooms, celery, chicken bouillon

Suggested Reading and/or Cookbooks

1. Berg, Frances M. *Afraid to Eat: Children and Teens I Weight Crisis*, Healthy Weight Journal, 1996, 310 pp.
2. Daum, Michelle, Lenmtey, Amy. *The Cano-Do Eating Plan for Overweight Kids and Teens: Helping Kids Control Weight, Look Better and Feel Great*, Avon Books, 1997, 204 pp.
3. Levine, Judith, Bine, Linda, Levine, Judi. *Helping Your Child Lose Weight the Healthy Way: A Family Approach to Weight Control*. Birch Land Publishing, 1986, 256 pp.
4. Jacobson, Michael, *Kitchen Fun for Kids*, 1991.
5. *American Heart Association Kids' Cookbook*, Times Books.
6. *Piscatella, Joseph C. Fat Proof Your Child*, Workman Publishing Company, June 1997.

Benefits of Physical Activity in Weight Control

Physical activity is necessary for effective, long term weight management. Research has determined the main reason people gain weight as they get older is due to loss of lean muscle tissue. Less muscle means less calorie input (food eaten) is needed. This is true because muscle is the main metabolizer of the food (calories) consumed. Over time one naturally will lose lean tissue if he/she does not keep using it. As this occurs, one's ability to eat the same as he/she did before becomes impossible because the need for energy lessens.

Each and every movement a person does is a positive step towards weight control in two ways:

1) Short movement sessions add up when looked at in a week's block of time. Example: Six 10-minute walks equal an hour of activity that week. 2) Biological and psychological systems are impacted every time large muscle groups are used.

Biological Benefits of Exercise

Benefit:	Explanation:
Burns calories	A person burns 20% more calories sitting as opposed to lying down. And it gets better with added movement! Burning (or expending) calories is important to balance out calories eaten.
Utilizes fat stores	Aerobic activity sustained longer than 20 minutes will tap into fat stores for energy.
Increases metabolism	Activity produces internal heat which increases the metabolic rate. One's metabolism remains elevated for a time after an activity session. This burns calories more efficiently.
Maintains or increases lean tissue	Research shows that the primary reason people gain weight over time is the loss of lean tissue. Lean tissue is alive and uses up the majority of calories and forms our shape. Lean tissue burns more calories and requires more calories to sustain itself than fat tissue.
Increases fat burning enzymes	Fat burning enzymes increase a person's ability to use fat for energy instead of glycogen stores, thus extending the workout. Activity improves the fat releasing mechanism.
Utilizes intramuscular fat	Fat is stored in muscle. This fat causes muscles to become soft and squat. Only through activity will the fat be burned so that the muscle can become lean and shapely again. Losing weight with lowered food intake alone will only burn subcutaneous fat (fat under the skin).
Improves fat releasing mechanisms	Fat releasing (lipolytic) improves with activity because the body senses a need to provide energy. When one fasts, the opposite happens because the fat cells gear up to store fat for survival.

Benefit:	Explanation:
Enhances oxygen consumption	Oxygen consumption has an effect on the body's ability to utilize and mobilize fat. Metabolic rate increases when more oxygen is utilized. Activity helps to promote higher oxygen usage by improving one's breathing mechanism (mitochondria and oxygen consumption). Often as one ages, oxygen consumption is reduced which contributes to the body's reduced ability to mobilize fat.

Psychological Benefits of Exercise

Benefit:	Explanation:
Enhances feeling of well-being	Sustained aerobic activity has been shown to stimulate the release of chemicals called monamines (neurotransmitters) and endorphins (pain controllers). These chemicals create a sense of well-being and euphoria which continues for a time beyond the activity session.
Relieves stress	Activity allows the muscles to feel massaged which helps to relieve tension.
Bestows a feeling of confidence	Because activity strengthens the muscles, an overall sense of feeling stronger physically and mentally occurs. This improves a person's self-esteem which in turn increases one's ability to withstand stress.

Other Health Benefits

Exercise is considered a preventive practice in regard to osteoporosis, heart disease, diabetes, and arthritis.

Getting Started

There are many ways to be physically active. Often when people begin considering an activity program they think it means training for a marathon or working out until one feels exhausted.

NOT SO.

When considering an activity program one should just think about moving more. Activity is nothing more than a movement done with a certain amount of repetitions. One option is to do short sessions of physical activity through the day. Examples:

Walking to the store
Gardening
Using stairs
Walking 10 minutes to work
Playing with the kids

A study compared two control groups for 8 weeks. In group one each person walked 10 minutes three times a day. Group two did a sustained 30-minute walk a day. Each group improved their cardiovascular system and lost an average of four pounds. The total amount of physical movement was the most important factor.

The second option is to incorporate a consistent physical activity program into one's weekly routine. This involves scheduling a time in which a chosen aerobic activity can be sustained at a moderate intensity, for 30-60 minutes per session, 3-5 times a week.

The best situation would be to combine both options. This might involve scheduling a 60-minute workout three times a week and a 10-minute walk on the other days. With consistency one becomes more active naturally because of feeling better and stronger.

A complete workout session should include:

- A warm-up
- Aerobic activity
- Muscle strength and endurance
- Stretching
- Cool-down

As a person becomes physically active, the intensity of the workout must be monitored. Two methods of determining intensity are "target heart rate" and "perceived exertion."

Target Heart Rate

To figure your *Predicted Maximum Heart Rate* (PMHR), use the formula below:

> 220 minus your age equals PMHR
> For example: a 40-year-old woman would be
> 220 - 40 = 180 beats per minute
> From this you can calculate your *Target Heart Rate Zone*, which is
> 60 - 80% of the PMHR
> .60 x 180 = 117
> .80 x 180 = 144

This woman would strive to work out at a pace that allows her to maintain a heart rate between 117 and 144 beats per minute.

Monitor your heart rate by finding your pulse at the radial artery (wrist) and count how many beats you feel in 10 seconds. The chart below shows where your heart rate should be during aerobic activity. Convert the 10-second count into beats per minute.

Heart rate training range

Age	Beginning Fitness Level (4-6 wks. min.) Beats Min.	Beats 10 Sec.	Intermediate Fitness Level (4-6 wks. min.) Beats Min.	Beats 10 Sec.	Advanced Fitness Level (Maintenance Level) Beats Min.	Beats 10 Sec.
19 and under	120-140	20-24	138-155	23-25	150-174	25-29
20-24	120-140	20-24	138-155	23-25	144-174	24-29
25-29	115-137	18-22	135-152	22-25	144-166	24-29
30-34	110-133	18-22	135-147	21-24	138-162	23-27
35-39	110-130	18-21	128-142	21-23	136-160	22-26
40-44	96-126	16-21	124-135	20-23	128-151	21-25
45-49	96-123	16-20	121-135	20-22	126-146	21-25
50-54	90-119	15-19	117-132	19-22	120-142	20-23
55-59	90-116	15-19	114-130	19-21	110-139	18-23
60 and older	90-112	15-18	110-127	18-21	110-134	16-22

Locate your level of fitness. Monitor your heart rate during and immediately after exercising.

Perceived exertion rate

This method uses a chart with numbers matched to perceptions of how strenuously you feel you are working.

6	13 Somewhat Hard
7 Very, Very Light	14
8	15 Hard
9 Very Light	16
10	17 Very Hard
11 Fairly Light	18
12	19 Very, Very Hard
	20

Perceived Exertion x 10 = the Predicted Heart Rate which corresponds to actual Heart Rate at the particular work intensity. Using the prior example of the 40-year-old woman from before, she feels she is working "Somewhat Hard," so we take the number that corresponds to that feeling, which is 13, and multiply it by 10. 13 x 10 = 130; 130 would be the Predicted Heart Rate. At 130, the woman would be working at the proper intensity because her target heart rate zone was 117-144.

However, some experts are moving away from using numbers or charts to identify intensity levels. Instead they are asking people to listen more to their bodies. For example, are you able to talk while working out?

Steps to success

- Vary activities.
- Be consistent.
- Begin slowly. Gradually increase the number of days and the rate of one's workout.
- Work first on completing a predetermined amount of time (duration).
- Once duration can be completed comfortably, consider increasing the speed used to move through the workout session.
- Add tension or hill climbs to an activity session for variety and as a way to incorporate resistance work within an aerobic workout.
- Exercise with a friend.

Five fitness components that influence weight management

Cardiovascular (aerobic):	Activity sustained for 5-20 minutes burns calories, builds muscle, affects aerobic enzymes. Activity sustained for beyond 20 minutes burns calories, builds muscle, greatly affects aerobic enzymes, and uses fat stores in muscles and under skin.
Muscle Endurance:	Improves the tone/shape of muscles.
Muscle Strength:	Increases the density of muscles. Improves strength which enhances self-esteem. Improves posture.

| Flexibility: | Improves posture. |
| | Movement is easier. |

| Agility/Coordination: | Improves performance of activities. |
| | Improves balance. |

Exercise component written by Marisa Cuneo, Fitness Director, IsoSystem, Inc.—health and weight management program.

References

1. Bailey, Covert. The New Fit or Fat. Boston: Houghton Mifflin, 1991.
2. Cooper, Robert K. Health and Fitness Excellence. Boston: Houghton Mifflin, 1989.
3. Bennim, Lynn M.D., Bierman, Edwin M.D., Ferguson, James M.D. Straight Talk About Weight Control. New York: Consumers Union of United States, Inc., 1991.
4. Vash, Peter M.D., Carlin Cris, Rak, Victoria. The Fat to Muscle Diet. New York: Berkley Book, 1988.
5. Quas, Vince. Lean Body Promise. Oregon: Synesis Press, 1990.

CHOLESTEROL AND FAT-CONTROLLED DIETS

Low-Saturated Fat, Low-Cholesterol Diet
General Description

The process of atherosclerosis begins in childhood and is directly related to elevated levels of blood cholesterol. Elevated blood cholesterol is the major cause of coronary artery disease in adults. Preventing or slowing the atherosclerotic process in childhood and adolescence could extend the years of healthy life for many Americans according to NIH's (National Institutes of Health) National Cholesterol Education Program (NCEP). The Academy of Pediatrics, NIH, and the American Heart Association recommend changes in nutrient intake and eating patterns for all healthy children over the age of two years and adolescents who are at the greatest risk of having elevated blood cholesterol and an increased risk of coronary heart disease into adulthood.

Basic Description of Lipids and Lipoproteins

Cholesterol is a fatlike substance (lipid) that is a key component of cell membranes and precursor of bile acids and steroid hormones. Cholesterol travels in the circulation as lipoprotein. The cholesterol level in blood plasma is determined partly by inheritance and partly by the fat and cholesterol content of the diet. Other factors such as obesity, physical inactivity and cigarette smoking also play a role.

Three major classes of lipoproteins can be measured in the serum of fasting individual: low density lipoproteins (LDL), high-density lipoproteins (HDL), and very low density lipoproteins (VLDL). The LDL are the major atherogenic class, and typically contain 60-70 percent of the total serum cholesterol. The HDL usually contains 20-30 percent of the total cholesterol, and their levels are inversely correlated with risk for coronary heart disease (CHD). The VLDL, which are largely composed of triglycerides, contain 10-15 percent of the total serum cholesterol.

Because most cholesterol in the serum is found in the LDL, the concentration of total cholesterol is closely correlated with the concentration of LDL-cholesterol. Thus, while LDL-cholesterol is the actual target of cholesterol-lowering efforts, total cholesterol can be used in its place in the initial stages of evaluating a patient's serum lipids. Testing for serum total cholesterol is more available, less expensive and does not require that a patient has fasted.

Cutpoints of Total and LDL-Cholesterol for Dietary Intervention in Children and Adolescents with Family History of Hypercholesterolemia or Premature Cardiovascular Disease

Category	Total Cholesterol (mg/dl)	LDL-Cholesterol (mg/dl)	Dietary Intervention
Acceptable	<170	<110	Recommended population eating pattern
Borderline	170-199	110-129	Step-One Diet prescribed, other risk factor intervention
High	$\geq$200	$\geq$130	Step-One Diet prescribed, then Step-Two Diet if necessary

Serum Triglyceride Levels in US Children and Adolescents (mg/dl)*

Males

Age, years	Number	Overall Means	Percentiles						
			5	10	25	50	75	90	95
0-4	238	58	30	34	41	53	69	87	102
5-9	1253	30	31	34	41	53	67	88	104
10-14	2278	68	33	38	46	61	80	105	129
15-19	1980	80	38	44	56	71	94	124	152

Females

Age, years	Number	Overall Means	Percentiles						
			5	10	25	50	75	90	95
0-4	186	66	35	39	46	61	79	99	115
5-9	1118	30	33	37	45	57	73	93	108
10-14	2087	78	38	45	56	72	93	117	135
15-19	2079	78	40	45	55	70	90	117	136

*All values have been converted from plasma to serum. Plasma value x 1.03 = serum value.
Source: Table 1-6, National Cholesterol Education Program, *Report of the Expert Panel on Blood Cholesterol Levels in Children and Adolescents.*

Serum HDL-Cholesterol Levels in US Children and Adolescents (mg/dl)*

Males

Age, years	Number	Overall Means	Percentiles						
			5	10	25	50	75	90	95
0-4	142	57	39	43	50	56	65	72	76
10-14	296	57	38	41	47	57	63	73	76
15-19	299	48	31	35	40	47	54	61	65

Females

Age, years	Number	Overall Means	Percentiles						
			5	10	25	50	75	90	95
5-9	124	55	37	39	48	54	63	69	75
10-14	247	54	38	41	46	54	60	66	72
15-19	295	54	36	39	44	53	63	70	76

*All values have been converted from plasma to serum. Plasma value x 1.03 = serum value.
Source: Table 1-5, National Cholesterol Education Program, *Report of the Expert Panel on Blood Cholesterol Levels in Children and Adolescents.*

Indications for Use

To lower blood cholesterol levels in children and adults, NIH's NCEP recommends using both a population and an individual approach. The **population approach** recommends the following changes for all healthy children over the age of two years and continuing through adolescence:

- Nutritional adequacy should be achieved by eating a wide variety of foods.
- Energy (calories) should be adequate to support growth and development and to reach or maintain desirable body weight.
- The following pattern of nutrient intake is recommended:
  -dietary cholesterol less than 300 mg/day.
  -total fat no more than 30% of total calories.
  -saturated fatty acids less than 10% of total calories.

The **individual approach** is indicated for children and adolescents who are at the greatest risk of having high cholesterol as an adult and an increased risk of coronary heart disease. This process would involve a screening of family history for premature cardiovascular disease at 55 years of age or less, or parental hypercholesterolemia where the blood cholesterol is 240 mg/dl or higher. *See Risk Assessment chart (page 250).*

Once this screening is completed and there is a positive risk factor, optional blood cholesterol testing of the child or adolescent can be obtained. If one parent has high blood cholesterol, a cholesterol test should be done. For a family history of premature heart disease, a young person should have a lipoprotein analysis done. *See Classification, Education, and Follow-up Based on LDL-Cholesterol figure (page 251).*

In the case of adolescents who smoke cigarettes, have high blood pressure, consume high amounts of saturated fatty foods or are overweight, a total cholesterol testing would be recommended.

The Step One and Step Two diets are designed to provide a progressive reduction of the intake of saturated fatty acids and cholesterol. If after three months the Step One diet does not achieve a reduction of lipoproteins to the desired goal, a Step Two diet should be implemented.

Special Groups
Secondary Hypercholesterolemia
Causes of secondary Hypercholesterolemia are listed in the table below. The health care provider will need to determine the type of diet plan desired and use of drug therapy if needed to lower blood lipid levels.

Causes of Secondary Hypercholesterolemia

Exogenous	Obstructive Liver Disease
Drugs: Corticosteroids, isotretinion (Accetane), thiazides, anticonvulsants, beta blockers, anabolic steroids, certain oral contraceptives	Biliary artesia Biliary cirrhosis
Alcohol	**Chronic Renal Diseases**
Obesity	Nephrotic syndrome
Endocrine and Metabolic	**Others**
Hypothyroidism	Anorexia nervosa
Diabetes mellitus	Progeria
Lipodystrophy	Collagen disease
Pregnancy	Klinefelter syndrome
Idiopathic hypercalcemia	
Storage Diseases	
Glycogen storage diseases	
Sphingolipidoses	

Hypertriglyceridemia
In some children and adolescents, highly elevated Triglycerides and low LDL levels may be found. This relationship is seen in familial dyslipoproteinemia. The provider should determine the type of diet plan needed and use of drug therapy if needed.

Obesity

Obesity in childhood and adolescence is increasing in the United States. According to NIH's NCEP, health studies suggest 27 percent of children ages 6 - 11, and 22 percent of adolescents ages 12 - 17 are obese in the United States. Obese children are at risk of becoming obese adults. Some of the health problems obesity can cause later in life are decreased work capacity, insulin resistance, and hypertension. Obesity in children is directly related to increased LDL and VLDL cholesterol, and decreased HDL cholesterol. The obese child should be encouraged to maintain a constant weight as they grow until their weight is at a desirable level for their height. Obese adolescents who have reached their maximum growth height should be monitored via an appropriate calorie restriction and regular aerobic exercise. The goal of treatment for obese children is to maintain a desirable weight and a lowering of blood lipids.

Nutritional Adequacy

The Step One and Step Two diets are planned to meet the Recommended Daily Allowances (RDA) for calories and all nutrients for healthy children over the age of two and adolescents. The diets are sage and consistent with normal growth and development. However, the diets are not recommended for infants from birth to two years of age whose fast growth requires a high percent of calories from fat.

Characteristics of Step-One and Step-Two Diets for Lowering Blood Cholesterol
Recommended Intake

Nutrient Diet	Step-One Diet	Step-Two Diet
Total Fat	Average of no more than 30% of total calories	Same
Saturated fatty acids	Less than 10% of total calories	Less than 7% of total calories
Polyunsaturated fatty acids	Up to 10% of total calories	Same
Monounsaturated fatty acids	Remaining total fat calories	Same
Cholesterol	Less than 300 mg/day	Less than 200 mg/day
Carbohydrates	About 55% of total calories	Same
Protein	About 15- 20% of total calories	Same
Calories	To promote normal growth and development and to reach or maintain desirable body weight	Same

Other Considerations
Drug Therapy

The NIH NCEP recommends drug therapy be implemented in children age 10 years or older if diet therapy has been in use for 6 months to one year and LDL-cholesterol remains above goal level. In the case of unusually high lipid levels, a provider may decide to start drug therapy at a younger age. A child or adolescent should be monitored six weeks after starting the medication and then every three months. At present, only bile acid sequestrants (cholestyramine, colestipol) have proven to be without serious side effects in children and adolescents.

The most common side effects of bile acids sequestrants are gastrointestinal, which include constipation, nausea, bloating, stomach fullness, and gas. In addition, the following parameters should be monitored if the drug is used:

- Close monitoring of height and weight
- Malabsorption of fat soluble vitamins (A,D,E) and folic acid may occur.
- Check the nutritional adequacy of the client's meal patterns.
- A multivitamin with iron for age may be needed with the use of a bile acid sequestrant.
- Niacin, HMG, CoA reductase inhibitors, producol, gemfibrozil, D-thyrozine, paraminosalicylic acid (PAS), and clofibrate are not recommended for children because of their side effects.

Professional References

1. American Heart Association. Diagnosis and Treatment of Primary Hyperlipidemia and Childhood - A Joint Statement for Physicians by the Committee on Atherosclerosis and Hypertension in Childhood and the Council on Cardiovascular Disease in the Young and the Nutrition Committee, American Heart Association. Circulation Vol. 74, No. 5, November, 1986.
2. National Cholesterol Education Program, Second Report of the Expert Panel on Detection, Evaluation, and Treatment of High Blood Cholesterol I Adults (Adult Treatment Panel II), National Institutes of Health, National Heart, Lung, and Blood Institute, NIH Publication No. 93-3095, September 1993.
3. Suskind, RM, Lewinter-Suskind, L. eds. Textbook of Pediatric Nutrition, New York City, Raven Press, 1993.
4. Timely Statement on NCEP Report on Children and Adolescents, Journal of the American Dietetic Association, 1991: 91. 983.
5. Weidenbach Wilson, DK, Lewis, NM. Weight for Height Measurements and Saturated Fatty Acid Intake Are Predicators of Serum Cholesterol Level in Children. Journal of the American Dietetic Association, 1992, 92, 192-196.

Client Resources

Booklets

A series of four, colorful, "hands on" booklets for children and their parents showing practical tips for eating a heart healthy diet is available from the National Cholesterol Education Program (NCEP).

1. *Eating with Your Heart in Mind* - for children 7 - 10 years of age, NIH Publication No. 92-3100.
2. *Heart Health...Your Choice* - for young teens 11 - 14 years of age, NIH Publication No. 92-3101.
3. *Hearty Habits, Don't Eat Your Heart Out* - for older teens 15-18 years of age, NIH Publication No. 92-3099.
4. *Cholesterol in Children - Healthy Eating Is a Family Affair* - parent's guide, NIH Publication No. 92-3099.

These publications can be ordered at:
>   National Cholesterol Education Program
>   NHLBI Information Center
>   P.O Box 30105
>   Bethesda, Maryland 208224-01015
>   Phone: (301)251-1222

Pamphlets

1. *Children, Cholesterol, and Diet - Answers to Questions Parents Often Ask*
>   The American Dietetic Association
>   216 West Jackson Boulevard
>   Suite 800
>   Chicago, Illinois 60606-6995
>   Phone: 1-800-877-1600

2. *Fast Food - Today's Guide to Healthy Choices* - a guide to how you can compare and find lower fat items at your favorite restaurant. Contact your state's Dairy Council, Inc.

Cookbooks

1. *Kids' Cookbook.* American Heart Association, ed. Winston, M. Random House, New York, 1993, 127 pages.
2. Hess, MA et al. *A Healthy Head Start: A Worry Free Guide to Feeding Young Children.* H.Holt Company, New York, 1990, 324 pages.

Low-Fat, Low-Saturated Fat, Low-Cholesterol Diets
Food Selection Guide (Step-One Diet)

Breads, cereals, pasta, rice, dried peas, and beans

These products are high in carbohydrates, and most are low in fat. Therefore, they can be increased in the diet as substitutes for fatty foods. However, they too contain calories and should not be eaten in excess. Cereals can be eaten for snacks as well as for breakfast. Dried peas and beans are good sources of protein. Combine larger quantities of pasta, rice, legumes, and vegetables with smaller amounts of lean meat, fish, or poultry to derive complete protein sources with less fat and calories.

Include foods that contain fiber (fruits, vegetables. whole grain, and legumes). Research indicates that fiber, either water-soluble or -insoluble, may be beneficial in lowering blood cholesterol levels.

Fruits and vegetables

It is wise to feature fruits and vegetables as an important part of each meal. Besides being sources of fiber, both are rich in vitamins and some minerals, and they contribute to achieving the recommended allowances of these nutrients. Fruits and vegetables can be used for snacks and desserts.

Meats

A reasonable approach to meat consumption is to limit intake of lean meat, chicken, turkey, and fish to **no more than six ounces** per day.

Beef, Pork and Lamb

Use lean cuts of beef, pork, and lamb. Lean cuts include:

- extra-lean ground beef
- sirloin tip
- round steak
- rump roast
- arm roast
- center-cut ham
- loin chops
- tenderloin

Trim all fat off the outside of meats before cooking. It is not necessary to severely decrease the intake of red meat, but lean choices should be made. Lean meat is rich in protein, and contains a highly absorbable form of iron. Premenopausal women, in particular, should avoid severe reduction of lean red meat because this could increase the risk for iron-deficiency anemia.

Processed Meats

Choose high-fat, processed meats - bacon, balogna, salami, sausage, and hot dogs infrequently. Processed meats contain large quantities of fat, and they are not rich in valuable nutrients.

Organ Meats

The organ meats - liver, sweetbreads, kidneys, and brain - are very rich in cholesterol, and they should be strictly limited.

Chicken and Turkey

These are good sources of protein. The in fat poultry should be reduced by removing the skin and underlying fat layers before cooking. Chicken and turkey can be substituted for lean red meat in the diet, but they do not contain as much iron. Poultry should not be fried or covered with high-fat sauces.

Fish and Shellfish

Fish are good sources of protein. Shellfish contain cholesterol, but usually are low in saturated fatty acids. The preparation of fish is important. Like chicken and turkey, they should not be fried or covered with fat-rich sauces.

Eggs

Egg yolks often are hidden in cooked and processed foods. Egg whites contain no fat or cholesterol, and they can be eaten often. Experiment with one to two egg whites instead of whole eggs in recipes, or use commercial egg substitutes that do not contain yolk.

Milk and dairy products

Use skim or one-percent milk instead of two-percent or whole milk. Decrease whole milk, natural and processed cheeses: substitute nonfat or low-fat (2 percent) cottage cheese or low-fat cheeses made from vegetable oils. Choose the nonfat or low-fat (1- to 2- percent) yogurt. Experiment with evaporated skim milk in recipes that call for heavy cream. Substitute low-fat yogurt, low-fat or nonfat sour cream, or low-fat cottage cheese for sour cream in dips and salad dressings. Have at least two to three servings of low-fat dairy products, such as two to three glasses of skim (or 1- percent) milk each day to help assure an adequate calcium intake.

Fats and oils

The general rule is to reduce the total intake of fats, especially saturated fat. Butter fat, lard, and beef fats are high in saturated fat and cholesterol, and should be avoided as much as possible. Vegetable fats do not contain cholesterol, but certain vegetable fats- coconut oil, palm oil, and palm kernel oil - are very high in saturated fats and should be limited. These fats are often used in bakery goods, processed foods, popcorn, oils, and nondairy creamers. Vegetables shortening and some peanut butters contain hydrogenated oils, which are also saturated fats. Read the labels on these foods to check for the use of saturated vegetable oils.

Unsaturated vegetable oils and fats do not raise blood cholesterol, but they should be limited because they are still fats and are high in calories. Total fat should still be limited to 20 to 30% of calories from fat. Desirable liquid vegetable oils are corn oil, cottonseed oil, olive oil, canola oil, safflower oil, soybean oil, and sunflower oil. Peanut oil is less desirable, but small amounts are acceptable. Margarine is made from partially hydrogenated vegetable oil, but is a better choice than butter or totally hydrogenated oil. Buy a margarine that has an allowed liquid oil as the first item on the package's ingredient list. Mayonnaise and salad dressings often are made from unsaturated fats, but they should also be limited because of their high calorie and fat content.

Seeds, nuts, peanut butter, olives, and avocados are high in fat, but the fat is mainly the unsaturated type. These foods should be limited to avoid excess calories and fat.

Other Eating Tips
Snacks

Most sweets should be limited as snacks. They tend to be rich in calories and fats, and their caloric content outweighs their nutritional value. Some good choices in snacks are graham crackers, Ry-Krisp® crackers, melba toast, soda crackers, bagels (non-egg), English muffins, fruits, and vegetables. These snacks are preferable to snack crackers, French fries, and chips. Popcorn should be air-popped or cooked in small amounts of liquid vegetable oil.

Desserts

Eat fruit, low-fat yogurt, and fruit ices instead of pastries, cake, and cookies. Also acceptable are sherbet, angel food cake, Jello-O®, frozen low-fat yogurt, or other frozen products that do not contain saturated fat (such as pure fruit juice bars or popsicles).

Cooking Methods

Choose those methods that use little or no fat. They include:
- Poaching
- Braising
- Steaming
- Grilling
- Baking
- Stir-frying
- Broiling
- Microwaving

Foods can be cooked in a nonstick pan without added fat, or use a nonfat cooking spray in regular cookware. Limit fried foods and avoid frying in saturated fat. Add moisture to lean meats by using water, broth, cooking wines, and other nonfat or low-fat sauces along with the cooking methods mentioned above.

Soups and stews should be chilled after cooking, and the congealed fat that forms on top after a few hours in the refrigerator should be skimmed off. When preparing meals, avoid using excess salt, which can contribute to raising blood pressure in some people.

Eating away from home

Order entrees, potatoes, and vegetables without sauces or butter. When meat exceeds the size of a deck of cards (three to four ounces), the rest can be taken home for another meal.

Choose vegetables or fruit salads, and ask for low-calorie salad dressings to be served on the side. Use dressings sparingly. Limit high-fat toppings such as bacon, crumbled eggs, cheese, sunflower seeds, and olives. Ask for margarine instead of butter, and limit amounts of margarine used.

General Counseling guidelines for reducing hyperlipidemia in children
1. Know what the child is eating. A three day diet record is extremely helpful prior to suggesting changes in the diet.
2. If the child is obese, reduce energy intake to that recommended for age.
3. Involve the family in adapting a lower cholesterol eating pattern. Try not to single out just the child affected with high cholesterol.
4. Use food models or pictures to review food groups and ways to avoid or limit high cholesterol foods.
5. Set realistic goals for changes in eating habits. To avoid discouragement in the diet, make gradual changes, e.g. from whole milk to 2% to 1% or skim milk in several weeks time rather than abrupt changes.
6. "Play-act" going to a restaurant or fast food place by using a restaurant menu to review ordering lower cholesterol foods.

Adapted from:

1. National Cholesterol Education Program, National Cholesterol Education Program, Second Report of the Expert Panel on Detection, Evaluation, and Treatment of High Blood Cholesterol I Adults (Adult Treatment Panel II), National Institutes of Health, National Heart, Lung, and Blood Institute, NIH Publication No. 93-3095, September 1993.

Low-Cholesterol Guidelines

What is cholesterol?

Cholesterol is a waxy, fat-like substance found only in animal fats. It is manufactured by the body and is essential to the functioning of the brain and many other organs. When eaten in excess, cholesterol can raise blood cholesterol levels or help form fatty deposits in blood vessel walls.

What is saturated fat?

Saturated fats occur naturally in all foods of animal origin and in a few vegetable products such as coconut oil, palm or palm kernel oil, and cocoa butter (chocolate). Hydrogenate (hardened) fats such as vegetable shortening are also highly saturated. They are solid at room temperature and can also have the same harmful effects on your circulatory system as cholesterol.

What are unsaturated fats?

Unsaturated fats are fats of plant origin and are liquid at room temperature. Monounsaturated fats such as peanut oil, olive oil, and fish oils tend not to raise blood cholesterol levels and may even be beneficial in lowering them when used in place of saturated fats.

Polyunsaturated fats such as safflower, sunflower, corn, soybeans, sesame, and canola oils tend not to raise blood cholesterol when used in moderate amounts.

How should I eat?

1. Eat more fish and poultry (with no skin, visible fat, or breaded and fried). Eat less red meat.
2. Buy lean meat and trim all visible fat. Eat no more than six ounces (total cooked weight) of any meat, fish, or poultry each day.
3. Limit intake of fried or fatty foods.
4. Use low-fat dairy products such as skim milk, low- or non-fat yogurt, and low-fat cheese.
5. Eat five or more servings of fruits and vegetables each day. Keep some ready to eat in your refrigerator for a healthy snack.
6. Use margarine or oils that are polyunsaturated rather than butter or vegetable shortening.
7. Avoid excessive use of foods known to be high in cholesterol, such as egg yolk, liver, shellfish, duck, and goose. Limit egg yolks to no more than 4 per week. Egg whites or egg substitute can be used in baking rather than whole eggs.
8. Include complex carbohydrate foods such as whole-grain breads and cereals, beans, rice, and pasta. They contribute needed fiber and are very low in fat.

FOOD GROUP	ALLOWED	USE SPARINGLY
VEGETABLES 3 servings or more*	All vegetables and vegetable juices.	Fried vegetables. Vegetables in cream, butter, or high-fat cheese sauces.
FRUIT 2 servings or more*	All fruits except coconut and avocado. Fruit juices.	Coconut or avocado. Fruit in cream or custard.

FOOD GROUP	ALLOWED	USE SPARINGLY
MEAT & SUBSTITUTES 2 servings or more (6 oz./day maximum)	Limit your intake of meat, seafood, and poultry to no more than 6 ounces (cooked weight) per day. All lean, well-trimmed beef, veal, pork, and lamb. All chicken and turkey without skin. All fish and shellfish (limit shrimp, lobster, and sardines to no more than 1 serving per week). Wild game: wild duck, rabbit, pheasant, venison. Meatless dishes: recipes with dried beans, peas, lentils, tofu (soybean curd).	Prime grade and other heavily marbled and fatty meats such as short ribs, spare ribs, rib eye roast or steak, frankfurters, sausage, bacon and high-fat luncheon meats; mutton. Caviar. Commercially fried fish. Domestic duck, goose; venison sausage. Organ meats: liver, gizzard, heart, chitterlings, brains, kidney, sweetbreads. Peanut butter.
(4 egg yolks/wk. maximum) (2 egg whites = 1 egg in recipes)	Limit egg yolks to no more than 4 per week, including those used in cooking. Egg whites or low-cholesterol egg substitutes may be used as desired. Low-fat cheeses: nonfat or low-fat cottage cheese (1% or 2% fat); cheeses made with part-skim milk, such as mozzarella, farmer's, string, or ricotta. (Cheeses should be labeled no more than 2-6 g fat per oz.) Seeds & nuts : all seeds and most nuts.	More than 3 egg yolks per week (including those used in cooking). Whole-milk-type cheeses, including colby, cheddar, muenster, monterey jack, havarti, brie, camembert, American, Swiss, and blue. Creamed cottage cheese; cream cheese. Seeds and nuts.
MILK 2 cups or the equivalent*	Skim (or 1%*) milk: liquid, powdered, or evaporated. Buttermilk made with skim milk; drinks made with skim or low-fat milk or cocoa. Chocolate milk or cocoa made with skim or low-fat (1%) milk. Nonfat or low-fat yogurt. * Skim milk and nonfat products are preferred. Low-fat refers to 1% milkfat.	Whole milk and whole milk products, including buttermilk or yogurt made from whole milk, drinks made from whole milk; condensed milk; evaporated whole milk, 2% milk.
SOUPS & COMBINATION FOODS	Low-fat soups: broth, bouillon, dehydrated soups, homemade broth, soups with the fat removed. Home-made cream soups made with skim or low-fat milk. Low-fat combination foods: spaghetti, lasagna, chili, and Spanish rice are examples of foods that can be low-fat if low-fat ingredients and low-fat cooking techniques are used.	Cream soups made with whole milk, cream, or high-fat cheese. All other soups. Combination foods high in fat or that contain types of fat not allowed.

FOOD GROUP	ALLOWED	USE SPARINGLY
DESSERTS & SWEETS **in moderation**	Sherbet, fruit ices, gelatins, meringues, angel food cake. Homemade desserts with recommended fats, oils, and milk products. (Use the weekly egg yolk allowances, or try egg whites in recipes, using two egg whites instead of one whole egg.) Jam, jelly, honey, marmalade, sugars and syrups. Pure sugar candy such as gum drops, hard candy, jelly beans, marshmallows, and non-chocolate mints.	Commercially prepared cakes, pies, cookies, frostings, and pudding or mixes for these products. Desserts containing whole milk products, egg yolk, chocolate, coconut, lard, palm oil, or palm kernel oil. Ice cream or ice cream drinks. Candy that contains chocolate, coconut, butter, hydrogenated fat, or unknown ingredients. Buttered syrups.
FATS & OILS **Up to 8 tsp./day maximum** **(use recommended oils)**	Vegetable oils: safflower, sunflower, corn, soybean, cottonseed, sesame, canola, olive, or peanut. Margarines: stick, tub, or squeeze, with one of the above oils listed as a LIQUID as the first ingredient. Salad dressing or mayonnaise: homemade or commercial, made with a recommended oil. Low- or non-fat salad dressing or mayonnaise. Limit added fats and oils to 6 to 8 tsp. per day (includes fats used on cooking, baking, salads, and spread on bread). Remember to count the "hidden fats" in foods. Avocado and olives: Use them only in small amounts, as they are high in fat.	Solid fats & shortenings: butter, lard, salt, pork, bacon drippings. Gravy containing meat fat, shortening, or suet. Margarines in which the first ingredient is NOT a liquid oil. Chocolate, cocoa butter, coconut. Coconut oil, palm oil, or palm kernel- these ingredients are often used in bakery products, nondairy creamers, whipped toppings, candy, and commercially fried foods. Read labels carefully. Salad dressings made of unknown oils, sour cream, or cheese, such as blue cheese, Green Goddess® , and Roquefort. Cream, all kinds: Half & Half, light, heavy, or whipping. Sour or cream cheese (even if "light" or low-fat). Nondairy cream substitutes, sour cream substitutes made with palm, palm kernel, or coconut oil.

FOOD GROUP	ALLOWED	USE SPARINGLY
BEVERAGES	Regular or diet carbonated beverages; mineral water. Check with your physician. Moderation is recommended.	Any beverage that contains avoided fats or egg yolks. Also see "MILK."
CONDIMENTS/ MISCELLANEOUS	All seasonings and condiments. Cocoa powder. "Cream" sauces made with recommended ingredients.	Carob powder made with hydrogenated fats.

* These amounts indicate the minimum number of servings needed each day from the Food Guide Pyramid to provide a variety of nutrients essential to good health. The word "maximum" is used if amounts of certain foods eaten must be controlled. Combination foods may count as full or partial servings from the food groups. Dark green, leafy, or orange vegetables are recommended 3 or 4 times weekly to provide vitamin A. A good source of vitamin C is recommended daily. Potatoes may be included as a serving of vegetables. The menu below is provided as a sample; your daily menus will vary.

SAMPLE MENU

Breakfast
1/2 cup orange juice
1/2 cup oatmeal
1 slice toast
1 tsp. margarine
1 cup skim milk

Noon Meal
Turkey sandwich with 2 oz.
    turkey, 2 slices bread
Lettuce and tomato slices
Fresh fruit
Carrot sticks
1 cup skim milk

Snack
Fresh fruit or low-fat crackers

Evening Meal
3 oz. lean ground beef
1 baked potato
1 tsp. margarine
1/2 cup green beans
Lettuce salad
1 tbsp. noncreamy dressing
1/2 cup peach slices
1 cup skim milk

Dietary Modifications to Lower Blood Cholesterol (Step-One Diet)

Increased blood cholesterol levels are related to an increased risk of coronary heart disease. Coronary risk rises progressively with cholesterol level. Part of a cholesterol-lowering treatment program includes diet modifications. They are designed to reduce intake of total fat, saturated fat, and cholesterol while maintaining a nutritionally adequate dietary intake. General guidelines are as follows:

1. Adjust calorie intake to promote normal growth and development and to achieve and maintain desirable body weight.
2. Limit total fat intake to less than 30 percent of total calories. Limit Meat and Substitutes to no more than six oz. per day and Fats & Oils to no more than eight tsp. per day.
3. Practice low-fat cooking techniques. Do not fry food; instead, broil, bake, boil, steam, grill, roast on a rack, stir-fry, or microwave it.
   - Remove the skin from poultry.
   - Remove all visible fat from meats.
   - Skim the fat off stews, soups, and gravies before serving them.
   - Steam vegetables in water or broth instead of sauteing them in fat.
4. Saturated fats are found in animal products and in some vegetable products. Saturated vegetable fats are found in many solid or "hydrogenated" shortenings, in coconut oil, cocoa butter, palm oil, and palm kernel oil. Read labels carefully to avoid these products as much as possible.
5. Cholesterol is found in all animal products. Cholesterol intake should be less than 300 mg per day. Limit high-cholesterol foods, such as egg yolks, liver, organ meats, and butterfat-containing dairy products. Plant foods do not contain cholesterol.
6. Increase intake of complex carbohydrates such as fruits, vegetables, whole grains, and legumes to replace foods high in fat.

FOOD GROUP	CHOOSE	USE SPARINGLY
BREADS/ STARCHES 6 servings or more*	Breads: All kinds (wheat, rye, raisin, white, oatmeal, Italian, French, and English muffin bread). Low-fat rolls: English muffins; frankfurter and hamburger buns; water (not egg) bagels; pita bread; tortillas (not fried). Pancakes, waffles, biscuits, and muffins made with recommended oil.	Products made with egg yolks or with avoided fats, oils, or whole milk products. Butter rolls, egg breads, egg bagels, cheese breads, croissants. Commercial doughnuts, muffins, sweet rolls, biscuits, waffles, pancakes, store-bought mixes.
Crackers:	Low-fat crackers & snacks: Animal, graham, rye, saltine (with recommended oil; no lard), oyster, and matzo crackers. Bread sticks, melba toast, rusks, and flatbread; pretzels; popcorn (with recommended fat); zwieback.	High-fat crackers: cheese crackers, butter crackers, and those made with coconut palm or oil. Buttered popcorn.
Cereals:	Hot or cold cereals: All kinds except granola-type cereals made with coconut or coconut oil.	Cereals containing coconut, hydrogenated vegetable fat, animal fat, or nuts.

FOOD GROUP	CHOOSE	USE SPARINGLY
Potatoes/ Pasta/ Rice:	All kinds of potatoes, rice, and pasta (such as macaroni, spaghetti, and noodles) except those listed to avoid.	Pasta or rice prepared with whole eggs, cream sauce, or high-fat cheese. Egg pasta; chow mein noodles, french fries.

Recommended Cookbooks:
Low-Cholesterol, Low-Fat, Low-Saturated Fat

1. American Dietetic Association. Cut the Fat! Harper Collins, 1996. Reducing fat and cholesterol.
2. American Dietetic Association. Skim the Fat: A Practical and Up-to Date Food Guide Chronimed, 1995.
3. American Heart Association. American Heart Association Cookbook. 5th ed. New York Times Books, 1992. An informative cookbook with nearly 600 recipes. It includes shopping tips, a discussion and a list of low-fat cheeses, and low-fat/low-cholesterol guidelines.
4. American Heart Association. American Heart Association Quick & Easy Cookbook. Times Books. Choose from over 200 options for truly appetizing meals, from breakfast treats to bedtime snacks, that can be made in minutes without giving up taste or nutrition.
5. American Heart Association. American Heart Association Kids' Cookbook. Times Books. Thirty recipes geared to eight- to twelve-year olds. Recipes are AHA approved, kid-tested, and include safety and nutrition basics.
6. American Heart Association. American Heart Association Around the World Cookbook: Healthy Recipes With International Flavor. Times Books. This cookbook offers delicious recipes from around the world that are low in fat, cholesterol, and sodium.
7. Brody, Jane. Jane Brody's Good Food Book-Living in the High Carbohydrate Way. New York: W.W. Norton, 1985. This combination cookbook/ nutrition guide emphasizes complex carbohydrates. The recipes are mainly vegetarian, fish, poultry, and pasta, with a few beef dishes. Nutrient analyses of recipes are not provided.
8. Connor, Sonja L.; Connor, William E. The New American Diet Cookbook: 250 All New Low-Fat/High-Flavor Recipes the creators of the bestselling New American Diet. Simon & Schuster, 1997.
9. Cooper, Nancy R.D. Joy of Snacks: Good Nutrition for People Who Like to Snack. 1991. This is an excellent book for those who love to snack. This book includes recipes and nutritional information on a great number of mouth watering dishes.
10. The Betty Crocker Editors. Betty Crocker's New Low-Fat, Low-Cholesterol Cookbook. Rev Edition. MacMillan General Reference. 1996.
11. Hachfeld, Linda; Eykyn, Betsy. Cooking A'La Heart. 1992. Offers a practical, hands-on guide to healthy eating, with up-to-date nutritional information and a wide variety of recipes with nutrient breakdowns.
12. Havala, Suzanne; Clifford, Mary. Simple, Lowfat & Vegetarian: Unbelievably Easy to Reduce the Fat in Your Meals! Vegetarian Resource Group. 1995. Tips on eating out at a variety of restaurants, plus low-fat tips
13. Jacobson, Michael. Kitchen Fun for Kids. 1991. A fun recipe book for children ages 7-12 with healthy recipes they can make and fun nutrition facts for children.

14. Moquette-Magee, Elaine. 200 Kid Tested Ways to Lower the Fat in Your Child's Favorite Foods (Child Nutrition). 1993. A step-by-step guide for cutting the fat in most popular brand names and homemade foods kids already eat.
15. Ponichetera, Brenda. Quick and Healthy Recipes and Ideas. 1991. Easy recipes that are low in fat, cholesterol and calories. Nutritional analysis of each recipe included and food exchanges for diabetes and weight control are included.
16. Smith, MJ. 60 Days of Low-Fat Low-Cost Meals in Minutes. 1990. An innovative and exciting cookbook helps to save you time , money, and still watch your fat intake. Over 150 low-fat and low-cost meals.
17. Spitler, Sue and Linda R. Yoakam. 1,001 Low Fat Recipes: Quick, Great-Tasting Recipes for the Whole Family. Surrey Books, 1995.
18. Tribole, Evelyn. Healthy Homestyle Cooking: 200 Favorite Family Recipes - With a Fraction of the Fat. Rodale Pr. December 1994.

What else can I do?

1. Bake, broil, or roast meat rather than frying them. Skip gravies and rich sauces. Don't buy self-basting turkeys, either!
2. Limit intake of rich pastries and desserts that are high in butter, eggs, cream, or shortening.
3. Choose a frozen fruit sorbet or low- or non-fat frozen yogurt rather than ice cream. (Some sherbets may contain whole milk, so check labels carefully.)

Remember to check all labels - many foods contain hidden fats!

4. Use a "nonstick" cooking spray or "nonstick" pans.
5. Chill and skim fat off of meat stock or drippings when making soup or sauces.
6. Check labels for the words "hydrogenated" or "hardened" fats or oils, and avoid these products.

Are there other terms you may have questions about?

HDL's (high-density lipoproteins) and LDL's (low-density lipoproteins) transport cholesterol in your blood. LDL's carry cholesterol into your cells and HDL's carry it away and dispose of it in the liver, having a protective effect on your circulatory system. High saturated fat, high cholesterol diets may increase the harmful LDL's. Not smoking, participating in aerobic activity, and losing weight if you are overweight may increase the beneficial HDL's.

Triglycerides (TG) are fatty compounds that are combination of three ("tri") fatty acids and glycerin. Body fat is made up of mostly stored triglycerides. Triglycerides also circulate in the bloodstream like cholesterol, and may have a link with heart disease. To lower triglycerides, maintain ideal body weight, limit intake of sugars and alcohol, and eat a low-fat diet.

Fat-Controlled Diet

Description

The Fat-Controlled Diet may be prescribed in disorders in which dietary fat is not used normally by the body. The diet limits total fat intake to approximately 30 percent of the total daily calories and restricts all types of fat.

Fat intake may be reduced even further during periods of acute fat intolerance by decreasing fat, egg, and meat allowances. For patients who require additional calories, medium- chain triglyceride (MCT) oil may be incorporated into foods. MCT oil has been effective in improving fat absorption and the palatability of the fat-restricted diet.

Indications for Use

1. Disorders of the liver, pancreas, or gallbladder in which digestion, absorption, or transport of dietary fat is impaired.
2. Malabsorption syndromes of the small intestine.
3. Hyperlipoproteinemia caused by abnormal metabolism of dietary fat.

Adequacy

This diet generally meets the Recommended Dietary Allowances of the National Research Council for adults when foods are supplied in the suggested amount daily. Iron may be inadequate for persons from ages 11 to 18 years. Restriction of fat to less than 30 grams a day may provide insufficient amounts of essential fatty acids.

Notes about Patient Education Material (Fat-Controlled Diet)

The 50-gram fat restriction may be modified to a 20-gram fat diet by:
- Omitting all egg yolks.
- Reducing the fat allowance to one serving per day.
- Reducing the meat allowances from 6 oz. to 3 oz., or by using 6 oz. of very lean meat.

To increase protein, 4 oz. of fat-free cottage cheese may be added to the diet.

NOTE: For patients who require a diet designed to lower blood cholesterol, see the Low-Cholesterol, Low-Fat, Low-Saturated Fat Diet.

Professional references

1. Anderson H. Low-fat diet in the short-gut syndrome (letter). Lancet 1983; 6:347.
2. Anderson H, Bosaeus I. Hyperoxaluria in malabsorptive states. Urol Int 1981; 36:1-9.
3. Bliss CM. Fat absorption and malabsorption. Arch Intern Med 1981; 141: 1213-15.
4. Boyar AP, Loughridge JR. The fat portion exchange list: A tool for teaching and evaluating low-fat diets. J Am Dietetic Assoc 1985; 85: 589-94.
5. Buzzard IM, et al. Diet intervention methods to reduce fat intake: Nutrient and food group composition of self-selected low fat diets. J Am Diet Assoc 1990; 90: 42-53.
6. Cerda JJ, Artnak EJ. Nutritional aspects of malabsorption syndromes. Comprehensive Therapy. 1983; 9(11): 35-46.
7. Dougherty RM, Fong AKH, Iacono JM. Nutrient content of the diet when fat is reduced. Am J Clin Nutr 1988; 48: 970-9.
8. Hallfrisch J, et al. Acceptability of a 7-day higher-carbohydrate, lower-fat menu: The Beltsville diet study. J Am Diet Assoc 1988; 88: 613-171.

245

9. Smith- Schneider LM, Sigmen-Grant MJ, Kris-Etherton PM. Dietary fat reduction strategies. J Am Diet Assoc 1992; 92: 34-8.

10. Tests for fat malabsorption. Nutrition and the M.D. 1986; 12(2): 3-4.

11. Ways to consume less fat: foods that do the job. Environmental Nutrition. March 1989.

Copyright © 1997, Twin Cities District Dietetic Association.

This information is to be used by a registered dietitian for the client education in cooperation with physician orders.
This educational material may be reproduced for the above purpose only.

246

FAT-CONTROLLED DIET
(APPROXIMATELY 50 GRAMS)

The main sources of fat in the diet are meats, some dairy products, and pure fats such as butter and margarine. There are also many "hidden" fats. This diet restricts the total amount of fat in your diet, but not the type of fat.

FOOD GROUP	ALLOWED/ RECOMMENDED	AVOID/ USE SPARINGLY
BREADS/ STARCHES 6 servings or more*	Enriched white, whole wheat, rye, oatmeal, French, or Italian breads. English muffins, plain bagels; plain dinner, hamburger, or hot dog rolls. Pita or pocket bread. Homemade baked products made with allowed foods.	Breads prepared with large amounts of fat, such as waffles, pancakes, muffins, biscuits, doughnuts, sweet rolls, party crackers, cornbread, or bread stuffing.
Crackers:	Saltines, graham crackers, matzo, melba toast, RyKrisp®, other plain breads or crackers that do not have a large amount of fat in them.	Most snack crackers such as Ritz®, Hi Ho's®.
Cereals:	Ready-to-eat cereal with 1 gram fat or less per serving.	Ready-to-eat cereal with more than 1 gram fat per serving such as wheat germ, granola, Cracklin Oat Bran®.
Potatoes/ Pasta/ Rice:	White or sweet potatoes. Creamed or mashed potatoes prepared with allowed fat. Rice or pasta products prepared without added fat (or with allowed amount of fat).	Fried potatoes. All prepared products containing fat, cream sauce, or cheese sauce. Potato or other snack chips. Chow mein noodles.
VEGETABLES 3 servings or more*	Prepared without added fat: Any fresh, frozen, or canned vegetables or vegetable juices.	Prepared with added fat: Buttered, with cream or cheese sauce, fried.
FRUIT 2 servings or more*	All fruits and fruit juices, except avocado and olives. Any prepared fruit products that do not have fat added to them.	Avocado and olives, except as allowed under "FATS & OILS." Prepared fruit products that have fat added to them.
MEAT & SUBSTITUTES 2 servings or more (up to 6 oz. total/day)	Limit to 6 oz. cooked weight per day. Prepare meat by baking, broiling, stewing, or simmering without addition of fat. Trim all visible fat from meat. Choose from lean-appearing, easily trimmed poultry, beef, veal, pork loin, lean ham, organ meats, fish, and shellfish. Low-fat luncheon meats. Meats and fish packed in water.	Prime grade, heavily marbled or fatty meats. Hot dogs, sausage, high-fat (regular) luncheon meats, bacon in excess of that allowed under "FATS & OIL." Fried meats. Dick and goose. Meats and fish packed in oil.

FOOD GROUP	ALLOWED/ RECOMMENDED	AVOID/ USE SPARINGLY
MEAT & **SUBSTITUTES**	One egg yolk daily, including that used in cooking. Egg whites. Uncreamed cottage cheese, 99% fat-free cheeses. 1/2 cup creamed cottage cheese or 1 oz. part-skim milk cheese can be substituted for 1 oz. of meat (as part of the 6 oz. per day). Dried beans or peas (if tolerated), prepared without fat. Chestnuts.	More than one egg yolk per day. Eggs prepared with fat in excess of that allowed under "FATS & OILS." All other cheeses. Nuts or peanut butter in excess of that allowed under "FATS & OILS."
MILK **2 cups or the equivalent**	Skim milk (including fluid, powdered, or evaporated), skim buttermilk. Other milk drinks that do not contain fat or chocolate syrup. NOTE: Beverages containing cocoa and skim milk are allowed, as are cocoa mixes with nonfat dry milk as the milk source. Skim milk (nonfat) yogurt. Yogurt beverages.	Whole milk or whole milk products, including fluid, condensed, evaporated, or chocolate milks (see below). 2% or 1% milks. Malted milks, eggnog, milk shakes. Drinks containing chocolate syrup or a milk source other that nonfat dry milk or skim milk. Whole, 2% or 1% yogurt.
SOUPS & **COMBINATION** **FOODS**	Broth, bouillon, dehydrated soups; homemade broth soups with the fat removed (cool soup; skim fat off). Homemade cream soups made with skim milk and no fat. Frozen or prepared dinners not containing any fried foods, gravies, cream sauces, or other fats.	All other soups. All other frozen or prepared dinners that contain fried foods, gravies, cream sauces, or other fats.
DESSERTS & SWEETS **in moderation**	Allowed fruits, fruit ices, sherbet made with skim milk, gelatins, meringues, frozen fruit bars with no fat added. Angel food cake, arrowroot cookies, vanilla wafers, fig bars, Rice Krispie® bars (limit to one portion per day). Pudding made with skim milk and egg whites or with egg yolk allowance. Frozen pudding made with skim milk. Nonfat frozen yogurt. Jam, jelly, honey, marmalade, molasses, sugars, and syrups. Sugar candies such as gumdrops, hard candies, jelly beans, marshmallows, non-chocolate mints. Sugar candies such as gumdrops, hard candies, jelly beans, marshmallows, non-chocolate mints.	All desserts made with fat in excess of the allowance. All desserts made with whole or 2% milk, butter, shortening, cream, egg yolk, chocolate, or nuts. Ice cream or frozen dairy desserts. Buttered syrups. Candies containing chocolate, nuts, coconut, cream, butter, shortening, or fat of any kind. Caramels.

FOOD GROUP	ALLOWED/ RECOMMENDED	AVOID/ USE SPARINGLY
FATS & OILS Up to 3 servings/day	Choose a total of 3 per day from the following list: 1 tsp. margarine or butter 1 tsp. oil, shortening, mayonnaise, or mayonnaise-type dressing 2 tsp. peanut butter 1 tbsp. salad dressing 2 tbsp. light coffee cream 1 strip crisp bacon 5 small ripe olives 1/8 small avocado 6 small nuts 1/4 cup gravy	Any fats in excess of the prescribed allowance
BEVERAGES	Coffee, tea, or herbal tea. Carbonated beverages. Any beverages without fat added	Any beverage that contains fat.
CONDIMENTS/ MISCELLANEOUS	All seasonings and condiments. Gravy prepared with fat-free broth. Cocoa powder. Fat-free salad dressings.	Nuts and peanut butter except as allowed under "FATS & OILS." Gravy except as allowed above.

* These amounts indicate the minimum number of servings needed from the Food Pyramid to provide a variety of nutrients essential to good health. A maximum amount (limit) is indicated when amounts of certain foods must be controlled. Combination foods may count as full or partial servings from the food groups. Dark green, leafy, or orange vegetables are recommended 3 or 4 times weekly to provide vitamin A. A good source of vitamin C is recommended daily. Potatoes may be included as a serving of vegetables. The menu following is provided as a sample; your daily menus will vary.

SAMPLE MENU

Breakfast		Noon Meal		Evening Meal	
Citrus fruit/juice	1/2 cup	Allowed soup	1 cup	Lean, trimmed meat	3 oz.
Cereal	1/2 cup	Lean, trimmed meat	3 oz.	Potato or substitute	1/2 cup
Skim milk	1/2 cup	Vegetable	1/2 cup	Vegetable	1/2 cup
Toast	1 slice	Bread	1 slice	Fruit or vegetable salad (no fat added)	1/2 cup
Peanut butter	2 tsp.	Butter or margarine	1 tsp.		
Jelly	1 tbsp	Jelly	1 tbsp.	French dressing	1 tbsp.
Coffee or tea	As desired	Fruit/ allowed dessert	1/2 cup	Plain dinner roll	1
		Skim milk	1 cup	Jelly	1 tbsp.
				Fruit or allowed dessert	1/2 cup
				Skim milk	1 cup

Blood Cholesterol Levels in Children and Adolescents: Risk Assessment

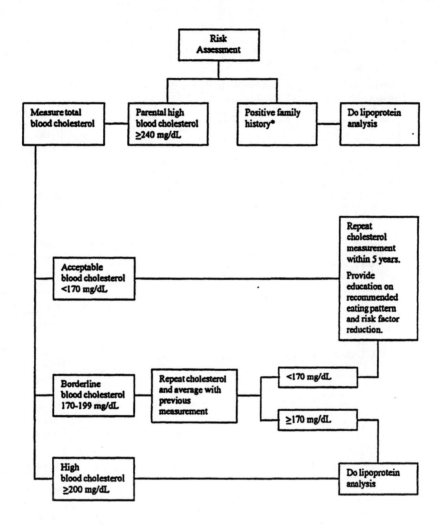

Defined as a history of premature (before age 55 years) cardiovascular disease in a parent or grandparent

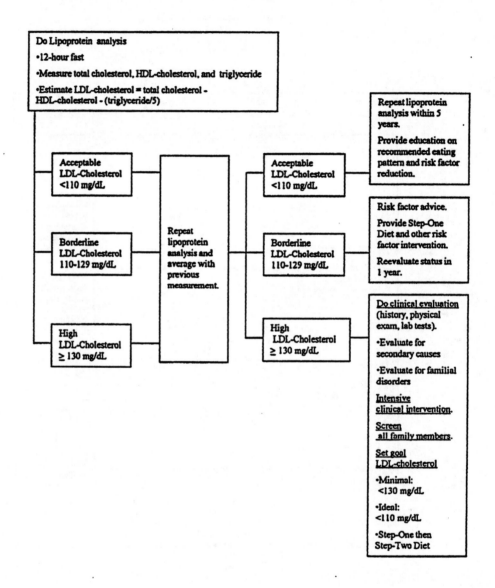

Calcium- and Phosphorus-Controlled Diet
Description
Low or high levels of total calcium or phosphorus can be achieved. If milligrams or milliequivalents are not specified, the following guidelines are suggested:

Calcium-controlled diets
1. 600 - 900 mg (30 - 45 meq) for children to adolescents (Low Calcium).
2. 1,000-1,500 mg (60-75 meq) for children to adolescents (High Calcium).

Phosphorus-controlled diets
1. 700-800 mg (45-52 mEq) Phosphorus-Controlled Diet.
   This level is recommended for use with Protein-Controlled Diets of fewer than 50 grams protein.
2. 800-1,200 mg (52-77 mEq) Phosphorus-Controlled Diet.
   This level is recommended for use with Protein-Controlled Diets of greater than 50 grams protein. This level is more applicable to a diet for dialysis. (See "Diets for Patients on Dialysis.")

Phosphorus-Controlled Diets usually require a simultaneous protein restriction.

Calcium and phosphorus points
One calcium point is equal to approximately 20 mg (1 mEq) of calcium.
One phosphorus point is equal to approximately 15.5 mg (1 mEq) of phosphorus.

Indications for use
The Calcium-Controlled Diet is used in the management of hypocalcemia, hypercalcemia, calcific nephrolithiasis, urinary calculi, and the prevention and treatment of osteoporosis.

The Phosphorus-Controlled Diet is used in the management of hyperphosphotemia, hypophosphotemia, and renal disease.

Adequacy
At a calcium level of 600 mg and a phosphorus level of 1,000 mg, the Calcium- and Phosphorus-Controlled Diet is inadequate in calcium, and may be inadequate in vitamin D, protein, B-complex vitamins, iron, and magnesium, according to the Recommended Dietary Allowances of the National Research Council.

Professional references
1. Allen LH. Calcium bioavailability and absorption: a review. Am J Clinical Nutr; 35(4):783-808; 1982.
2. Delmez JA, et al. Hyperphosphatemia: its consequences and treatment in patients with chronic renal disease. Am J Kidney Dis 19(4):303-17; 1992.
3. Food and Nutrition Board. Recommended dietary allowances. 10th ed. Washington, D.C.: National Research Council, 1989.
4. Friedman NE, et al. Effects of calcitriol and phosphorus therapy on the growth of patients with x-linked hypophosphatemia. J Clin Endocrinol Met: 76(4):839-44; 1993.
5. National Dairy Council. Calcium: a summary of current research for the health professional (0147N). Rosemount, Ill.: National Dairy Council, 1984:21.

6. National Institutes of Health Consensus Development Conference Statement. Osteoporosis. Washington, D.C.: Government Printing Office, 5(3): 1984.

7. Orwoll E, et al. Effects of dietary protein deficiency on mineral metabolism and bone mineral density. Am J Clin Nutr 56(2):314-9: 1992.

8. Osteoporosis: cause, treatment, prevention (Publ. no. [NIH] 86-2226). U.S. Department of Health and Human Services. Washington, D.C.: Government Printing Office, 1986.

9. Slatopolsky E, Martin K. Monograph: management of hypocalcemia and secondary hyperparathyroidism in patients with chronic renal disease. Chicago: Abbott Laboratories Renal Care, 1987:16-17.

10. Stamp T, et al. Metabolic balance studies of mineral supplementation in osteoporosis. Clin Sci 81(6):799-802; 1991.

11. Subcommittee on Nonpharmacological Therapy, 1984 Joint National Committee on Detection, Evaluation, and Treatment of High Blood Pressure. Nonpharmacological approaches to the control of high blood pressure. Hypertension; 8:451-2; 1984.

12. Walser M, Chandler EC. Phosphorus. In: Walser M, Imbembo AL, Margolis S, Elfert GA. Nutritional management: the Johns Hopkins handbook. Philadelphia: W.B. Saunders, 1984:226-9.

13. Wetstein L. Dietary considerations in the treatment of renal disease. In: Mitch WE, Klahr S, eds. Nutrition and the kidney. Boston: Little, Brown, and Company, 1988:300.

Calcium- and phosphorus-controlled diet

Calcium and phosphorus are minerals that are found naturally in many foods. Foods containing less than one point of calcium or phosphorus may be consumed in moderate amounts.

1 point (Pt.) = 1 milliequivalent (mEq)

(1 mEq Calcium=20 mg; 1 mEq Phosphorus=15.5 mg)

Foods containing calcium may be selected until you reach _____ points.

Foods containing phosphorus may be selected until you reach _____ points.

Note: Milligrams were rounded off to the nearest whole numbers; calcium and phosphorus points were rounded off to the nearest 1/2 point.

	Portion	Ca Mg	Ca Pt.	Phos Pt.	Phos mg
BEVERAGES					
Carbonated beverages					
Cola	12 oz.	11	1/2	4	61
Cola, diet	12 oz.	0	0	4	61
Non-cola, diet	12 oz.	14	1	1	14
Others	12 oz.	12	1/2	0	0
Coffee, tea	4-6-oz. cups	18	1	1-1/2	23
Milk					
2%	1/2 cup	149	7	7	116
Buttermilk, 1% fat	1/2 cup	142	7	7	109
Skim, fortified	1/2 cup	151	8	8	124
Whole, chocolate skim	1/2 cup	145	7	8	120
Soybean milk	1/2 cup	28	1	4	63
Goat Milk	1/2 cup	158	8	8	129
Yogurt-Juice blend drinks	1/2 cup	145	7		
BREADS AND STARCHES					
Bagel, egg	1 average	9	1/2	2	37
Biscuit, muffin (except corn or bran)	1 average	55	3	3	49
Bread					
Cracked wheat	1 slice	22	1	2	32
Pumpernickel or rye	1 slice	7	0	3	42
Raisin	1 slice	15	1	1	20
Whole wheat	1 slice	25	1	4	65
White	1 slice	30	1	2	25
White, calcium enriched	1 slice	300	15	2	25
Doughnut, plain cake	1 average	31	1-1/2	2	33
French bread	1 slice	25	1	1	23
Graham cracker, 2-1/2" square	2	6	0	1	21
Lefse	1 piece	8	0	1	21
Pancake, plain (4-5" diameter)	1	50	2-1/2	8	125
Roll, hard, soft, or hamburger (small)	1	28	1	2	33
Rye wafer, 3-1/2" x 1-7/8" x 1/4"	1 triple cracker	3	0	2	25
Saltines	6 saltines	3	0	1	15
Waffle (5-1/2" diameter)	1	150	7-1/2	16-1/2	257

	Protein	Ca Mg	Ca Pt.	Phos Pt.	Phos mg
CEREALS					
Bran cereals (All Bran® type)	1 cup	63	3	49	761
Bran flakes	1 cup	25	1	16	252
Chex®, rice and corn	1 cup	3	0	1	11
Corn grits, cooked	1 cup	0	0	3	53
Cream of rice, cooked in water	1 cup	5	0	2	32
Cream of wheat (mix & eat)	1 cup	28	1	2	28
Cream of wheat, regular, cooked in water	1 cup	49	2	6	98
Granola	1 cup	111	6	24	378
Grape-Nuts®	1 cup	43	2	18	285
Kix®, corn flakes, or Rice Krispies®	1 cup	1	0	1	14
Oat bran, cooked	1 cup	19	1	14	213
Oats, instant, mixed with water	1 packet	215	11	12	190
Oats, regular, quick, instant, cooked	1 cup	19	1	11	178
Product 19®	1 cup	4	0	3	47
Puffed rice	1 cup	1	0	1	14
Puffed wheat	1 cup	3	0	3	43
Shredded wheat®	1 biscuit	9	1/2	5	83
Special K®	1 cup	6	0	3	41
Total®	1 cup	56	3	9	137
Wheaties® or Cheerios®	1 cup	44	2	6	100
POTATO OR SUBSTITUTE					
Macaroni, cooked	1/2 cup	7	0	3	42
Noodles, spaghetti, cooked	1/2 cup	8	0	3	47
Popcorn, popped	1 cup	1	0	1	17
Potato chips	10	5	0	2	31
Potato, baked or boiled	1/2 cup	8	0	3	44
Rice, brown, cooked	1/2 cup	9	1/2	4	55
Rice, regular and instant, cooked	1/2 cup	1	0	2	29
Rice, wild, cooked	1/2 cup	5	0	6	90
Sweet potato or yams, cooked, fresh	1/2 cup	35	2	5	70
VEGETABLES					
Asparagus (cooked)	1/2 cup	22	1	3	54
Beans					
Green, Italian, yellow (cooked)	1/2 cup	29	2	1	24
Kidney, canned	1/2 cup	37	2	9	139
Lima, baby (cooked)	1/2 cup	25	1	7	101
Navy or pinto (cooked)	1/2 cup	45	2	9	133
Beets (cooked)	1/2 cup	9	1/2	2	26
Broccoli (cooked)	1/2 cup	89	4-1/2	2-1/2	37
Broccoli, raw	1/2 cup	21	1	2	29
Brussels sprouts (cooked)	1/2 cup	28	1	3	44
Cabbage, raw, shredded	1/2 cup	16	1	1/2	8
Carrots (cooked)	1/2 cup	24	1	1-1/2	24
Carrot, raw	1, 4" long	10	1/2	1	16
Carrots, raw, shredded	1/2 cup	15	1	1-1/2	24
Cauliflower (cooked)	1/2 cup	17	1	1	22
Cauliflower, raw	1/2 cup	14	1	1-1/2	23
Celery, raw	1/2 cup	22	1	1	16
Corn, cooked	1/2 cup	2	0	5	84
Cucumber, raw, sliced	1/2 cup	7	0	1/2	9
Eggplant (cooked)	1/2 cup	3	0	1	11

Vegetables, continued	Protein	Ca Mg	Ca Pt.	Phos Pt.	Phos mg
Kohlrabi (cooked)	1/2 cup	20	1	2	37
Lettuce, iceberg	1/2 cup	6	0	0	6
Mushrooms (cooked)	1/2 cup	4	0	4	68
Mushrooms, raw, sliced	1/2 cup	2	0	2	36
Onions, chopped, raw	1/4 cup	10	1/2	1	12
Parsley, raw	1 tbsp.	5	0	0	2
Parsnips (cooked)	1/2 cup	29	1-1/2	3	54
Peas, green (cooked)	1/2 cup	22	1	6	94
Peppers, sweet, green, and red (raw)	1/4 cup	2	0	0	6
Radishes	10	9	1/2	1/2	8
Rutabagas (cooked)	1/2 cup	36	2	3	42
Spinach (cooked)	1/2 cup	122	6	3	50
Spinach, raw, all varieties	1/2 cup	28	1	1	14
Squash, summer, all varieties (cooked)	1/2 cup	24	1	2	35
Squash, summer, all varieties (raw)	1/2 cup	13	1	1-1/2	23
Squash, winter, all varieties (cooked)	1/2 cup	14	1	1	20
Tomato juice, canned	1/2 cup	10	1/2	1-1/2	23
Tomato, raw	1/2 cup	6	0	1	21
Tomatoes (cooked)	1/2 cup	10	1/2	2	23
Turnips (cooked)	1/2 cup	18	1	1	35

FRUIT AND FRUIT JUICES

	Protein	Ca Mg	Ca Pt.	Phos Pt.	Phos mg
Apple juice	1/2 cup	8	0	1/2	9
Apple, raw (with skin)	1 medium	10	1/2	1	10
Applesauce	1/2 cup	4	0	1/2	9
Apricot nectar	1/2 cup	9	1/2	1	16
Apricots, canned	1/2 cup	15	1	2	25
Apricots, dried	5 halves	8	0	1	21
Banana, raw	1 medium	7	0	1	22
Blueberries, raw	1 cup	9	1/2	1	15
Cantaloupe, raw	1/6 melon	9	1/2	1	15
Cherries, raw	1 cup	21	1	2	28
Cranberry juice	1/2 cup	4	0	0	2
Cranberry sauce, canned	1/2 cup	5	0	1/2	8
Fruit cocktail	1/2 cup	10	1/2	1	17
Grapefruit juice, canned, unsweetened	1/2 cup	9	1/2	1	14
Grapefruit, raw	1/2 medium	14	1	1	10
Grape juice	1/2 cup	4	0	0	4
Grapes, raw	1 cup	15	1	1	15
Honeydew	1/10 melon	8	0	1	13
Kiwifruit, raw	1 medium	20	1	2	31
Lemon juice	1/2 cup	9	1/2	1/2	7
Lemon, raw, with peel	1 medium	66	3	1	16
Nectarine, raw	1 medium	6	0	1	22
Orange juice, frozen, diluted	1/2 cup	11	1/2	1	20
Orange juice, calcium fortified	1/2 cup	140	7	1	20
Orange, raw	1 medium	52	3	1	18
Peach, canned	1/2 cup	8	0	1	22
Peach, raw	1 medium	5	0	1	11
Pear, raw	1 medium	19	1	1	18
Pears, canned	1/2 cup	11	1/2	1	15
Pineapple juice, canned	1/2 cup	21	1	1	10
Pineapple, canned	1/2 cup	17	1	1/2	8
Pineapple, raw	1/2 cup	6	0	0	6

	Protein	Ca Mg	Ca Pt.	Phos Pt.	Phos mg
Fruit, continued					
Plum, raw	1 medium	2	0	1/2	7
Plums, canned	1/2 cup	13	1	1	20
Prunes, dried	1/2 cup	41	2	4	64
Prune juice	1/4 cup	8	0	1	16
Raisins	1/4 cup	18	1	2	35
Raspberries, raw	1 cup	27	1	1	15
Rhubarb, frozen, cooked	1/2 cup	174	9	1	10
Rhubarb, raw, diced	1/2 cup	52	3	1/2	9
Strawberries, raw	1 cup	21	1	2	28
Tangerine, raw	1 medium	12	1	1/2	8
Watermelon, cubed	1 cup	13	1	1	14
FISH					
Cod, broiled	3 oz.	27	1	15	234
Crab, canned	1/2 cup	31	2	8	124
Fish sticks, frozen (4"x1"x1/2")	2 sticks or 2 oz.	6	0	6	94
Halibut, broiled	3 oz.	15	1	14	210
Lobster, cooked	1/2 cup	47	2	9	139
Oysters, canned	1/2 cup	108	5	11	178
Salmon, pink, canned	1/2 cup	82	4	14	212
Sardines, canned and drained	1 medium	52	3	4	60
Scallops, cooked	3 oz.	98	5	19	287
Shrimp, canned (cooked)	4 medium or 1 oz.	91	5	5	77
Tuna, canned	1/2 cup	8	0	6	148
MEAT AND SUBSTITUTES					
Beef (varies with cut of meat), cooked	3 oz.	9	1/2	11	165
Beef, chipped or dried	1 oz.	5	0	7	115
Beef, corned	1 oz.	1	0	2	29
Cheese:					
Borden's Lite-Line®	1 oz.	125	6	14	214
Cheddar, natural	1 oz.	204	10	9	145
Cottage, 2% fat	1/2 cup	77	4	11	170
Cream	1 oz. (2 tbsp.)	11	1/2	1	19
Kraft Lite & Lively®	1 oz.	202	10	11	175
Mozzarella, part skim	1 oz.	207	10	10	149
Parmesan	1 tbsp.	69	3	3	40
Process American	1 oz.	175	9	14	211
Spreads	1 tbsp.	91	5	6	94
Swiss	1 oz.	272	14	11	172
Chicken, turkey, Cornish hen, cooked (light or dark meat)	3 oz.	18	1	11	169
Egg	1 large	28	1	6	90
Frankfurter, beef	2 oz.	7	0	3	46
Lamb (cooked)	3 oz.	10	1/2	10	161
Liver, beef or pork (cooked)	3 oz.	9	1/2	21	324
Peanut butter	1 tbsp.	9	1/2	4	61
Pheasant, wild duck, with or without skin	3 oz.	42	2	17	264
Pork, fresh (cooked)	3 oz.	8	0	13	208
Pork, smoked	3 oz.	8	0	11	178
Tofu	4 oz.	145	7	9	143
Veal (cooked)	3 oz.	9	1/2	13	207
Venison (cooked)	3 oz.	24	1	16	247

	Protein	Ca Mg	Ca Pt.	Phos Pt.	Phos mg
DESSERTS					
Angel food cake	1/16 cake	38	2	3	48
Brownie	1 (2"x2"x1")	8	0	2	30
Cake, chocolate, white, or yellow	1 piece (2"x3"x2")	33	2	2	37
Cinnamon roll	1 average	16	1	4	55
Cookie, sandwich type	4 (2" diameter)	10	1/2	6	96
Custard, baked	1/2 cup	159	8	10	158
Flavored gelatin	1 cup	0	0	0	0
Fruit ice or 1 popsicle	1 cup	0	0	0	0
Ice cream (10% fat)	1/2 cup	88	4	4	67
Pie					
Apple	1/6 of 9" pie	13	1	2	35
Blueberry	1/6 of 9" pie	17	1	2	36
Cherry	1/6 of 9" pie	22	1	3	40
Peach	1/6 of 9" pie	16	1	3	46
Pumpkin	1/6 of 9" pie	78	4	7	105
Raisin	1/6 of 9" pie	28	1	4	63
Rhubarb	1/6 of 9" pie	101	5	3	41
Pudding					
Commercial (no chocolate)	1/2 cup	130	7	17	266
Commercial, chocolate	1/2 cup	138	7	22	339
Tapioca	1/2 cup	107	5	7	106
Yogurt, unflavored, 1 to 2% fat	1/2 cup	136	7	7	107
FATS AND OILS					
Almonds	2 tbsp.	38	2	3	43
Bacon, fried crisp	1 strip	1	0	1	21
Coffee creamer (liquid or powder)	1 tbsp.	1	0	1	10
Dressing, French, Italian, or mayonnaise	1 tbsp.	2	0	0	2
Half & Half	1/2 cup	127	6	7	115
Margarine or butter	1 tsp.	1	0	0	1
Oil, cooking	1 tbsp.	0	0	0	0
Sour cream	1 tbsp.	16	1	1	14
MISCELLANEOUS					
Beef broth, bouillon, or consommé	1 cup (diluted)	10	1/2	2	32
Chocolate sauce, fudge type	2 tbsp.	48	2	4	60
Honey	1 tbsp.	1	0	0	1
Jam or jelly, assorted flavors	1 tbsp.	4	0	0	1
Milk chocolate bar (without nuts)	1 oz.	65	3	4	65
Molasses, blackstrap	1 tbsp.	137	7	1	17
Mustard	1 tbsp.	13	1/2	1	11
Pickle, dill (4" long, 1/4" diameter)	1 large	35	2	2	28
Soy sauce	1 tbsp.	3	0	2	38
Syrup, maple (real)	1 tbsp.	22	1	0	2
Tartar sauce	1 tbsp.	3	0	0	5
Tomato catsup	1 tbsp.	4	0	1/2	9
Vinegar, cider	1 tbsp.	1	0	0	1
Yeast, Brewer's	1 tbsp.	5	0	19	288

High Calcium Foods

Foods highest in calcium - These foods provide 100-300 mg.

Item	Portion	Ca(mg)
Milk	1/2 cup	150
Yogurt	1/2 cup	136
Tofu	4 oz.	145
Cheese: Swiss	1 oz.	272
Cheddar/Mozzarella	1 oz.	175
American	1 oz.	208
Yogurt-Juice blend drinks	1 cup	290
Orange juice, calcium fortified	1 cup	280
Bread, calcium fortified	1 slice	300
Oatmeal, instant	1 packet	215
Waffle, from mix	1 (5 1/2")	179
Spinach, cooked	1/2 cup	122
Collard greens, boiled	1 cup	148
Blackstrap Molasses	1 tbsp.	137
Oysters, canned	1/2 cup	108
Soybeans, mature, boiled	1 cup	175
Soymilk, calcium fortified	1 cup	200-300

Foods moderately high in calcium - These foods provide 50-100 mg.

Item	Portion	Ca(mg)
English muffin	1	92
Cream of wheat, regular	1 cup	49
Total® brand cereal	1 cup	56
Salmon, pink, canned	1/2 cup	82
Frozen yogurt	1/2 cup	100
Ice cream	1/2 cup	88
Pancake, from mix	1 (4")	50
Shrimp, canned	4 medium	91
Scallops, cooked	3 oz.	98
Sardines, canned	1 medium	52
Biscuit	1	55
Broccoli, cooked	1/2 cup	89
Orange, raw	1 medium	52
Parmesan cheese	1 Tbsp.	69
Cottage cheese	1/2 cup	77
Almonds	3 Tbsp.	57

High Phosphorus Foods

Foods highest in phosphorus - These foods provide 100-350 mg.

Item	Portion	Phos(mg)
Beef, cooked	3 oz.	165
Chicken, turkey, cornish hen, light or dark meat, cooked	3 oz.	169
Pork, fresh, cooked	3 oz.	208
smoked	3 oz.	178
Veal, cooked	3 oz.	207
Venison, cooked	3 oz.	247
Lamb, cooked	3 oz.	161
Liver, cooked	3 oz.	324
Pheasant, wild duck, cooked	3 oz.	264
Fish: Cod, halibut / salmon	3 oz. / 1/2 cup	220
Crab, lobster, tuna	1/2 cup	130
Scallops	3 oz.	287
Beans: Kidney, navy, pinto, lima	1/2 cup	135
Tofu	4 oz.	143
Cheese:Cheddar	1 oz.	145
Mozzarella, part skim	1 oz.	149
Swiss	1 oz.	172
Lite, Kraft®	1 oz.	175
American, processed	1 oz.	211
Cottage	1/2 cup	170
Milk	1/2 cup	120
Pudding	1/2 cup	300
Yogurt	1/2 cup	107
Custard	1/2 cup	158
Waffle	1 (5 1/2 ")	257
Pancake	1 (4")	125
Bran cereals	1 cup	761
Bran flakes/ Grape Nuts® brand	1 cup	252
Total® / Wheaties® brand cereals	1 cup	115
Granola	1 cup	378
Oats, instant, prepared	1 cup	180

Foods moderately high in phosphorus - These foods provide 50-100 mg.

Item	Portion	(mg)
Fishsticks	2 sticks (2 oz.)	94
Sardines, canned	1 medium	60
Shrimp, canned-4 medium (1 oz.)	1 oz.	77
Cola soda, regular and diet	12 oz.	61
Rice, wild, cooked	1/2 cup	90
Sweet potatoes, cooked	1/2 cup	70
Corn/Peas, cooked	1/2 cup	85
Spinach, cooked	1/2 cup	50
Ice cream	1/2 cup	70
Pie, pumpkin	1/6 of 9" pie	100
Chocolate fudge sauce	2 Tbsp.	60

High-Iron Diet
Description

The General Diet of an individual should provide 10 to 15 mg of iron, depending on the person's age, sex, and nutritional needs. High-iron foods must be eaten in order to:

- Provide amounts of iron needed for growth in childhood and pregnancy.
- Achieve or maintain normal body iron stores.
- Replace losses that occur through the gastrointestinal tract.
- Replace iron lost due to significant blood loss.

Indications for use

1. For treatment of iron deficiency or microcytic, hypochromic anemia due to loss of iron stores.
2. Deficiency of iron in the diet during a period of accelerated demand.
3. Inadequate absorption of iron or nutritional deficiencies, such as in severe protein depletion.
4. Various vegetarian dietary practices (e.g. individuals who eat little or no animal protein).
5. To compensate for diets low in ascorbate due to prolonged heating and/or storage of food.

Adequacy

The High-Iron Diet is nutritionally adequate in all the Recommended Dietary Allowances, according to the National Research Council.

Absorption capacity of iron

1. Chelating agents in the intestinal lumen can affect the absorption of iron.
2. Iron is more readily absorbed in the ferrous form.
3. Ascorbic acid, the amino acids histidine, lysine, and methionine, and reducing sugars (primarily fructose) enhance iron absorption.
4. The amount of dietary iron does not reflect the net amount of iron absorbed and utilized by the body.
5. Heme-iron versus non-heme-iron is less affected by other dietary components in meals and at least partly by-passes intestinal mucosal control.
6. Iron absorption is dependent on individual iron status.

Professional references

1. Brittin HC, Nossaman CE. Iron content of food cooked in iron utensils. J Am Dietetic Assoc 1986; 86:897-901.
2. Dallman PR, et al. Iron deficiency in infancy and childhood. Am J Clinical Nutr 1980; 33:86-118.
3. Food and Nutrition Board. Recommended dietary allowances. 10th ed. Washington, D.C.: National Academy of Sciences, 1989:195-205.
4. Melki IA, Bulus NM, Abumrad NN. Trace elements in nutrition. Nutr in Clinical Practice 1987; 2(Dec): 230-
5. Mertz W. Mineral elements: new perspectives. J Am Dietetic Assoc 1980; 77:258.
6. Monsen ER, et al. Estimation of available dietary iron. Am J Clinical Nutr 1978; 31:134-41.
7. Monsen ER, Balintfy JL. Calculating dietary iron bioavailability: refinement and computerization. J Am Dietetic Assoc 1982; 80(4):307-11.
8. Walser M. Iron. In: Walser M, Imbembo AL, Margolis S, Elfert GA. Nutritional management: the John Hopkins handbook. Philadelphia: W.B. Saunders, 1984;229-34.

High-Iron Food List

Choose a minimum of _____ milligrams (mg) of iron per day from the chief, moderate, and minor sources. When shopping for foods, it is necessary to choose bread products, cereals, and pastas that have been enriched or fortified with iron. These words must appear on the label.

CHIEF SOURCES OF IRON (Greater than 4 milligrams)

Foods	Average Serving (approximate measure)	Iron (mg)
Bran Buds® or All Bran®-type cereals, dry	1/2 cup	6.7
Bran flakes, dry	1/2 cup	5.5
Blood sausage	3 oz.	5.4
Braunschweiger	3 oz.	7.9
Buckwheat groats, dry	1 cup	4.6
Carob stars or chips	1/2 cup	20.1
Cereals, fortified with 100% of the U.S. RDA for iron	1 oz.	18.0
Cornmeal, dry	1 cup	5.9
Cream of Wheat, Ralston®, farina, Malt-O-Meal® (cooked)	1 cup	10.0
Duck, wild, with or without skin	3 oz.	7.1
Heart, beef (cooked)	3 oz.	6.3
Kidney, beef (cooked)*	3 oz.	6.2
Liver, beef (cooked)*	3 oz.	5.7
Liver, chicken (cooked)*	3 oz.	7.2
Liver, calf (cooked)*	3 oz.	12.0
Liver sausage, liverwurst	3 oz.	5.4
Oysters	6 med.	5.6
Pheasant, with or without skin	3 oz.	7.1
Venison, rabbit, squirrel, moose, elk (cooked)	3 oz.	6.6

MODERATE SOURCES OF IRON (2 to 4 milligrams)

Foods	Average Serving (approximate measure)	Iron (mg)
Almonds, dried, unbalanced	1/2 cup	2.6
Apricots, dried	1/2 cup	3.0
Asparagus, canned, drained solids	1/2 cup	2.2
Dried beans:		
Baked beans, no pork	1/2 cup	2.2
Northern, navy, red, or dry beans (cooked)	1/2 cup	2.4
Soybeans, cooked	1/2 cup	2.4
Beef, cooked (varies with cut of meat)	3 oz.	2.2
Figs, dried	1/2 cup	2.2
Goose, domestic, with or without skin (cooked)	3 oz.	2.3
Oatmeal, dry	1 cup	3.6
Peaches, dried	1/2 cup	3.2
Prunes, dried (uncooked)	1 cup	4.0
Salmon, canned	1/2 cup	2.1
Sardines, canned and drained.	8 med.	2.8
Scallops	3 oz.	2.5
Shrimp, moist heat	3 oz.	2.6
Tuna, light meat, canned	3 oz.	2.7
Veal, cooked (varies with cut)	3 oz.	3.0

MINOR SOURCES OF IRON (Less than 2 milligrams)

Foods	Average Serving (approximate measure)	Iron (mg)
Black-eyed peas, cow peas (cooked)	1/2 cup	1.1
Bread, whole wheat	2 slices	1.4
Chard, Swiss (cooked)	1/2 cup	1.9
Chicken, with or without skin (cooked)	3 oz.	1.5
Dates, dried	1/2 cup	1.0
Dried beans and peas:		
Green peas (cooked)	1/2 cup	1.2
Lentils, split peas (cooked)	1/2 cup	1.7
Lima beans, Fordhook (cooked)	1/2 cup	1.1
Egg, large*	1	1.0
Eggstro'dnaire®, Liquid Egg Substitute	1-3/4 oz.	0.23
Greens, beet, mustard, or turnip (cooked)	1/2 cup	0.5
Lamb, cooked	3 oz.	1.2
Macaroni, spaghetti, noodles, white, enriched (cooked)	1/2 cup	0.7
Molasses, blackstrap	1 tsp.	1.6
Muffin, English, whole wheat	1 whole	1.3
Oat bran (cooked)	1/2 cup	0.9
Peanuts, roasted without shells	1/2 cup	1.3
Pork, cooked, smoked or fresh (varies with cut of meat)	3 oz.	1.2
Prune juice	1/2 cup	1.5
Raisins, dried (seedless)	1/4 cup	0.8
Rice, long grain or instant	1/2 cup	0.9
Rice, wild (cooked)	1/2 cup	1.1
Simply Eggs®, reduced cholesterol	1-3/4 oz.	0.9
Spinach, frozen (cooked)	1/2 cup	1.4
Spinach, raw	1 cup	1.5
Tomato juice, canned	1 cup	1.4
Turkey, with or without skin, dark meat (cooked)	3 oz.	1.5
Wheat germ	3 tbsp.	1.8
Yeast, Brewer's	1 tbsp.	1.3

* These foods contain 250 mg or more of cholesterol in the portion listed.

Nutrition and Lead Exposure
Description

Beginning in the early 1970s, researchers began to identify metabolic changes associated with blood lead levels greater than 60 mcg/dl. Further studies suggest that even lower blood lead levels of 10-15 mcg/dl prenatally and in the infant can result in impaired cognitive and behavior development.

The new Centers for Disease Control (CDC) guidelines, released in the fall of 1991, reflect these studies, and the intervention level has been revised downward to 10 mcg/dl. (1)

Many references are available defining the clinical signs and symptoms, and adverse health effects of lead poisoning and will not be included in this discussion.

Incidence

Estimates of the number of children with elevated blood lead levels come from projections based on data from the Second National Health and Nutrition Examination Survey (NHANES II). These data reveal that 3-4 million children age 6 months to 5 years in the United States have blood levels greater than 15 mcg/dl. (1) The new CDC guidelines call for universal screening but especially for children who live in a house built before 1960, and/or whose family is low income and lives in an urban area. These children are at highest risk.

Sources of lead

Although lead-based paint was banned in 1977, it continues to be the most common source of lead exposure in children. It also contributes significantly to the other most common pathways through which children become exposed, lead contaminated household dust and soil. Other possible sources of lead include:

- lead contaminated skin or clothing from a family member's place of work (demolition, auto repair, lead refinery, battery manufacture)
- lead containing cookware or pottery glaze
- airborne lead (refineries, smelters, combustion of leaded gasoline)
- metallic lead (fishing weights, curtain weights)
- water contaminated by lead solder in pipes

Although these sources contribute to children's lead exposure they are less likely to be the primary source of elevated blood lead levels requiring intervention.

Intervention and treatment of lead poisoning

Once a child is assessed to have a blood lead level of 10-15 mcg/dl or higher, some type of intervention is indicated. The most important intervention is identification of the lead source, and environmental modification to eliminate continued exposure to and absorption of lead.

Environmental Intervention

The new CDC guidelines support environmental inspection and modification for all children with lead levels of 20 mcg/dl or higher, as well as for children whose blood lead levels remain at 15 mcg/dl or higher for a prolonged time.

The primary environmental interventions are:

- Lead paint abatement which many states are requiring be done by licensed workers and during which the family must leave the home.
- Control of household dust as best as is possible through frequent wet mopping and dusting with a damp cloth.

Dietary Intervention

All children with elevated lead levels should be assessed for iron deficiency. Children with iron deficiency should receive supplemental iron. For children who are not assessed to be iron deficient, it may be appropriate to give daily prophylactic doses of iron if a dietary history suggests inadequate iron intake.

- For all children with blood lead levels 15 mcg/dl and greater, a diet rich in iron, calcium and zinc, and lower in fat is recommended because gastrointestinal lead absorption is increased with deficiencies of these minerals, and enhanced by high fat foods.
- See the high-calcium and high-iron food lists for foods to encourage.
- Foods high in zinc include: Meats, eggs, liver, seafood, nuts, legumes,
- dried beans and peas, whole grain breads and cereals, and cheese
- Limit fat in the diet by limiting butter, margarine, vegetable oils and shortening, bacon and sausage, fat from meats, fried foods, peanut butter, nuts and seeds. (Children less than 2 years of age should have whole milk.)

Lead Chelation Therapy

Chelation Therapy is used for significantly elevated lead levels. The guidelines for choice of chelating agent and its administration are described in therapeutic guidelines manuals as well as in information available from state and county health departments.

Any child undergoing chelation therapy warrants a diet history and evaluation of diet adequacy. Adequacy of calcium, iron, and zinc intakes should be determined due to the depletion of these minerals during lead chelation possibly superimposed upon already existing deficiencies.

References

1. Weitzman M, Glotzer D: Lead Poisoning. Ped in Rev Dec. 1992 13(12): 461-468.
2. Centers for Disease Control. Preventing Lead Poisoning in Young Children: A Statement by the Centers for Disease Control. Atlanta, GA: US Dept. of Health and Human Services/Public Health Service; 1991.

Potassium-Controlled Diet

Potassium is a mineral that is found naturally in most foods. Foods containing less than one point may be consumed in moderate amounts.

Foods containing potassium may be selected until you reach _____ points.

1 potassium point = 1 milliequivalent (39 milligrams)

Note: Milligrams were rounded off to the nearest whole numbers; potassium points were rounded off to the nearest 1/2 point.

Item	Amount	Potassium Points	mg
BEVERAGES			
Beer	12 oz.	3	115
Carbonated beverages			
Cola	8 oz.	0	5
Cola, diet	8 oz.	0	7
Lemon-lime, gingerale, tonic	8 oz.	0	2
Non-cola, diet	8 oz.	0	5
Fruit-flavored	8 oz.	0	5
Coffee (decaffeinated)	8 oz.	2	96
Coffee, instant, prepared	8 oz.	2	96
Coffee, regular, brewed	8 oz.	4	156
Eggnog, commercial	8 oz.	11	429
Hot chocolate, from mix	6 oz.	5	202
Limeade, lemonade	8 oz.	1	23
Milk shake, malted milk, soft serve, or ice milk			
Nonchocolate	8 oz.	17	672
Chocolate	8 oz.	13	529
Milk			
Buttermilk, 1%, low-fat	8 oz.	9	370
Chocolate skim milk	8 oz.	11	423
Condensed, sweetened	1 tbsp.	2	71
Dry skim powder	1/4 cup	14	538
Evaporated (whole)	2 tbsp.	2	95
Skim, fortified	8 oz.	10	407
Whole, 3-4% fat	8 oz.	10	370
2% low fat	8 oz.	10	377
Postum®, instant	1 tsp.	3	98
Tea, brewed or instant	8 oz.	1-1/2	58
Tea, herbal	8 oz.	1	38
Wine, table or dessert	4 oz.	2-1/2	100
Bagel, egg or water	1	1	41
Baking powder biscuit	2" diam.	1	33

Item	Amount	Potassium Points	mg
BREAD			
Cracked wheat	1 slice	1	34
Crumbs	1/4 cup	1	38
French or Italian	1 slice	1/2	15
Pumpernickel	1 slice	1	51
Raisin	1 slice	1-1/2	60
Rye	1 slice	1	42
White	1 slice	1	27
Whole wheat	1 slice	1	44
Corn bread	2" square	2	80
Crackers			
Graham	2 squares	1/2	23
Rye wafer (triple cracker)	1 cracker	1	32
Saltines, soda	6 crackers	1/2	24
Matzoth	1 piece	1	46
Doughnut, cake or raised	1 average	1	27
Flour, enriched	2-1/2 tbsp.	1/2	17
Hamburger or hot dog bun	1 average	1	38
Lefse	1 serving	3	103
Muffin	1 average	1	50
Muffin, bran	1 average	4	172
Muffin, English	1 whole	4	159
Pancake	1 (4" diam.)	1	55
Popcorn	2 cups	1	30
Popover	1 average	2	75
Rice cake	1 serving	1	27
Roll, hard or soft	1	1	29
Sweet roll	1 small	1	39
Tortilla, corn	1 medium	1	52
Waffle	1 (5-1/2" diam.)	1	39
Zwieback toast	3 pieces	1	33
CEREALS			
Hot			
Cream of wheat, Malt-O-Meal®, Ralston®	1/2 cup	1	44
Oats, regular, quick, instant (cooked)	1 cup	3	131
Oats, instant (mixed with water)	1 packet	2-1/2	100
Ready-to-serve cereals			
All-Bran®, Bran Buds®	1 oz.	9	350
Cheerios®, Wheaties®	1 cup	3	108
Corn flakes, puffed wheat, Rice Krispies®			
Special K®	1 cup	1	26
40% Bran® Flakes	1 cup	6	248
Grape-nuts®	1/4 cup	2	95
Puffed rice	1 cup	1/2	16
Raisin Bran®	1/2 cup	5	184
Barley, pearled (2 tbsp. dry or 1/2 c. cooked)	1 serving	1	45

Item	Amount	Potassium Points	mg
Macaroni, noodles, spaghetti (cooked)	1/2 cup	1	43
Potatoes			
Au gratin, home prepared	1/2 cup	7	287
Baked, 2-1/3" diam.	1/2	13	503
Boiled	1/2 cup	7	285
French-fried	10 (1/2" x 1/2" x 2")	11	427
Hashed brown, frozen, prepared	1/2 cup	8	315
Mashed, dehydrated (no milk), prepared	1/2 cup	9	350
Mashed with milk, home prepared	1/2 cup	6	250
Potato chips	10 (2" diam.)	6	226
Rice, white (cooked)	1/2 cup	1	29
Rice, wild, (cooked)	1/2 cup	1-1/2	58
Sweet potatoes, baked in skin	1, 5" x 2" diam.	10	397
Canned	1/2 cup	8	313
Yam, cooked, baked	1/2 cup	12	468

VEGETABLES

Item	Amount	Potassium Points	mg
Artichokes (cooked)	1/2 cup hearts	6	221
Asparagus (cooked)	1/2 cup	7	279
Canned	1/2 cup	5	186
Frozen (cooked)	4 medium spears	3	131
Bamboo shoots (cooked)	1/2 cup	8	320
Beans			
Dry, white or red (cooked)	1/2 cup	10	374
Lima, canned	1/2 cup	9	334
Lima, baby, frozen (cooked)	1/2 cup	9	370
Beans, green, Italian, yellow (cooked)	1/2 cup	5	185
Canned	1/2 cup	2	74
Frozen (cooked)	1/2 cup	2	76
Bean sprouts	1/2 cup	2	77
Beets (cooked)	1/2 cup	7	266
Canned	1/2 cup	4	175
Broccoli			
Cooked	1/2 cup	3	127
Frozen, chopped (cooked)	1/2 cup	4	166
Raw, chopped	1/2 cup	4	143
Brussels sprouts (cooked)	1/2 cup	6	247
Frozen (cooked)	1/2 cup	7	254
Cabbage			
Cooked	1/2 cup	4	154
Raw	1/2 cup, shredded	2	86
Carrots			
Canned	1/2 cup	3	131
Cooked	1/2 cup	5	177
Raw	1 (4" long)	3	117
Raw, shredded	1/2 cup	5	178
Cauliflower			
Cooked	1/2 cup	5	200
Frozen (cooked)	1/2 cup	3	125
Raw	1/2 cup	5	178

Item	Amount	Potassium Points	mg
Vegetables, continued			
Celery			
Cooked	1/2 cup, diced	7	266
Raw	1/2 cup, diced	4	170
	1 stalk 7" long	3	114
Corn (cooked)	1/2 cup	5	204
Canned	1/2 cup	5	195
On cob	1 ear (4" long)	4	158
Frozen (cooked)	1/2 cup	3	114
Cucumber, raw, peeled, sliced	1/2 cup	2	78
Dandelion greens (cooked)	1/2 cup	3	121
Eggplant (cooked)	1/2 cup, diced	3	119
Endive, raw	1/2 cup	2	79
Kale (cooked)	1/2 cup	4	148
Lettuce, chopped, iceberg, crisphead	1/2 cup	1	45
Mushrooms			
Cooked	1/2 cup	7	277
Raw	1/2 cup	3	130
Mustard greens (cooked)	1/2 cup	4	141
Onions			
Cooked	1/2 cup	4	159
Raw, chopped	1/4 cup	2	62
Parsley, raw	1 tbsp.	1/2	20
Parsnips (cooked)	1/2 cup, diced	7	287
Pea pods	1/2 cup	4	144
Peas, green (cooked)	1/2 cup	6	217
Canned	1/2 cup	4	147
Frozen (cooked)	1/2 cup	3	134
Peppers, sweet, green, red (raw)	1/4 cup	1	49
Pumpkin, canned	1/2 cup	6	251
Radishes, red	10 small	3	104
Rutabaga (cooked)	1/2 cup, cubed	6	244
Sauerkraut, canned	1/2 cup	5	201
Spinach, all varieties			
Cooked	1/2 cup	11	419
Raw	1/2 cup	4	156
Squash, summer, all varieties			
Cooked	1/2 cup	4	173
Raw	1/2 cup	3	126
Squash, winter			
Baked	1/2 cup	11	445
Boiled, mashed	1/2 cup	8	321
Frozen, mashed (cooked)	1/2 cup	4	160
Tomatoes			
Canned	1/2 cup	7	265
Cooked	1/2 cup	8	312
Raw, chopped	1/2 cup	5	186
Raw, whole	1, 2-3/5" diam.	6	254
Tomato juice, canned	1/2 cup	7	268
Tomato paste, canned	1/4 cup	16	611
Tomato puree, canned	1/4 cup	7	263
Turnip (cooked)	1/2 cup, diced	3	106
Vegetables, mixed, frozen (cooked)	1/2 cup	4	154
Vegetable juice cocktail	1/2 cup	6	234

Item	Amount	Potassium Points	mg
FRUITS			
Apple, raw	2" diam.	4	159
Apple juice	1/2 cup	4	148
Applesauce	1/2 cup	2	91
Apricots, raw	3 medium	8	313
Canned	3 medium halves	4	161
Dried	5 halves	6	241
Nectar	1/2 cup	4	144
Banana, raw	1 (6" long)	12	451
Blackberries	1/2 cup	3-1/2	141
Blueberries, raw	1 cup	3	129
Frozen	1 cup	2	83
Cantaloupe, raw	1/6 melon (5" diam.)	7	275
Cherries, raw or canned (sweet)	1/2 cup	4	163
Cranberry juice	1/2 cup	1	31
Cranberry sauce, canned	1/2 cup	1	35
Dates	5 medium	7	271
Figs	1 medium	3	116
Fruit cocktail	1/2 cup	3	118
Grapefruit, raw	1/2 medium	4	167
Juice, canned, unsweetened	1/2 cup	5	189
Segments, canned	1/2 cup	4	164
Grapes, raw	20 grapes	4	139
Canned	1/2 cup	3	132
Grape juice, canned	1/2 cup	4	168
Frozen, sweetened (diluted)	1/2 cup	1	28
Honeydew melon	1/10 (5" diam.)	9	350
Kiwi	1 medium	6	252
Lemon, raw	1 medium	4	157
Juice	1/2 cup	3	124
Lime, raw	1 medium	2	68
Juice (from raw lime)	1/2 cup	3	134
Nectarine, raw	1 medium	7	288
Orange, raw	1 medium	6	237
Juice, frozen (diluted)	1/2 cup	6	237
Peach, raw	1 medium	4	171
Canned	1/2 cup or 2 halves	4	152
Nectar	1/2 cup	1	51
Pear, raw	1 medium	5	208
Canned	2 halves	3	114
Nectar	1/2 cup	1/2	17
Pineapple, raw	1/2 cup	2	87
Juice-packed, canned	1/2 cup	4	152
Juice, canned	1/2 cup	4	170
Plum, raw	1 medium	3	113
Canned	1/2 cup	4	157
Prunes, canned with sugar	5 fruits	5	194
Dried	5 fruits	8	313
Dried, cooked	1/2 cup	9	354
Juice, canned	1/4 cup	5	176
Raisins	1/4 cup	7	272
Raspberries, raw	1 cup	5	187
Rhubarb (cooked)	1/2 cup	3	115

Item	Amount	Potassium Points	mg
Fruits, continued			
Strawberries, raw	1 cup	6	247
Frozen, unsweetened	1 cup	6	220
Tangerine, raw	1 large	3	132
Watermelon, diced	1 cup	5	186

MEATS & CHEESE

Item	Amount	Potassium Points	mg
Beef, ham, lamb, pork	1 oz.	3	123
Bologna	1 oz.	1	51
Canadian bacon	1 slice	2	84
Cheese			
American, cheddar, and natural cheeses	1 oz.	1	28
Cottage cheese, 2% fat	1/2 cup	3	109
Farmer	1 oz.	1	35
Mozzarella, part-skim	1 oz.	1	27
Process American	1 oz.	1	46
Egg	1 large	2	65
Eggbeaters®, prepared per directions	1/4 cup	4	159
Fish and Shellfish			
Clams, mussels (cooked)	1 oz.	2-1/2	90
Cod, haddock (cooked)	1 oz.	3	110
Crab (cooked)	3 oz.	2-1/2	100
Flounder, sole (cooked)	1 oz.	3	104
Halibut (cooked)	1 oz.	4	157
Lobster	1 oz.	1/2	16
Oysters	2 medium	1	39
Salmon, pink, canned	1/2 cup	11	451
Sardines	4 medium	7	280
Scallops	1 oz.	3	135
Shrimp, raw	1 oz.	2	75
Tuna, canned	1/2 cup	5	210
Frankfurter, beef or pork	1 average	2	75
Liver, beef or pork	1 oz.	2	71
Luncheon meat	1 oz. slice	1-1/2	57
Nuts, mixed	1/4 cup	5	206
Peanut butter	1 tbsp.	3	123
Poultry	1 oz.	2	74
Sausage	1 oz. or 2 links	2	64
Veal	1 oz.	4	142

Item	Amount	PotassiumPoints	mg
SOUPS			
Bouillon cube	1 tsp.	0	15
Soups (diluted or reconstituted with water)			
Bean, split pea	3/4 cup	8	298
Beef broth, bouillon, consommé	3/4 cup	2-1/2	97
Beef noodle	3/4 cup	2	75
Cream of asparagus, made with water	3/4 cup	3	130
Cream of celery, made with water	3/4 cup	2	92
Cream of chicken, made with water	3/4 cup	2	66
Cream of mushroom, made with water	3/4 cup	2	75
Chicken broth, bouillon	3/4 cup	4	157
Chicken noodle	3/4 cup	1	41
Chicken rice	3/4 cup	2	75
Clam chowder, Manhattan	3/4 cup	5	196
Minestrone	3/4 cup	6	234
Onion	3/4 cup	1	51
Tomato	3/4 cup	5	198
Vegetable beef	3/4 cup	3	130
Vegetarian vegetable	3/4 cup	4	157
DESSERTS			
Apple crisp	1/2 cup	2	79
Boston cream pie	1/8 of 8" cake	2	92
Brownie	3" x 3" x 2"	1	40
Cake			
Angel food, sponge	3" x 3" x 2"	1/2	59
Chocolate	3" x 3" x 2"	3	129
Fruit cake	3" x 3" x 1"	5	198
Pound cake	3" x 3" x 2"	1	23
Yellow or white	3" x 3" x 2"	1	35
Cookies			
Sandwich type, shortbread, sugar (no chocolate)	1	0	8
Chocolate, chocolate chip, oatmeal raisin	1	1	22
Ginger snaps	5 small	2	92
Sugar wafers, vanilla wafers	6 wafers	1/2	19
Custard	1/2 cup	5	205
D'Zerta® gelatin	1/2 cup	1	44
Gelatin, flavored or unflavored	1 cup	0	0
Ice cream (10% fat)	1/2 cup	3	128
Ice milk (5% fat)	1/2 cup	3	132
Ices, popsicles	1 cup or 1	0	4
Pie			
Apple, blueberry	1/6 of 9" pie	2-1/2	100
Cherry, strawberry, pecan	1/6 of 9" pie	4	162
Chocolate, custard	1/6 of 9" pie	4	162
Lemon meringue	1/6 of 9" pie	2	70
Mince, rhubarb	1/6 of 9" pie	7	266
Pumpkin, raisin	1/6 of 9" pie	6	240
Pudding			
Cornstarch, commercial or mix (no chocolate)	1/2 cup	5	185
Chocolate	1/2 cup	5	205
Tapioca, homemade or canned	1/2 cup	4	147

Item	Amount	Potassium Points	mg
Desserts, continued			
Sherbet	1/2 cup	3	99
Yogurt, plain, unflavored (1-2% fat)	1/2 cup	4	175
Sweets			
Caramel	1 oz.	1/2	17
Chocolate, bitter	1 oz. (1 square)	6	235
Milk chocolate, Hershey® Kisses	1 oz.	3	115
Semi-sweet chocolate	1 oz. (1 square)	2	90
Fondant, hard candy, sugar mint,			
jelly beans, gum drops, lollipops	any amount	0	0
Marshmallows	any amount	0	3
Honey	3 tbsp.	1	30
Jam, jelly, preserves	3 tbsp.	1	45
Maple syrup, real	1 tbsp.	1	26
Molasses, light	1 tbsp.	8	300
Blackstrap	1 tbsp.	15	586
Sugar			
Brown	1 tbsp.	1	32
White	1 tbsp.	0	0
Syrup			
Chocolate sauce	2 tbsp.	1	48
Maple-flavored, corn	1 tbsp.	0	0

FATS

Bacon	2 strips	1-1/2	62
Butter, margarine, or oil	1 tsp.	0	0
Cream cheese	1 tbsp.	0	16
Cream, Half & Half	1 oz.	1	38
Salad dressings, various	1 tbsp.	0	0
Sour cream	1 tbsp.	0	0

MISCELLANEOUS

Chili powder, paprika	1 tsp.	1	50
Cocoa powder	1 tbsp.	2	89
Coconut, shredded, sweet	2 tbsp.	1	36
Curry powder	1 tsp.	1	31
Morton® Lite Salt	1/2 tsp.	19	750
Mustard, prepared	1 tbsp.	1/2	19
Salt substitute, No Salt®	1/2 tsp.	32	1244
Seasonings and spices (other than those listed)	1 tsp.	0	7-33
Soy sauce	1 tbsp.	2	64
Tartar sauce	2 tbsp.	1	22
Tomato catsup, chili sauce, Heinz 57®	1 tbsp.	1-1/2	62
Turmeric, ground	1 tsp.	1	55
Vinegar	1 tbsp.	0	15
Yeast, Brewer's	1 tbsp.	5	189
Wheat germ	1 tbsp.	2	69

High-Potassium Foods

Foods containing a high amount of potassium
(over 10 milliequivalents or 390 milligrams):

Avocado	½ cup mashed or ½ fruit
Banana, raw	1 (6" long)
Eggnog	1 cup
Molasses, blackstrap	1 tbsp.
Orange juice, frozen (diluted)	1 cup
Potato, baked	1 (2-1/3" diam.)
Potatoes, French-fried	10 strips
Prune juice, canned	3/4 cup
Squash, winter, all varieties (cooked)	1/2 cup
Tomato juice, canned	1 cup
Vegetable juice, canned	1 cup

Foods containing a moderately high amount of potassium
(7-10 milliequivalents or 275-390 milligrams):

All Bran®	1 oz.
Apricot nectar	1 cup
Apricots (canned, raw, or dried)	3 whole
Beans, white or red (cooked)	1/2 cup
Bran Buds®	1/4 cup
Cantaloupe (5" diam.)	1/6 melon
Honeydew melon (5" diam.)	1/10 melon
Dates	6 medium
Figs (dried)	3 medium
Grapefruit juice, canned, unsweetened	1 cup
Lima beans	1/2 cup
Milk (whole, skim, 2%, or buttermilk)	1 cup
Mushrooms (raw)	10 small
Orange, raw	1 large
Parsnips (cooked)	1/2 cup
Pineapple juice, canned	1 cup
Plums, raw	3 fruits
Potatoes, mashed, hash browns	1/2 to 3/4 cup
Prunes, dried	5 medium
Raisins	1/4 cup
Spinach, raw, chopped	1 cup
Tomatoes, raw, whole	1 to 1-1/2 medium
Yams, baked in skin	1 small
Yogurt, 1-2% fat, unflavored	1 cup

References for Tables

The following references were used for the values of milliequivalents (points) and milligrams in the tables "Calcium- and Phosphorus-Controlled Diet" and "High Iron Diet," and "Potassium-Controlled Diet."

1. Nutrition Coordinating Center, University of Minnesota, 1993. (2829 University Avenue S.E., Suite 526, Minneapolis, MN 55414). Used with permission.
2. Agricultural Research Service, United States Department of Agriculture. Nutritive value of American foods in common units (agriculture handbook no. 456). Washington, D.C.: Government Printing Office, 1975.
3. Nutrition Monitoring Division, United States Department of Agriculture. Composition of foods: beef products (agriculture handbook no. 8-13). Washington, D.C.: Government Printing Office, 1986.
4. Consumer Nutrition Center, United States Department of Agriculture. Composition of foods: fruits and fruit juices (agriculture handbook no. 8-9). Washington, D.C.: Government Printing Office, 1982.
5. Nutrition Monitoring Division, United States Department of Agriculture. Composition of foods: vegetables and vegetable products (agriculture handbook no. 8-11). Washington, D.C.: Government Printing Office, 1984.
6. Consumer Nutrition Center, United States Department of Agriculture. Composition of foods: sausages and luncheon meats (agriculture handbook no. 8-7). Washington, D.C.: Government Printing Office, 1980.
7. Consumer and Food Economics Institute, United States Department of Agriculture. Composition of foods: soups, sauces, gravies (agriculture handbook no. 8-6). Washington, D.C.: Government Printing Office, 1980.

Sodium-Controlled Diets
Description
Sodium-Controlled Diets are used in clinical situations to:

1. Prevent, control, and/or eliminate edema and ascites
2. Control hypertension

Indications for use
1. Cardiovascular disorders and severe cardiac failure
2. Edema
3. Hypertension
4. Impaired liver function and cirrhosis of the liver
5. Renal insufficiency and chronic renal failure

Adequacy
Sodium-Controlled Diets providing >500 mg Na/day are nutritionally adequate according to the Recommended Dietary Allowances of the National Research Council. The 250 and 500 mg sodium diets can be inadequate in some nutrients and therefore need to be carefully planned. These two levels of sodium restriction are recommended **only** for tests and short term use.

Notes about diet instruction material for sodium-controlled diets:

1. The Sodium-Controlled Diets are referred to in terms of milligrams or sodium points (milliequivalents). Each sodium point is equal to 23 milligrams. Patients may be given instruction about the total number of points or milligrams they are allowed each day.
2. The General Diet contains 6000 mg (260 mEq) or more of sodium daily. Sodium-controlled diets have been developed as follows:

Milligrams	Sodium Points
500	22
1,000	45
2,000	90
3,000-5,000	135-225

500 milligram (22 MEQ) Education Sheet

Sodium, a mineral, is abundant in many foods. Sodium may be found naturally, or it may be added during the processing of a food. The most common form is salt, which is composed of sodium and chloride. Reducing your sodium intake involves changing your eating behavior.

The following guidelines will help you reduce the sodium in your diet:
1. Stop using the salt shaker.
2. Omit salt in cooking and in baking.
3. Substitute sodium-free seasonings and spices.
4. Use a salt substitute (potassium chloride) only with a doctor's permission.
5. Include a variety of fresh, unprocessed foods in your diet.
6. Use low-sodium commercial products.
7. Use the general guidelines listed below, or monitor your sodium intake using the milligram (mg) or the point system listed in the Sodium Counter (available from your dietitian).

FOOD GROUP	ALLOWED/RECOMMENDED	AVOID/USE SPARINGLY
BREADS/STARCHES *6 servings or more**	Salt-free breads, rolls, crackers.	Sodium-containing breads, rolls, or crackers. Bread products made with salt, self-rising flour, or baking powder.
Cereals:	Cooked cereal prepared without salt or sodium, or any cereal prepared without the addition of salt	Any cereal containing salt. Sodium-free dry cereals.
Potatoes/Pasta/ Rice:	Fresh, frozen, or canned without salt or sodium added: white or sweet potatoes, rice, spaghetti, noodles, barley, macaroni, etc., prepared without salt. Salt-free potato chips or other snacks. Unsalted popcorn.	Prepared potato products or substitutes containing salt or sodium, or any prepared with the addition of salt. Salted snack foods. Salted popcorn.
VEGETABLES *3 servings or more*	Fresh, frozen, or canned without salt or sodium. Peas or Lima beans must be fresh or canned without salt (not frozen). Tomato and vegetable juices without salt or sodium. Tomato sauce, paste, or puree without salt or sodium.	Any vegetables or vegetable juices containing salt or sodium, including those prepared in cream or cheese sauces. Vegetables with high natural sodium content: beets & beet greens; celery, dandelion, kale, & mustard greens; spinach; Swiss chard, sauerkraut, white turnips. Tomato sauce, paste, or puree canned with salt or sodium.

FOOD GROUP	ALLOWED/RECOMMENDED	AVOID/USE SPARINGLY
FRUIT *2 servings or more*	All fruits & juices.	None.
MEAT & SUBSTITUTES *2 servings or more* *(5 oz. maximum/day)*	5 oz. (cooked weight) per day of any meat, poultry, or fish prepared without salt or sodium. Dried peas or beans, prepared or processed without salt. One egg may be used in place of one ounce of meat. Low-sodium cheese or cottage cheese. Low-sodium peanut butter or unsalted nuts.	Salted, smoked, cured, pickled, or canned meats, poultry, or fish (such as bacon, ham, corned or chipped beef, frankfurters, luncheon meats, meats Koshered by salting, salt pork, sausage, anchovies, herring, caviar, sardines, canned tuna, canned salmon). All other cheese. Regular (salted) peanut butter or salted nuts.
MILK *Limit to 2 cups*	Not more than two cups per day of milk, including reconstituted dry or evaporated milks. Use low-sodium milk. Cocoa may be used as part of milk allowance.	Buttermilk, malted milk, sweetened condensed milk. Milk shakes and other milk mixes.
SOUPS & COMBINATION FOODS	Low-sodium broth; low-sodium cream soups made from milk allowance and allowed foods. Commercial low-sodium (not reduced-sodium) soups.	Soups, broth, bouillon, or consommé containing salt or sodium. Prepared entrées containing salt or sodium.
DESSERTS & SWEETS *in moderation*	Gelatin desserts using plain gelatin or gelatin made without sodium; tapioca, rice, or cornstarch pudding or custard made with allowed ingredients. Ice cream or ice milk used as part of the milk allowance. Sugar, honey, molasses, syrup, jam, jelly, marmalade, candy without nuts, marshmallows. Fruit ice, sorbet, popsicles.	Desserts containing salt, baking powder, baking soda, or any other sodium-containing ingredient. Pudding or custard mixes. All sweets containing salt or sodium. Artificial sweetener containing sodium.
FATS & OILS *in moderation*	Salt-free butter or margarine; vegetable shortening or oil; lard; low-sodium salad dressings. Not more than 1/4 cup of cream or sour cream daily.	Salted butter or margarine; sodium-containing salad dressings. Bacon fat; mayonnaise; tartar sauce; liquid or dry cream substitutes. Gravy or sauces prepared or canned with salt or sodium. Chip dips.

FOOD GROUP	ALLOWED/RECOMMENDED	AVOID/USE SPARINGLY
BEVERAGES	Fruit drinks, cereal beverages, coffee (regular or decaffeinated), tea.	Water treated with a water softener.
CONDIMENTS/ MISCELLANEOUS	Herbs, spices, flavoring extracts, cream of tartar, vinegar, and yeast. Semisweet & baking chocolate; cocoa. Low-sodium baking powder; low-sodium baking soda (potassium bicarbonate). Low-sodium catsup, mustard, chili sauce, or soy sauce. Sweet pickles.	Salt, flavored salts, mono-sodium glutamate, poultry seasoning. Prepared horse-radish, meat tenderizers, dill pickles, relish, olives, soy sauce. Dutch-processed cocoa. Regular catsup, meat sauces, mustard, chili sauce, salsa. Baking powder or baking soda. Worcestershire sauce.

* These amounts indicate the **minimum** number of servings needed from the basic food groups to provide a variety of nutrients essential to good health. A maximum amount (limit) is indicated when amounts of certain foods must be controlled. Combination foods may count as full or partial servings from the food groups. Dark green, leafy, or orange vegetables are recommended 3 or 4 times weekly to provide vitamin A. A good source of vitamin C is recommended daily. Potatoes may be included as a serving of vegetables. The menu below is provided as a sample; your daily menus will vary.

SAMPLE MEAL PLAN

Breakfast:
6 oz. fruit juice, 1/2 cup canned fruit, or 1 serving fresh fruit
1 cup low-sodium cereal or 1 egg
1 slice salt-free toast
1 tsp. salt-free margarine or butter
1 cup low-sodium milk
Coffee, tea

Noon Meal:
2 oz. lean, unsalted ground beef
Salt-free hamburger bun
Low-sodium catsup and mustard
1 cup tossed salad
1 tbsp. low-sodium salad dressing
1 serving fresh fruit or 1/2 cup canned fruit
Coffee, tea

Evening Meal:
3 oz. unsalted baked chicken
1/2 cup unsalted potato, pasta, or grain
1 tsp. salt-free margarine or butter
1/2 cup allowed vegetables
1 cup low-sodium milk
Coffee, tea

1,000 milligrams (45 mEq) Education Sheet
Special notes

Sodium, a mineral, is abundant in many foods. Sodium may be found naturally, or it may be added during the processing of a food. The most common form is salt, which is composed of sodium and chloride. Reducing your sodium intake involves changing your eating behavior.

The following guidelines will help you reduce the sodium in your diet:
1. Stop using the salt shaker.
2. Omit salt in cooking and in baking.
3. Substitute sodium-free seasonings and spices.
4. Use a salt substitute (potassium chloride) only with a doctor's permission.
5. Include a variety of fresh, unprocessed foods in your diet.
6. Use low-sodium commercial products.
7. Use the general guidelines listed below, or monitor your sodium intake using the milligram (mg) or the point system listed in the Sodium Counter (available from your dietitian).

FOOD GROUP	ALLOWED/RECOMMENDED	AVOID/USE SPARINGI
BREADS/STARCHES *6 servings or more**	Up to three slices of regular bread (or the equivalent) per day. Salt-free breads, rolls, and crackers. Biscuits, pancakes, waffles, and cornbread made with low sodium baking powder.	More than three slices per da of sodium-containing breads, rolls, or crackers. Self-rising flours; mixes containing salt/ sodium. Regular bread and cracker crumbs. Commercial bread stuffing mixes. Products made with regular baking powder.
Cereals:	Any cooked cereal prepared without salt. Dry cereals: Puffed Wheat®, Puffed Rice®, Shredded Wheat®, Sugar Smacks®.	Any cereal containing salt or sodium, or any cereal prepared with the addition of salt. Instant hot cereal packets.
Potatoes/Pasta/Rice:	Fresh, frozen, or canned without salt or sodium: white or sweet potatoes, rice, spaghetti, macaroni, or other pastas, barley. Salt-free potato chips or other snacks. Unsalted popcorn.	Prepared potato products or substitutes containing salt or sodium, or any prepared with the addition of salt. Salted snack foods. Salted popcorn.
VEGETABLES *3 servings or more*	Fresh, frozen, or canned without salt or sodium. Peas or lima beans must be fresh or canned without salt (not frozen). Not more than 1/2 cup per day of: beets, beet greens, carrots, celery, dandelion greens, kale, mustard greens, spinach, Swiss chard, white turnips, frozen peas, or frozen lima beans. Tomato (or vegetable) juices, sauce, paste, or puree without salt or sodium.	Any vegetables or vegetable juices containing salt or sodium, including those prepared in cream or cheese sauces. Sauerkraut.

FOOD GROUP	ALLOWED/RECOMMENDED	AVOID/USE SPARINGLY
FRUIT *2 servings or more**	All fruits & juices.	None.
MEAT & **SUBSTITUTES** *Up to 6 oz. total*	6 oz. (cooked weight) per day of any meat, poultry, fish or shellfish prepared without salt or sodium. One egg may be used for 1 oz. of meat. Dried peas or beans, processed and prepared without salt or ·sodium. Low-sodium tuna and salmon. Low-sodium cheese. Low-sodium peanut butter or unsalted nuts.	Salted, smoked, cured, pickled, or canned meats, poultry, or fish (such as bacon, ham, corned beef, chipped beef, frankfurters, luncheon meats, meats Koshered by salting, salt pork, sausage, anchovies, herring, caviar, sardines, canned tuna, canned salmon). Other shellfish. All other cheeses. Regular (salted) peanut butter or salted nuts.
MILK *Limit to 2 cups per day*	Not more than two cups per day of regular milk (including reconstituted dry or evaporated). Low-sodium milk. Yogurt or cocoa used as part of the milk allowance.	Buttermilk, malted milk, and milkshake.
SOUPS & **COMBINATION** **FOODS**	Low-sodium broth; low-sodium cream soups made from milk allowance and allowed foods. Commercial low-sodium soups.	Soups, broth, bouillon, or consommé containing salt or sodium. Prepared entrées containing salt or sodium.
DESSERTS & **SWEETS** *in moderation*	Gelatin desserts using plain gelatin or gelatin made without sodium; tapioca, rice, or cornstarch pudding or custard made with allowed milk and egg. Ice cream, ice milk, or sherbet used as part of the milk allowance. Fruit ice, sherbet, popsicles. Baked goods made from allowed ingredients. Sugar, honey, molasses, syrup, jam, jelly, marmalade, candy without nuts, marshmallows.	Desserts containing salt, baking powder, baking soda, or any other sodium-containing ingredient. All sweets containing salt or sodium. Artificial sweeteners containing salt or sodium. Desserts made with rennin and rennin tablets.

FOOD GROUP	ALLOWED/RECOMMENDED	AVOID/USE SPARINGI
FATS & OILS *Up to 3 tsp. salted*	Three teaspoons per day of salted butter, margarine, or mayonnaise. Salt-free butter or margarine. Vegetable shortening, oil, lard, low-sodium salad dressing or mayonnaise. Not more than 1/4 cup cream or sour cream daily. Unsalted gravy.	More than three teaspoons of salted butter, margarine, or mayonnaise. Sodium-containing salad dressing; bacon fat; tartar sauce. Chip dip. Liquid or dry cream substitutes. Gravy mixes or canned gravy.
BEVERAGES	All fruit juices or fruit drinks. Cereal beverages, coffee, decaffeinated coffee, tea.	Water treated with a water softener.
CONDIMENTS/ MISCELLANEOUS	Herbs, spices, flavoring extracts, cream of tartar, vinegar, and yeast. Semi-sweet and baking chocolate; cocoa. Low-sodium catsup; low-sodium baking powder; low-sodium baking soda; low-sodium chili sauce; low-sodium mustard; low-sodium soy sauce.	Salt, flavored salts, "light" salt, monosodium glutamate, poultry seasoning. Pre-pared horseradish, meat sauces, meat tenderizers, dill pickles, relish, olives, soy sauce, Dutch pro-cessed cocoa. Regular meat sauces, catsup, mustard, chili sauce, salsa. Baking powder or baking soda. Worcestershire sauce.

- These amounts indicate the **minimum** number of servings needed from the basic food groups to provide a variety of nutrients essential to good health. A maximum amount (limit) is indicated when amounts of certain foods must be controlled. Combination foods may count as full or partial servings from the food groups. Dark green, leafy, or orange vegetables are recommended 3 or 4 times weekly to provide vitamin A. A good source of vitamin C is recommended daily. Potatoes may be included as a serving of vegetables. See menu provided as a sample; your daily menus will vary.

Breakfast:	1/2 cup fruit juice, 1/2 cup canned fruit, or 1 serving fresh fruit
	1 cup low-sodium cereal or 1 egg
	1 slice salt-free or regular toast
	1 tsp. margarine or butter
	1 cup low-fat milk
	Coffee, tea
Noon Meal:	2 oz. lean, unsalted ground beef
	Hamburger bun
	Low-sodium catsup and mustard
	1 cup tossed salad
	1 tbsp. low-sodium salad dressing
	1 serving fresh fruit or 1/2 cup canned fruit
	Coffee, tea
Evening Meal:	3 - 4 oz. unsalted, baked chicken
	1/2 cup unsalted potato, pasta, grain, or rice
	1 slice regular bread
	1-2 tsp. margarine or butter
	1/2 cup allowed vegetables
	1 cup low-fat milk
	Coffee, tea

Consumer references for sodium-restricted diets are available from your dietitian.

2,000 milligram (90 mEq) Education Sheet

Sodium, a mineral, is abundant in many foods. Sodium may be found naturally, or it may be added during the processing of a food. The most common form is salt, which is composed of sodium and chloride. Reducing your sodium intake involves changing your eating behavior.

The following guidelines will help you reduce the sodium in your diet:

1. Stop using the salt shaker.
2. Omit salt in cooking and in baking.
3. Substitute sodium-free seasonings and spices.
4. Use a salt substitute (potassium chloride) only with a doctor's permission.
5. Include a variety of fresh, unprocessed foods in your diet.
6. Use low-sodium commercial products.
7. Use the general guidelines listed below, or monitor your sodium intake using the milligram (mg) or the point system listed in the Sodium Counter (available from your dietitian).

FOOD GROUP	ALLOWED/RECOMMENDED	AVOID/USE SPARINGLY
STARCHES/BREADS 6 servings or more*	Three slices regular bread (or the equivalent) per day. Salt-free breads, rolls, and crackers.	More than three slices per day of sodium-containing breads, rolls, or crackers. Self-rising flours; mixes containing salt or sodium.
Cereals:	Any cooked cereal prepared without salt. Dry cereals: any.	Do not add salt when cooking hot cereal.
Potatoes/Pasta/Rice:	Fresh, frozen, or canned without salt or sodium, potatoes rice, spaghetti, noodles, barley, macaroni, etc. Salt-free potato chips or other snacks. Unsalted popcorn.	Prepared potato products or substitutes containing salt or sodium, or any prepared with the addition of salt. Salted snack foods. Salted popcorn.
VEGETABLES *3 servings or more*	Fresh, frozen, and low-sodium canned vegetables. Low-sodium vegetable juices	Any vegetables or vegetable juices canned with salt or sodium, including those prepared in cream or cheese sauces. Sauerkraut. Pickled vegetables.
FRUIT *2 servings or more*	All fruits & juices.	None.

FOOD GROUP	ALLOWED/RECOMMENDED	AVOID/USE SPARINGLY
MEAT & SUBSTITUTES *2 servings* *(up to 6 oz. total)*	6 oz. (cooked weight) per day of any fresh or frozen meat, poultry, fish, or shellfish prepared without salt, sodium or breading. Low sodium canned tuna and salmon.	Salted, smoked, cured, pickled, or canned meats, poultry, or fish (such as bacon, ham, corned or chipped beef, frankfurters, luncheon meats, meats Koshered by salting, salt pork, sausage, anchovies, herring, caviar, sardines, canned tuna, canned salmon). Breaded meat, poultry, fish, and shellfish.
	One egg may be used for 1 oz. of meat. Low-sodium cheese. Low-sodium peanut butter or unsalted nuts. Dried peas and beans-no salt added.	All other cheeses. Regular (salted) peanut butter or salted nuts.
MILK *2 cups or the equivalent*	Skim, low-fat, whole, chocolate, milk. Cocoa, eggnog, yogurt.	Buttermilk, malted milk, and milkshake.
SOUPS & COMBINATION FOODS	Low-sodium broth; low-sodium cream soups made from milk allowance and allowed foods. Commercial low-sodium soups.	Soups, broth, bouillon, or consommé containing salt or sodium. Prepared entrées containing salt or sodium.
DESSERTS & SWEETS *in moderation*	Gelatin desserts; sherbet; fruit ice. Baked goods made from allowed ingredients. Not more than one serving per day of sodium-containing pudding, custard, cake, cookies, pie, or ice cream. Sugar, honey, molasses, syrup, jam, jelly, marmalade, candy, marshmallows.	More than one serving per day of sodium-containing desserts. All sweets containing salt or sodium.
FATS & OILS *Up to 5 tsp. salted*	Up to 5 teaspoons per day of salted butter, margarine, or mayonnaise. Salt-free butter or margarine. Vegetable shortening, oil, lard, low-sodium salad dressing. Cream, sour cream, liquid or dry cream substitutes.	More than 5 teaspoons of salted butter, margarine, or mayonnaise. Sodium-containing salad dressing; bacon fat; tartar sauce. Gravy mixes or canned gravy. Chip dips.
BEVERAGES	Fruit drinks, cereal beverages, coffee (regular or decaffeinated) tea, herbal tea. Carbonated beverages.	None.

FOOD GROUP	ALLOWED/RECOMMENDED	AVOID/USE SPARINGLY
CONDIMENTS/ MISCELLANEOUS	Herbs, spices, flavoring extracts, cream of tartar, vinegar, and yeast. Semi-sweet & baking chocolate; cocoa. Low-sodium catsup; low-sodium baking powder; low-sodium baking soda, low-sodium chili sauce. Low-sodium mustard; low-sodium soy sauce.	Salt, flavored salts, mono-sodium glutamate, poultry seasoning. Prepared horseradish, meat sauces, meat tenderizers, pickles, relish, olives, soy sauce, Dutch processed cocoa. Regular catsup, mustard, chili sauce, salsa. Baking powder or baking soda. "Light" salt.

* The amounts listed on the diet list indicate the **minimum** number of servings needed from the basic food groups to provide a variety of nutrients essential to good health. A maximum amount (limit) is indicated when amounts of certain foods must be controlled. Combination foods may count as full or partial servings from the food groups. Dark green, leafy, or orange vegetables are recommended 3 or 4 times weekly to provide vitamin A. A good source of vitamin C is recommended daily. Potatoes may be included as a serving of vegetables. The menu above is provided as a sample; your daily menus will vary.

SAMPLE MEAL PATTERN

Breakfast: 6 oz. fruit juice, 1/2 cup canned fruit, or 1 serving fresh fruit
1 cup cereal or 1 egg
1 slice toast
1 tsp. margarine or butter
1 cup low-fat milk
Coffee, tea

Noon Meal: 2 oz. lean, unsalted ground beef
Hamburger bun
Low-sodium catsup and mustard
1 cup tossed salad
1 tbsp. low-sodium salad dressing
1 serving fresh fruit or 1/2 cup canned fruit
Coffee, tea

Evening Meal: 3-4 oz. unsalted baked chicken
1/2 cup unsalted potato, rice, or pasta
1 slice bread
1-2 tsp. margarine or butter
1/2 cup vegetables, fresh, frozen, or low-sodium canned
1 cup low-fat milk
Coffee, tea

Consumer references for sodium-restricted diets are available from your dietitian.

3,000-4,000 milligrams (135-175 mEq) Education Sheet
No-Added Salt Diet

Sodium, a mineral, is abundant in many foods. Sodium may be found naturally, or it may be added during the processing of a food. The most common form is salt, which is composed of sodium and chloride. Reducing your sodium intake involves changing your eating behavior.

The following guidelines will help you reduce the sodium in your diet:

1. Stop using the salt shaker.
2. Use salt sparingly in cooking and baking.
3. Substitute sodium-free seasonings and spices.
4. Do not use a salt substitute (potassium chloride) without your doctor's permission.
5. Include a variety of fresh, unprocessed foods in your diet.
6. Limit the use of processed and convenience foods high in sodium.
7. Use the general guidelines listed below, or monitor your sodium intake using the milligram (mg) or the point system listed in the Sodium Counter (available from your dietitian).

FOOD GROUP	AVOID/USE SPARINGLY
BREADS/STARCHES *6 servings or more**	Commercial bread stuffing; commercial pancake or waffle mixes; coating mixes; waffles. Croutons. Prepared (boxed or frozen) potato, rice, or noodle mixes that contain salt or sodium. Salted French fries or hash browns. Salted popcorn, breads, crackers, chips, or snack foods.
VEGETABLES *3 servings or more*	Vegetables canned with salt* or prepared in cream, butter, or cheese sauces. Sauerkraut. Tomato or vegetable juices canned with salt. *Allowed if rinsed thoroughly.
FRUIT *2 servings or more*	None.
MEAT & **SUBSTITUTES** *2 servings or more* *(4 to 6 oz. total/day)*	Salted or smoked meats such as bacon or Canadian bacon; chipped or corned beef; hot dogs; salt pork; luncheon meats; pastrami; ham; sausage. Canned or smoked fish, poultry, or meat; processed cheese or cheese spreads; blue or Roquefort cheese; battered, frozen fish products; prepared spaghetti sauce; baked beans; Reuben sandwiches. Salted nuts. Caviar.
MILK *2 cups or the equivalent*	Limit buttermilk to 1 cup per week.

FOOD GROUP	AVOID/USE SPARINGLY
SOUPS & COMBINATION FOODS	Bouillon cubes; canned or dried soups; broth; consommé (prepared with salt or sodium). Convenience (frozen or packaged) dinners with more than 600 mg sodium, pot pies; pizza; Oriental food. Fast food cheeseburgers and specialty sandwiches.
DESSERTS & SWEETS *in moderation*	More than 1 serving per day of regular (salted) desserts; pie; commercial fruit snack pies; commercial snack cakes; canned puddings.
FATS & OILS *in moderation*	Gravy mixes or canned gravy. No more than 1 to 2 tbsp. of salad dressing (French or Thousand Island type). Chip dips.
BEVERAGES	None except as listed under vegetable and milk groups.
CONDIMENTS/ MISCELLANEOUS	Salt, flavored salts, monosodium glutamate, poultry seasoning. Bacon-flavored bits, BBQ sauce, chili sauce, catsup, mustard, meat sauces, salsa, regular (salted) soy sauce or mustard, dill pickles, olives, meat tenderizer. Prepared horseradish or pickle relish. Dutch processed cocoa; baking powder or baking soda used medicinally. Worcestershire sauce. "Light" salt. Salt substitute unless approved by physician.

* These amounts indicate the **minimum** number of servings needed from the basic food groups to provide a variety of nutrients essential to good health. A maximum amount (limit) is indicated when amounts of certain foods must be controlled. Combination foods may count as full or partial servings from the food groups. Dark green, leafy, or orange vegetables are recommended 3 or 4 times weekly to provide vitamin A. A good source of vitamin C is recommended daily. Potatoes may be included as a serving of vegetables.

Dining Out on a Sodium-Controlled Diet

There are several ways to help reduce your sodium intake while eating out. Choices will vary with the type of eating situation. Successful sodium control will come by taking the following steps to lower your sodium intake while dining out:

Ordering from a menu

- Request that your food be prepared without salt. Carry your own spice blend, salt-free seasoning, or salt substitute.
- Choose food that requires minimal preparation, such as broiled, baked, or roasted meats made without sauces, breadings, or batters. Order sauces and au jus "on the side," and use them sparingly.
- Try lemon juice or vinegar and oil for salad dressing, or request that regular salad dressings be served "on the side," and use them sparingly. Carry your own low-sodium salad dressings, available in individual packets.
- Choose fresh fruit or fruit juice for an appetizer.
- Choose beverages lower in sodium such as coffee, tea, milk, soda pop, or lemonade. Avoid buttermilk, tomato juice, and vegetable juice.
- Choose lean, fresh meats for sandwich fillings rather than processed meats and meat salads. Request fresh fruit, unsalted French fries, lettuce, tomato, and onion for sandwich accompaniments in place of dill pickles and potato chips.
- Choose ice cream, sherbet, gelatin, or fruit for dessert rather than higher sodium items such as pies and pastries.

Fast food restaurants

- Order a plain sandwich—hold the pickles, catsup, mustard, cheese, and special sauces. Request lettuce, tomato, and onion for garnish.
- Order unsalted French fries.

Salad bars

- Choose fresh vegetables or canned or fresh fruits as a major part of your meal.
- Choose vinegar and oil or lemon juice for salad dressing.
- Limit use of higher sodium ingredients such as bacon bits, pickles, cheese, and meat salads.

Ethnic foods

- For Oriental dining, choose menu items that are made to order. Request that food be prepared without salt, soy sauce, or MSG (monosodium glutamate).
- Choose menu items that do not include sauces. Mexican entrées such as tacos, burritos, and tostadas are lower sodium choices.
- Other ethnic foods, such as German and Italian, are difficult to control since these foods may be prepared ahead of time. Compensate for your meal out by consuming foods low in sodium at home (prior to and after the ethnic meal).

Banquets

- Request a low-sodium meal from the banquet organizer as soon as possible. If this is not possible, adjust your portion size according to the sodium content of the food. Compensate by choosing foods as low in sodium as possible prior to and following the meal.

Parties

- Choose more fresh fruits, fresh vegetables, and natural cheeses.
- Limit your portion size of sauced and pickled foods.

Air travel

- Order a low-sodium airline meal by calling the airline reservation office at least 24 hours prior to take-off. Upon boarding, notify the seat reservationist and/or flight attendant of your request.

Guest in a home

- Notify host or hostess and explain your diet needs.
- Decrease portion sizes of foods higher in sodium. Compensate by choosing more foods lower in sodium (prior to and after the meal).

Fast Food Restaurants

Sodium Counter

Food Item	Amount	mg	Points
Arby's			
Regular Roast Beef®	1	1009	44
Junior Roast Beef®	1	779	34
Roast Beef Light Deluxe®	1	829	36
French Dip®	1	1411	61
Roast Chicken Light Deluxe®	1	777	34
Turkey Light Deluxe®	1	1262	55
Potato Cakes®	1 serving	397	17
Burger King			
Hamburger®	1	530	23
Cheeseburger®	1	770	33
Whopper®	1	870	38
Whopper with Cheese®	1	1350	59
BK Broiler Chicken Sandwich®	1	480	34
BK Big fish™ Sandwich	1	980	43
French fries® ,medium	1 serving	240	10
Croissan'wich with sausage, egg & cheese®	1	1140	50
Biscuit with bacon, egg & cheese®	1	1530	67
French Toast Sticks®	1 serving	490	21
Dairy Queen			
Hamburger ®	1	630	27
Cheeseburger®	1	850	37
Chili Dog®	1	870	38
Fish Fillet sandwich®	1	630	27
Grilled Chicken Breast Fillet sandwich®	1	1040	45
French fries®, regular	1 serving	160	7
Banana split®	1	180	8
Buster Bar®	1	280	12
Dilly Bar®	1	75	3
Dipped cone, regular®	1	200	9
DQ sandwich®	1	115	5
Heath Blizzard, regular®	1	580	25
Mr. Misty, regular®	1	30	1
Malt, chocolate, regular ®	1	500	22
Peanut Buster Parfait ®	1	400	17
Domino's Pizza			
Cheese, 12" diam.® (hand tossed)	2 slice	622	27
Pepperoni, 12" diam.® (hand tossed)	2 slice	799	35
Veggie, 12" diam.® (hand tossed)	2 slice	967	42

Sodium Counter

Food Item	Amount	mg	Points
Hardee's			
Hamburger ®	1	670	9
Cheeseburger ®	1	890	39
Cravin Bacon™ cheeseburger®	1	1150	50
Chicken Fillet ®	1	1280	56
Fisherman's Fillet ®	1	1330	58
Rise'n'shine Biscuit®	1	1000	43
Apple Cinnamon 'n' Raisin Biscuit®	1	350	15
Canadian Sunrise Biscuit®	1	1340	58
Hash Rounds®	1 serving	560	24
Kentucky Fried Chicken			
<u>Original Recipe Chicken®</u>			
breast	1	1116	49
drumstick	1	422	18
thigh	1	747	32
wing	1	414	18
<u>Extra Tasty Crispy Chicken®</u>			
breast	1	930	40
drumstick	1	260	11
thigh	1	540	23
wing	1	290	13
<u>Hot & Spicy Chicken®</u>			
breast	1	1110	48
drumstick	1	300	13
thigh	1	570	25
wing	1	340	15
<u>Tenderoast Crispy Chicken®</u> (without skin)			
breast	1	797	35
drumstick	1	259	11
thigh	1	312	14
Chicken sandwich®	1	782	34
Mashed potatoes & gravy®	1 serving	440	19
Buttermilk biscuit ®	1	560	24
McDonald's			
Hamburger ®	1	530	22
Cheeseburger ®	1	770	32
Quarter Pounder ®	1	730	31
Quarter Pounder with Cheese®	1	1200	53
Big Mac®	1	880	43
Grilled Chicken Deluxe™	1	970	42
Chicken McNuggets®	1 serving (6)	510	22
Fish Fillet Deluxe	1	1200	49
Chef Salad without dressing®	1	490	21
Chunky Chicken Salad without dressing®	1	230	10
Egg McMuffin®	1	710	31

Sodium Counter

Food Item	Amount	mg	Points
Rax			
Regular Rax Sandwich®	1	705	31
Deluxe Roast Beef®	1	865	38
Philly Melt®	1	1055	46
Grilled Chicken Breast Sandwich®	1	870	38
Country Fried Chicken Breast Sandwich®	1	1080	47
Grilled Chicken Garden Salad without dressing®	1	745	32
Taco Bell			
Bean burrito®	1	1140	50
Burrito Supreme®	1	1220	53
Soft taco®	1	530	23
Taco®	1	280	12
Taco salad with salsa®	1	1670	73
Tostada®	1	700	30
Mexican pizza®	1 serving	1050	46
Nachos Bellgrande®	1 serving	1200	52
Wendy's			
Hamburger ®	1	510	22
Jr. Cheeseburger ®	1	770	33
Bacon cheeseburger ®	1	770	33
Big Bacon Classic®	1	1500	65
Chicken Club Sandwich®	1	990	43
Chili ®, large	1 serving	1000	43
Baked potato with broccoli & cheese®	1	440	19
Baked potato with chili & cheese®	1	700	30
Grilled Chicken sandwich	1	720	31

A Dash of Flavor

Re-educate your taste buds and enjoy the unsalted flavor of foods, or try some of these salt-free seasoning suggestions:

Basil	Soups, tomato dishes, vegetables, chicken, eggs.
Bay leaves	Soups, stews, meat dishes, vegetable dishes, fish.
Cardamom	Coffee cakes, Scandinavian pastries, curries, soups.
Cayenne pepper	Meats, fish, sauces, Mexican and Asian dishes.
Celery seed	Salad dressings, fish, cole slaw, meat loaf, salads.
Chili pepper	Tomato sauces, soups, chili, meat sauces, Spanish rice.
Chives	Soups, salads, cheese dishes, potatoes, rice.
Cilantro	Use like parsley, Asian cooking.
Coriander	Curries, baked products.
Cumin	Mexican, Middle Eastern & Asian dishes; stews, soups, curries.
Curry	Fish, lamb, veal, vegetable dips, chicken, rice dishes.
Dill	Chicken, cucumber, fish, potato salad, tomato juice, vegetables.
Fennel seed	Italian, Swedish, and Asian cookery.
Garlic	Fish, meat, poultry, potatoes, vegetables, sauces, salads.
Lemon juice	Vegetables, salads, fish, puddings, desserts.
Mace	Fish, baked products, pastries, tomato juice, apples, carrots.
Marjoram	Soups, tomatoes, spinach, cottage cheese, salad dressings.
Mint	Carrots, fruit, fruit juices, tea, peas, tomatoes.
Mustard	Salad dressings, potatoes, broccoli, chicken, fish.
Nutmeg	Cauliflower, French toast, chicken, fish, meat loaf, apple dishes.
Onion	Meats, vegetables, soups, stews.
Oregano	Tomatoes, vegetable salads, beans, peas, hamburgers.
Paprika	Chicken, fish, tomatoes, soups, stuffings, salad dressings.
Pepper	Sauces, fish, stews, pork, chicken, stuffing, cheese, sauces.
Saffron	Rice, Asian and Spanish cooking.
Summer savory	Poultry, meats, creamed potatoes, green beans.
Thyme	Stews, meats, fish, lima beans, soups, stuffing, beets.
Tarragon	Vinegar, salad dressings, sauces, mustard, poultry.

Professional references

1. Recommended Dietary Allowances. 10th ed. Washington, D.C.: National Academy Press, 1989.
2. Snetselaar, LG. Nutrition counseling skills, assessment, treatment, and evaluation. Rockville, MD: ASPEN Publication, 1983: Chapters 1, 2, 3, 8 and 10.
3. Supplement to hypertension: The National Heart, Lung and Blood Institute Workshop on Salt and Blood Pressure. (17I): 1991.
4. Pennington, J. Food values of portions commonly used. 15th ed. New York: Harper and Row, 1989.
5. Mahan LK, Arlin MT. Krause's food, nutrition and diet therapy. 8th ed. Philadelphia: W.B. Saunders Co. 1992.

Cookbooks

1. Cooking without your salt shaker. American Heart Association, AHA. Northeast Ohio Affiliate, Inc., 1978.
2. Hachfeld L, Eykyn B. Cooking a la Heart, 2nd ed. Mankato: Apple Tree Press, Inc., 1992.
3. Starke RD, Winston M. American Heart Association Low Salt Cookbook: A complete guide to reducing sodium and fat in the diet. New York: Times Book Random House, 1990.
4. McThuen M. Microwaving on a diet. Minnetonka: Cy DeCosse Inc., 1981.

References

1. Byerly's grocery stores. Sodium restricted shopping guide.
2. Lund's grocery stores. Good foods—good choices. 1989.
3. Reader D, Franz M. Pass the pepper please. Minneapolis: Chronimed Publishing, 1988.
4. The Barbara Kraus sodium guide to brand name and basic foods, 1983 ed. New York: The New American Library, Inc., 1983.

Associations and organizations

1. American Heart Association—Minnesota Affiliate
   4701 West 77th Street
   Minneapolis, MN 55435
   612-835-3300

2. Minnesota State Department of Health
   717 Delaware Street S.E.
   Minneapolis, MN 55440
   612-623-5774

3. National Kidney Foundation of the Upper Midwest, Inc.
   920 South 7th Street
   Minneapolis, MN 55415
   612-337-7300

4. U.S. Department of Health and Human Services
   National Institutes of Health
   National Heart, Lung, and Blood Institute
   National High Blood Pressure Education Program
   120/80
   4733 Bethesda Avenue, Suite 530
   Bethesda, MD 20814

Label Reading for a Sodium-Controlled Diet

The Food & Drug Administration has established the following guidelines for sodium terms used on food labels:

Sodium Free	Less than 5 mg (0 points) per serving
Very Low Sodium	35 mg (2 points) or less per serving
Low Sodium	140 mg (6 points) or less per serving
	Meals or main dishes 140 mg or less per 100 grams
Reduced or Less Sodium	25% reduction in sodium content
Lite, Light, Lightly	50% reduction in sodium content
Unsalted, No Salt Added, Without Added Salt	Foods processed without salt that are usually processed with salt

Follow these steps when reading the nutrition information on the label:

1. Check the serving size.
2. Nutrient values are expressed per serving. Compare your serving size to the serving size listed.
3. Check the milligrams of sodium per serving.
4. Divide the number of milligrams by 23 to convert to sodium points.
5. Check the ingredient list.

Look for the following sodium-containing ingredients: salt, sodium, brine, baking soda, baking powder, soy sauce.

Label Reading Example

Cream of Mushroom Soup

Nutrition Information per Serving

1. —> **Serving Size**	**4 oz. condensed**
Serving Size —>	*(8 oz. as prepared)*

Servings per container	2-3/4
Calories	100
Protein (grams)	2
Carbohydrate (grams)	8
Fat (grams)	7
Cholesterol	less than 5 mg/serving
Sodium	**820 mg/serving**

2.
Sodium
Content
—>

3.
Ingredient
Listing —>

Ingredients: water, mushrooms, vegetable oil, wheat flour, cream, **salt,** cornstarch, dried dairy blend (whey calcium caseinate), modified food starch, whey, **monosodium glutamate,** soy protein isolate, natural flavoring, yeast extract and dehydrated garlic.

Associations and affiliated organizations

1. American Heart Association—Minnesota Affiliate
   4701 West 77th Street
   Minneapolis, MN 55435
   612-835-3300

2. National Kidney Foundation of the Upper Midwest, Inc.
   920 South 7th Street
   Minneapolis, MN 55415
   612-337-7300

3. U.S. Department of Health & Human Services
   National Institutes of Health
   National Heart, Lung, and Blood Institute
   National High Blood Pressure Education Program
   120/80
   4733 Bethesda Ave., Suite 530
   Bethesda, MD 20814

4. Minnesota State Department of Health
   717 Delaware Street SE
   Minneapolis, MN 55440
   612-623-5774

Sodium Counter
(Sodium Point System)

Sodium is a mineral that is measured in terms of weight. Two measurements are commonly used: **milligrams** (mg.) or **sodium points** (pt.). Milligrams are the measurement used on food labels. To convert milligrams to sodium points (for example, if you see a sodium value on a food label in milligrams and need to convert it to points), the following equation is used:

milligrams ÷ 23 = points

Your diet prescription is _____ of sodium.

Food containing sodium may be selected from the following Sodium Counter until you reach

_____ mg or _____ points.

Food Item	Amount	Sodium mg	Poin
BEVERAGES			
Coffee, Tea, Cocoa			
Coffee, regular, decaffeinated	8 oz.	5	0
Tea, regular, decaffeinated	8 oz.	5	0
Iced tea, instant	8 oz.	10	0
Cocoa mix, powder, sweetened	6 oz.	150	7
Cocoa mix, powder, sugar-free	6 oz.	175	8
Fruit Drinks			
Fruit Punch, canned	6 oz.	40	2
Hi-C® Orange Drink	6 oz.	60	3
Koolaid®	8 oz.	10	0
Lemonade	8 oz.	10	0
Tang®	6 oz.	0	0
Fruit & Vegetable Juices			
Apple juice	4 oz.	5	0
Apricot nectar	4 oz.	5	0
Carrot juice	4 oz.	25	1
Cranberry juice	4 oz.	5	0
Grape juice	4 oz.	5	0
Grapefruit juice	4 oz.	0	0
Lemon juice	1 tbsp.	5	0
Lime juice	1 tbsp.	0	0
Orange juice	4 oz.	5	0
Pineapple juice	4 oz.	0	0
Prune juice	4 oz.	5	0
Tomato or vegetable juice (V-8®)	6 oz.	660	29
Tomato or vegetable juice (V-8®), no added salt	6 oz.	40	2

Food Item		Amount	Sodium mg	Points
Soft Drinks, Mixers, Water				
Soft drinks, regular		12 oz.	25	1
Soft drinks, diet		12 oz.	10	0
Club soda		12 oz.	75	3
Mineral water		12 oz.	0	0
Seltzer water		8 oz.	50	2
Tonic water		12 oz.	15	1
Tap water, Twin Cities		8 oz.	0	0
Softened tap water, Twin Cities		8 oz.	10	0
Alcohol				
Beer		12 oz.	20	1
Beer, Lite, nonalcoholic		12 oz.	10	0
Gin, Rum, Vodka, Whiskey, etc.		1-1/2 oz.	0	0
Malt liquor		12 oz.	15	1
Wine, dessert		3 oz.	10	0
Wine, table, regular		5 oz.	10	0
Wine, table, lite		5 oz.	0	0
Wine cooler		12 oz.	40	2
Miscellaneous				
Alba 77®		8 oz.	160	7
Carnation Instant Breakfast®		1 pkg.	135	6
Carnation® Slender		10 oz.	500	22
Eggnog		8 oz.	140	6
Gatorade®		8 oz.	125	5
Postum®		6 oz.	5	0
BREADS, MUFFINS, ROLLS				
Bagel		1	200	9
Biscuit		1	230	10
Bread:	white	1 slice	125	5
	whole wheat	1 slice	160	7
	multi-grain	1 slice	150	7
	oat bran	1 slice	160	7
	rye	1 slice	175	8
	challah (egg bread)	1 slice	140	6
	French	1 slice	165	7
	cinnamon raisin	1 slice	140	6
	lite, light, reduced calorie	1 slice	100	4
	low sodium, white or whole wheat	1 slice	5	0
Bread crumbs, unseasoned		1 cup	735	32
Bread crumbs, seasoned		1 cup	2115	92
Bread cubes, unseasoned		1 cup	205	9
Bread cubes, seasoned		1 cup	390	17
Bread dressing		1/2 cup	505	22
Bun, hamburger, hot dog		1	240	10
Cinnamon roll		1	150	7
Coffee cake (snack cake)		2 oz.	200	9
Cornbread		2" square	265	12
Cornbread dressing		1/2 cup	570	25

Food Item	Amount	Sodium mg	Poin
Croissant	1	230	10
Danish	1	105	5
Dinner roll	1	230	10
Doughnut, cake, old-fashioned	1	185	8
Doughnut, yeast	1	145	6
English Muffin	1	365	16
French toast	1 slice	230	10
Hush puppy	1	110	5
Lefse	12" diam.	300	13
Matzo ball	1	200	9
Muffin: various flavors	1" diam.	55	2
	2-1/2" diam.	170	7
	3" diam.	205	9
	4" diam	340	15
Pancake	4" diam.	235	10
Pocket or pita bread	4" diam.	135	6
Pocket or pita bread	6" diam.	280	12
Popover	1	115	5
Quick bread	1 slice	190	8
Roll, kaiser	1	310	13
Roll, hoagie	1	785	34
Scone	2-1/2" diam.	300	13
Taco shell, hard	1	65	3
Toaster pastries	1	230	10
Tortilla, corn	6" diam.	40	2
Tortilla, flour	6" diam.	110	5
Turnover	1	275	12
Waffle	7" diam.	515	22

Crackers

Food Item	Amount	Sodium mg	Poin
Bread sticks	1	95	4
Goldfish crackers	10	55	2
Graham crackers	2	105	5
Matzoth crackers	1	0	0
Melba rounds, plain	10	5	0
Oyster crackers	10	85	4
Rice cake	1	0-10	0
Ritz®	1	30	1
RyKrisp®, seasoned	1	90	4
Saltine	1	35	2
Saltine, unsalted tops, low salt	1	25	1
Saltine, salt free	1	0	0
Soda cracker	1	75	3
Triscuits®	1	30	1
Wheat Thins®	8	120	5
Wheatsworth® Stone Ground Wheat crackers	1	40	2
Zwieback toast	1	20	1

Food Item	Amount	Sodium mg	Points
CEREALS			
Ready-to-Eat			
All Bran®	1/3 cup	320	14
Bran Chex®	2/3 cup	300	13
Bran Flakes®	3/4 cup	265	12
Cheerios®	1-1/4 cup	290	13
Corn Chex®	1 cup	295	13
Cornflakes®	1-1/4 cup	350	15
Frosted Flakes®	3/4 cup	230	10
Frosted Mini Wheats®	4	10	0
Fruit Squares, Fruit Wheats®	1/2 cup	5	0
Granola	1/2 cup	150	7
Grape-nuts®	1/4 cup	165	7
Life®	2/3 cup	150	7
Oat Bran Flakes®	1 cup	260	11
Oat Squares®	1/2 cup	200	9
Product 19®	3/4 cup	325	14
Puffed Rice®, Puffed Wheat®	1 cup	0	0
Raisin Bran®	3/4 cup	270	12
Rice Krispies®	1 cup	340	15
Shredded Wheat®, Spoon-size	2/3 cup	0	0
Shredded Wheat®, large biscuit	1	0	0
Special K®	1-1/3 cup	265	12
Team Flakes®	1 cup	175	8
Total®	1 cup	280	12
Wheat Chex®	2/3 cup	200	9
Wheaties®	1 cup	270	12
Cooked			
Cream of wheat or rice, cooked without salt	1 cup	0	0
Cream of Wheat, Mix-n-Eat	1 pkg.	240	10
Grits, instant	1 pkg.	345	15
Grits, cooked without salt	1 cup	0	0
Oat bran, dry	1/3 cup	0	0
Oatmeal, instant	1 pkg.	230	10
Oatmeal, cooked without salt	1 cup	0	0
DAIRY PRODUCTS			
Cheese			
American	1 oz.	405	18
Baby Swiss	1 oz.	25	1
Blue or Roquefort	1 oz.	395	17
Bonbel, mini	1 oz.	230	10
Brick	1 oz.	160	7
Brie	1 oz.	180	8
Camembert®	1 oz.	240	10
Caraway	1 oz.	195	8
Cheddar	1 oz.	175	8
Cheese Spread	1 tbsp.	260	11

Food Item		Amount	Sodium mg	Poin
Cheshire®		1 oz.	200	9
Colby		1 oz.	170	7
Cottage cheese:	4% fat	1/2 cup	425	18
	2% fat	1/2 cup	460	20
	1% fat	1/2 cup	460	20
	Nonfat	1/2 cup	220	10
	2% fat, no salt added	1/2 cup	25	1
Cream cheese		1 tbsp.	45	2
Edam		1 oz.	275	12
Farmers		1 oz.	45	2
Feta		1 oz.	315	14
Gjetost		1 oz.	170	7
Gouda		1 oz.	230	10
Havarti®		1 oz.	145	6

Cheese

Food Item	Amount	Sodium mg	Poin
Jarlsberg	1 oz.	140	6
Limburger	1 oz.	225	10
Monterey jack	1 oz.	150	7
Mozzarella, string cheese, part-skim	1 oz.	150	7
Muenster	1 oz.	180	8
Neufchatel	1 tbsp.	55	2
Parmesan, grated	1 tbsp.	95	4
Port du Salut	1 oz.	150	7
Provolone	1 oz.	250	11
Ricotta cheese, lowfat	1 oz.	40	2
Romano	1 oz.	340	15
Samsoe	1 oz.	205	9
Swiss, natural	1 oz.	75	3
Swiss, processed	1 oz.	390	17
Swiss Lace, Alpine, Oberlander	1 oz.	35	2

Cream

Food Item	Amount	Sodium mg	Poin
Creamer, nondairy, liquid	1 tbsp.	10	1
Half & Half®	1 tbsp.	5	0
Sour cream	1 tbsp.	5	0
Sour cream, reduced fat	1 tbsp.	15	1
Sour cream dips	1 tbsp.	105	5
Whipped topping, nondairy, regular, lite	1 tbsp.	0	0
Whipped cream	1 tbsp.	5	0

Milk

Food Item	Amount	Sodium mg	Poin
Skim, 1%, 2%, whole, Lactaid®	8 oz.	125	5
Buttermilk	8 oz.	255	11
Chocolate milk, skim, lowfat, whole	8 oz.	150	7
Condensed milk, sweetened	8 oz.	390	17
Evaporated milk, whole	8 oz.	265	12
Evaporated milk, low-fat	8 oz.	275	13
Evaporated milk, skim	8 oz.	295	13
Milk powder, nonfat, dry	1/2 cup	185	8
Soy milk	8 oz.	30	1

Food Item		Amount	Sodium mg	Points
Yogurt				
Yogurt, whole milk	fruit-flavored	8 oz.	140	6
	plain	8 oz.	115	5
Yogurt, lowfat	fruit-flavored	8 oz.	145	6
	plain	8 oz.	170	7
Yogurt, nonfat	fruit flavored	8 oz.	110	5
	plain	8 oz.	185	8

DESSERTS

Food Item		Amount	Sodium mg	Points
Cakes				
Angel food cake, 1/12 of 10" diam.		1 piece	120	5
Boston cream pie, 1/16 of 8" diam.		1 piece	280	12
Bundt cake, 1/16		1 piece	280	12
Cake, layer with frosting, 1/16 of 8" diam.		1 piece	130	6
Cake, sheet with frosting, 3"x3"x2"		1 piece	190	8
Carrot cake with cream cheese frosting		1 piece	200	9
Cheesecake, 1/8 of 9" diam.		1 piece	355	15
Cakes				
Cupcake, with frosting, 2-1/2" diam.		1	105	5
Fruitcake, 3-1/2"x2"x1/2"		1 piece	70	3
Gingerbread, 2-1/2"x2-1/2"x1"		1 piece	190	8
Poundcake, 2-1/2"x3"x1"		1 piece	130	6
Shortcake, 2" diam.		1 piece	265	12
Snack cake, commercial		1 piece	135	6
Sponge cake, 1/12 of 12" diam.		1 piece	165	7
Cookies and Bars				
Animal crackers		10	80	3
Brownies & bars with frosting, 2"x2"		1	120	5
Cookies, various kinds	2" diam.	1	45	2
	3" diam.	1	95	4
	4" diam.	1	170	7
Fig bar		1	45	2
Gingersnap		1	20	1
Sandwich		1	70	3
Vanilla wafers		2	20	1
Frozen Desserts				
Frozen yogurt, regular, lowfat		1/2 cup	55	2
Fruit juice bar		1	5	0
Ice cream		1/2 cup	60	3
Ice cream bar		1	35	2
Ice cream sandwich		1	55	2
Ice milk		1/2 cup	55	2
Malt		10 oz.	435	19
Milkshake		10 oz.	175	8
Popsicle®		1	0	0
Pudding Pops®		1	105	5
Sherbet		1/2 cup	45	2
Sorbet		1/2 cup	10	0

Food Item	Amount	Sodium mg	Poin
Gelatin and Pudding			
Bread pudding	1/2 cup	285	12
Custard	1/2 cup	90	4
Gelatin	1/2 cup	60	3
Pudding, from mix	1/2 cup	160	7
Pudding, ready-to-eat	1/2 cup	160	7
Pies (pc = 1/6 of 9" diam.)			
Cream, custard	1 piece	350	15
Fruit, double crust	1 piece	400	17
Lemon meringue	1 piece	260	11
Mincemeat	1 piece	785	34
Pecan	1 piece	480	21
Pumpkin	1 piece	280	12
Snack pie, fruit, commercial	1	450	20
Egg, whole, large	1	70	3
Egg, scrambled with milk & fat	1	155	7
Egg, substitute	1/4 cup	120	5
Omelet, plain, 3 eggs	1	700	30
Omelet, cheese, 3 eggs	1	1065	46

FATS AND OILS

Bacon fat	1 tbsp.	125	5
Butter, salted, stick	1 tsp.	40	2
Butter, lightly salted, stick	1 tsp.	40	2
Butter, unsalted, stick	1 tsp.	0	0
Butter, whipped	1 tsp.	30	1
Butter Buds®, dry	2 tsp.	170	7
Lard	1 tbsp.	0	0
Margarine, salted, stick	1 tsp.	45	2
Margarine, unsalted, stick	1 tsp.	0	0
Margarine, diet	1 tsp.	35	2
Margarine, liquid, squeeze	1 tsp.	30	1
Margarine, tub	1 tsp.	50	2
Margarine, extra light, tub	1 tsp.	15	1
Margarine, butter blend, stick, salted	1 tsp.	30	1
Molly McButter®	1/2 tsp.	90	4
Oil, vegetable, all varieties, spray	1 tbsp.	0	0
Salt pork, raw	1 oz.	405	18
Shortening, vegetable	1 tbsp.	0	0

FRUIT, FRESH, CANNED, DRIED

Apple	1	0	0
Applesauce	1/2 cup	5	0
Apples, dried, rings	10	55	2
Apricots, fresh	3	0	0
Apricots, canned	1/2 cup	5	0
Apricots, halved, dried	10 medium	5	0
Banana	1	0	0
Blueberries, fresh, frozen	1/2 cup	5	0
Cantaloupe	1 cup	15	

Food Item	Amount	Sodium mg	Points
Cherries, fresh	10	0	0
Cherries, canned	1/2 cup	5	0
Cherry, maraschino	1	0	0
Cranberries	1 cup	0	0
Cranberry sauce	1/4 cup	20	1
Dates	5	0	0
Figs	3	5	0
Fruit cocktail	1/2 cup	5	0
Grapefruit, fresh	1/2	0	0
Grapefruit, canned	1/2 cup	0	0
Grapes, fresh	1/2 cup	0	0
Honeydew melon	1 cup	35	2
Kiwi	1	5	0
Mandarin oranges, canned	1/2 cup	10	0
Nectarine	1	0	0
Orange	1	0	0
Peach, fresh	1	0	0
Peaches, canned	1/2 cup	15	1
Peaches, dried	5 halves	5	0
Pear, fresh	1	0	0
Pears, canned	1/2 cup	5	0
Pineapple, fresh	1/2 cup	0	0
Pineapple, canned	1/2 cup	0	0
Plum, fresh	1	0	0
Plums, canned	3	0	0
Prunes, canned	5	0	0
Prunes, dried	5	0	0
Raisins	1/4 cup	10	0
Raspberries	1/2 cup	0	0
Rhubarb	1/2 cup	0	0
Strawberries	1/2 cup	0	0
Tangerine	1	0	0
Watermelon	1 cup	5	0

MEAT, POULTRY, FISH, SEAFOOD

Beef, lean cuts prepared without salt

Food Item	Amount	Sodium mg	Points
Ground beef, lean	1 oz.	20	1
Prime rib	1 oz.	20	1
Roast, chuck, rib, round	1 oz.	20	1
Steak, filet, porterhouse, round, sirloin	1 oz.	20	1
Liver	1 oz.	20	1
Tongue	1 oz.	15	1

Chicken

Chicken, roasted, broiled without salt

Food Item	Amount	Sodium mg	Points
— breast	1	60	3
— drumstick	1	40	2
— thigh	1	45	2
— wing	1	15	1

Chicken, fried, with breading

Food Item	Amount	Sodium mg	Points
— breast	1	655	28
— drumstick	1	270	12
— thigh	1	515	22
— wing	1	390	17
Chicken, canned	1 oz.	145	6
Chicken liver	1 oz.	0	0

Food Item	Amount	Sodium mg	Points
Fish			
Fish, fresh, frozen	1 oz.	15	1
Fish, breaded, fried	1 oz.	85	4
Fishsticks	1	165	7
Gefilte fish	1 piece	220	10
Herring, pickled	1 piece	130	6
Lox	1 oz.	550	24
Salmon, canned	1 oz.	155	7
Sardines, canned in oil	1	60	3
Smoked fish	1 oz.	220	10
Tuna, water-packed, oil-packed	1 oz.	100	4
Tuna, low sodium	1 oz.	68	3
Tuna, no salt added	1 oz.	14	1
Lamb, lean cuts, prepared without salt			
Leg, shoulder roasts	1 oz.	20	1
Loin, rib chop	1	35	2
Pork, lean cuts, prepared without salt			
Pork chop	1 oz.	20	1
Ground pork	1 oz.	10	0
Ham	1 oz.	425	18
Liver	1 oz.	15	1
Roast: loin, rib, sirloin, shoulder blade	1 oz.	20	1
Spare ribs	1 oz.	15	1
Seafood			
Clams, fresh, frozen	1 oz.	15	1
Clams, breaded, fried	1 oz.	105	5
Clams, canned	1 oz.	30	1
Crab, fresh, frozen	1 oz.	235	10
Crab legs, imitation	1 oz.	240	10
Lobster, fresh, frozen	1 oz.	110	5
Oysters, raw, fresh	6 med.	95	4
Oysters, breaded, fried	6 med.	355	15
Oysters, canned	1 oz.	30	1
Scallops, fresh	1 oz.	45	2
Scallops, breaded, fried	1 large	70	3
Shrimp, fresh	1 oz.	40	2
Shrimp, breaded, fried	1 oz.	95	4
Shrimp, canned	1 oz.	50	2
Squid (calamari), fresh	1 oz.	15	1
Turkey, lean cuts, prepared without salt			
Turkey, fresh, white and dark meat	1 oz.	10	0
Turkey, pre-basted	1 oz.	45	2
Ground turkey	1 oz.	25	1
Turkey roll, light meat	1 oz.	140	6
Turkey roll, light and dark meat	1 oz.	165	7
Giblets	1 oz.	15	1
Gizzard	1 oz.	15	1
Heart	1 oz.	15	1
Liver	1 oz.	20	1

Food Item	Amount	Sodium mg	Points
Veal, lean cuts, prepared without salt			
Chuck, leg	1 oz.	15	1
Loin, rib, round	1 oz.	20	1
Venison, lean cuts, prepared without salt	1 oz.	15	1
Cured & Deli Meats			
Bacon	1 slice	100	4
Bacon, lower salt	1 slice	65	3
Canadian bacon	1 oz.	440	19
Chipped beef	1 oz.	985	43
Ham, deli	1 oz.	265	12
Hot dog	1	505	22
Hot dog, reduced sodium	1	300	13
Jerky, beef	1 oz.	290	13
Cured & Deli Meats			
Luncheon meat	1 oz.	315	14
Pastrami, corned beef	1 oz.	350	15
Roast beef, deli	1 oz.	290	13
Sausage:			
— Bratwurst, Polish	1	635	28
— Links	2	370	16
— Liver sausage	1 oz.	325	14
— Pepperoni	1 oz.	580	25
— Pork sausage	1 oz.	365	16
— Salami	1 oz.	525	23
— Summer sausage	1 oz.	300	13
Turkey ham	1 oz.	280	12
Turkey, deli	1 oz.	280	12
Turkey, deli, low sodium	1 oz.	20	1
Turkey, smoked	1 oz.	260	11

MIXED DISHES

Food Item	Amount	Sodium mg	Points
Beef stew, canned	1 cup	1010	44
Cabbage roll	1	385	17
Chicken a la king, canned	1 cup	725	32
Chili, canned	1 cup	1030	45
Chop suey, canned	1 cup	1055	46
Chow mein, canned	1 cup	720	31
Corned beef hash, canned	1 cup	1160	50
Lasagna, 4"x2-1/2"x1-1/2"	1 piece	1465	64
Macaroni and cheese, box mix	1 cup	870	38
Meat loaf	3 oz.	495	22
Pizza, thin crust, cheese, 1/8 of 12" diam.	1 piece	395	17
Pizza, thick crust, cheese, 1/8 of 12" diam.	1 piece	635	28
Quiche, bacon, 1/8 of 9" diam.	1 piece	465	20
Ravioli	1 cup	780	34
Sloppy Joe filling	1/3 cup	345	15
Spaghetti, canned, with meat or cheese sauce	1 cup	1175	51
Spanish rice	1 cup	940	41
Taco	1	460	20
Tuna noodle casserole	1 cup	1210	53

Food Item	Amount	Sodium mg	Poin
NOODLES, PASTA, RICE			
Noodles, pasta, rice cooked without salt	1 cup	5	0
Noodles and pasta cooked with salt	1 cup	215	9
Rice cooked with salt	1 cup	765	33
Ramen Noodles®	1 cup	980	43
Nuts, roasted, salted	1/4 cup	230	10
Nuts, roasted, unsalted	1/4 cup	5	0
Nuts, dry roasted, salted	1/4 cup	290	13
Nuts, dry roasted, unsalted	1/4 cup	5	0
Peanut butter	1 tbsp.	75	3
Peanut butter, unsalted	1 tbsp.	5	0
Seeds, salted	1 tbsp.	60	3
Seeds, unsalted	1 tbsp.	0	0
SALADS			
Carrot raisin	1/2 cup	150	7
Chef salad	2 cups	1020	44
Chicken salad	1/2 cup	460	20
Coleslaw, creamy	1/2 cup	130	6
Fruit salad	1/2 cup	5	0
Gelatin with fruit	1/2 cup	40	2
Ham salad	1/2 cup	1300	57
Pasta salad	1/2 cup	320	14
Potato salad, German	1/2 cup	175	8
Potato salad	1/2 cup	555	24
Three-bean salad	1/2 cup	305	13
Tossed salad without dressing	1 cup	5	0
Tuna and macaroni salad	1/2 cup	365	16
Tuna salad	1/2 cup	350	15
Waldorf salad	1/2 cup	130	6
Salad Dressings			
Mayonnaise	1 tbsp.	80	3
Mayonnaise, light	1 tbsp.	100	4
Mayonnaise, fat free	1 tbsp.	190	8
Salad dressing	1 tbsp.	85	4
Salad dressing, light	1 tbsp.	105	5
Salad dressing, fat free	1 tbsp.	210	9
Salad dressings:			
— Blue cheese	1 tbsp.	165	7
— French	1 tbsp.	215	9
— Italian	1 tbsp.	115	5
— Ranch	1 tbsp.	130	6
— Russian	1 tbsp.	135	6
— reduced-calorie, all kinds	1 tbsp.	145	6
— fat free or oil free, all kinds	1 tbsp.	145	6
— vinegar and oil	1 tbsp.	0	0

Food Item	Amount	Sodium mg	Points
Salad Bar Trimmings			
Bacon bits	1 tbsp.	135	6
Beets, pickled	1/4 cup	150	7
Cheese, shredded	1 tbsp.	55	2
Croutons	2 tbsp.	60	3
Garbanzo or kidney beans	1 tbsp.	25	1
Olives, black	1	50	2
Olives, green	1	155	7
Sprouts, alfalfa or bean	1/4 cup	0	0
Sunflower seeds	1 tbsp.	60	3
Sauces & Condiments			
Au jus	1/4 cup	265	12
Barbecue sauce	1 tbsp.	125	5
Catsup	1 tbsp.	170	7
Catsup, no added salt	1 tbsp.	5	0
Cheese sauce	1 tbsp.	100	4
Chili sauce	1 tbsp.	190	8
Cocktail sauce	1 tbsp.	160	7
Gravy, canned, from mix	1/4 cup	300	13
Gravy, homemade	1/4 cup	165	7
Hollandaise sauce	1/4 cup	280	12
Horseradish	1 tsp.	5	0
Mustard	1 tsp.	65	3
Pickle, dill, 4" long	1	1885	82
Pickle, dill, slice	1	95	4
Pickle, sweet, slice	1	45	2
Pickle relish	1 tbsp.	105	5
Pizza sauce, canned	1/4 cup	350	15
Salsa	1 tbsp.	155	7
Soy sauce	1 tsp.	345	15
Soy sauce, reduced-sodium	1 tsp.	200	9
Spaghetti sauce	1/2 cup	560	24
Spaghetti sauce, low-sodium	1/2 cup	20	1
Steak sauce	1 tbsp.	275	12
Sweet & sour sauce	1/4 cup	195	8
Tabasco	1 tsp.	35	2
Taco sauce	1 tbsp.	155	7
Tartar sauce	1 tbsp.	100	4
Teriyaki sauce	1 tbsp.	690	30
Tomato paste	1 tbsp.	130	6
Tomato paste, no added salt	1 tbsp.	10	0
Tomato sauce	1/4 cup	370	16
Tomato sauce, no added salt	1/4 cup	20	1
White sauce	1/4 cup	210	9
Worcestershire sauce	1 tsp.	60	3

Food Item	Amount	Sodium mg	Poin
Seasonings			
Accent®	1 tsp.	615	27
Garlic salt	1 tsp.	2050	89
Garlic salt, light	1 tsp.	340	15
Kitchen Bouquet®	1 tsp.	20	1
Lemon pepper	1 tsp.	575	25
Meat tenderizer	1 tsp.	1760	77
Onion salt	1 tsp.	1585	69
Onion salt, light	1 tsp.	305	13
Salt	1 tsp.	2300	100
Salt, lite	1 tsp.	975	42
Salt substitute	1 tsp.	0	0
Sea salt	1 tsp.	2300	100
Seasoned salt	1 tsp.	1485	65
Wine, cooking	1/4 cup	5	0
Baking Ingredients			
Baking powder	1 tsp.	425	18
Baking soda	1 tsp.	950	41
Bisquick®	1 cup	1705	74
Brewer's yeast	1 tbsp.	10	0
Chocolate, baking, unsweetened	1 oz.	0	0
Chocolate chips, milk chocolate	1/2 cup	105	5
Chocolate chips, semi-sweet	1/2 cup	10	0
Coating mix	1 pkg.	30	2
Cornmeal, self-rising	1 cup	1755	76
Flour	1 cup	0	0
Flour, self-rising	1 cup	1310	57
Oat bran	1 tbsp.	0	0
Rice bran	1 tbsp.	0	0
Wheat bran	1 tbsp.	0	0
Wheat germ	1 tbsp.	0	0
SNACK FOODS			
Chex Cereal Party Mix®	1 cup	360	16
Cheese puffs (1 oz = 36 puffs)	1 oz.	330	14
Corn chips (1 oz = 14 chips)	1 oz.	200	9
Corn chips, unsalted	1 oz.	30	1
Popcorn:			
— airpopped, unbuttered, no added salt	1 cup	0	0
— caramel corn	1 cup	105	5
— commercial, butter with salt added	1 cup	80	3
Popcorn, microwaved			
— natural, butter-flavored	1 cup	115	5
— light	1 cup	55	2
— salt-free	1 cup	0	0
Popcorn, popped in oil, salted	1 cup	130	6
Potato chips (1 oz = 16 chips)	1 oz.	250	11
Potato chips, light	1 oz.	155	7
Potato chips, unsalted	1 oz.	20	1
Shoestring potatoes	3/4 cup	70	3
Pretzels, sticks	10	60	3
Pretzels, twists	1	80	3
Pretzels, unsalted	1 oz.	30	1

Food Item	Amount	Sodium mg	Points
SOUPS			
Beef bouillon cube	1	865	38
Chicken bouillon cube	1	1150	50
Bouillon granules	1 tsp.	960	42
Bouillon granules, low sodium	1 tsp.	5	0
Broth, diluted with water	1 cup	640	28
Onion soup mix, dry	1 pkg.	3495	152
Soups, canned			
— broth-based, diluted with water	1 cup	895	39
— cream-based, diluted with water	1 cup	970	42
— cream-based, diluted with milk	1 cup	1025	45
— reduced-sodium (1/3 less salt) diluted with water	1 cup	540	23
— low sodium, ready-to-serve	1 cup	35	2
— condensed cream soup, undiluted	1 can	2245	98
SWEETS			
Candy			
Candy bar	2 oz.	115	5
Candy bar, snack size	1	45	2
Caramels	4	85	4
Chocolate covered cream	1/2 oz.	25	1
Fudge, 1" cube	1	25	1
Granola bar®	1	80	3
Hard candy	5	10	0
Hershey Kisses®	4	20	1
Jelly beans	10	5	0
Licorice, 7" long	1	30	1
M&M's®, plain	1 pkg.	35	2
M&M's®, peanut	1 pkg.	30	1
Mints, chocolate covered	1	20	1
Sweeteners			
Honey	1 tbsp.	0	0
Jam, jelly, preserves, regular, unsweetened	1 tsp.	0	0
Molasses	1 tbsp.	5	0
Sugar, white, brown, powdered	1 tsp.	0	0
Sugar substitutes	1 pkg.	0	0
Syrup			
Corn	1 tbsp.	15	1
Maple	1 tbsp.	0	0
Pancake or waffle	1 tbsp.	15	1
Pancake or waffle, reduced-sugar	1 tbsp.	35	2
Toppings			
Caramel	1 tbsp.	30	1
Chocolate	1 tbsp.	10	0
Fudge	1 tbsp.	40	2
Strawberry	1 tbsp.	5	0

Food Item	Amount	Sodium mg	Poi
VEGETABLES, FRESH, FROZEN, CANNED			
Artichoke, fresh	1	80	
Asparagus spears	4	0	
Asparagus, canned	1/2 cup	470	2
Avocado	1	20	
Bamboo shoots	1/2 cup	5	
Beans, green, yellow, Italian	1/2 cup	10	
Beans, green or waxed, canned	1/2 cup	170	
Beets	1/2 cup	40	
Beets, regular, canned	1/2 cup	115	
Beets, pickled, canned	1/2 cup	300	1
Broccoli	1/2 cu	15	
Brussels sprouts	1/2 cup	20	
Cabbage	1/2 cup	5	
Carrots	1/2 cup	35	
Carrots, canned	1/2 cup	175	
Cauliflower	1/2 cup	10	
Celery, diced	1/2 cup	55	
Corn	1/2 cup	5	
Corn-on-the-cob	1	15	
Corn, whole kernel, canned	1/2 cup	265	1
Corn, cream-style, canned	1/2 cup	365	1
Cucumber	1/2 cup	0	
Eggplant	1/2 cup	0	
Endive	1/2 cup	5	
Escarole	1/2 cup	5	
Greens: collard, kale, mustard, etc.	1/2 cup	20	
Jicama	1/2 cup	5	
Lettuce	1/2 cup	0	
Lima beans	1/2 cup	45	
Mixed vegetables, frozen, no sauce	1/2 cup	30	
Mixed vegetables, canned	1/2 cup	120	
Mushrooms, fresh	1/2 cup	0	
Mushrooms, canned	1/2 cup	330	1
Okra	1/2 cup	5	
Onions	1/2 cup	5	
Onions, canned	1/2 cup	415	1
Parsnips	1/2 cup	10	
Peas, fresh	1/2 cup	5	
Peas, frozen	1/2 cup	70	
Peas, canned	1/2 cup	185	
Peapods	1/2 cup	5	
Peppers, green, red, yellow	1/2 cup	0	
Peppers, chili	1/2 cup	5	
Pumpkin	1/2 cup	5	
Pumpkin, canned	1/2 cup	5	
Pumpkin pie filling, canned	1/2 cup	280	1
Radishes	1/2 cup	15	
Rutabaga	1/2 cup	15	
Sauerkraut	1/2 cup	780	3
Spinach, raw	1/2 cup	20	
Spinach, frozen	1/2 cup	80	
Spinach, canned	1/2 cup	210	
Squash, summer	1/2 cup	0	

Food Item	Amount	Sodium mg	Points
Squash, winter	1/2 cup	0	0
Succotash, canned	1/2 cup	285	12
Sweet potatoes, fresh	1/2 cup	15	1
Sweet potatoes, candied, canned	1/2 cup	220	10
Swiss chard	1/2 cup	155	7
Tomatoes, fresh	1	5	0
Tomatoes, whole, canned	1/2 cup	195	8
Tomatoes, stewed, canned	1/2 cup	325	14
Turnips, fresh	1/2 cup	40	2
Water chestnuts	1/2 cup	10	0
Zucchini	1/2 cup	0	0

Potatoes

Potatoes, fresh

— Baked or boiled, prepared without salt	1 medium	5	0
— French fries	20	10	0
— Hash browns	1/2 cup	5	0
— Mashed, without salt	1/2 cup	20	1
— Mashed, with salt	1/2 cup	310	13

Potatoes, frozen

— Cottage fries	1/2 cup	40	2
— French fries	10 pieces	70	3
— Hash browns	1/2 cup	55	2
— Tater Tots	10	590	26

Potato Mixes

— Au gratin	1/2 cup	600	26
— Hash browns	1/2 cup	460	20
— Mashed potatoes	1/2 cup	340	15
— Scalloped potatoes	1/2 cup	465	20

BEANS, LENTILS, PEAS, FRESH

Beans, cooked from dry, all kinds	1/2 cup	5	0
Black-eye peas, cooked	1/2 cup	5	0
Lentils, cooked	1/2 cup	0	0
Split peas, cooked	1/2 cup	0	0

Beans & peas, canned

Baked beans, with meat	1/2 cup	555	24
Baked beans, without meat	1/2 cup	215	9
Beans, kidney or chili	1/2 cup	215	9
Black-eye peas	1/2 cup	360	16
Refried beans	1/2 cup	535	23
Tofu (soybean curd)	1/2 cup	10	0

NUTRITIONAL CONSIDERATIONS FOR SPECIFIC PEDIATRIC CONDITIONS

Cystic Fibrosis

Cystic Fibrosis (CF) is an inherited genetic disease with clinical symptoms due to altered function of the exocrine glands. The saliva, sweat, and mucus producing glands produce a thick, sticky mucus instead of normal thin secretions while the sweat contains an abnormally high concentration of salt. Complications develop due to the obstruction of body organs and ducts by the thick mucus. Primary complications are caused by obstructions of the pulmonary system leading to chronic obstructive lung disease and chronic and acute lung infections, and obstruction of the pancreas and gastrointestinal tract which results in maldigestion and malabsorption, particularly of fat-soluble vitamins, and nitrogen.

Treatment is directed toward control of the 1) pulmonary obstructive process; 2) pulmonary infection, and 3) pancreatic and nutritional deficiencies. Treatment consists of chest physical therapy, aerosol inhalation, antibiotics, exercise, pancreatic enzyme replacement, vitamin supplementation, and a high calorie, high protein diet.

Nutrition is of prime importance in the treatment of the CF patient. Malnutrition contributes to pulmonary complication, susceptibility to infection, poor growth and decreased energy and motivation.

A well balanced diet with increased calorie, protein and vitamin intake is need to offset malabsorption losses, a general increase in metabolic rate, and an increase expenditure of energy during chest therapy, labored respiration, and periods of infection and fever.

Good nutritional habits as well as consistent growth, weight gain and/or weight maintenance are the primary goals of nutrition therapy for the CF patient. Normal ranges on the NCHS growth curves are used as guidelines for the CF infant and child while ideal weights for height are the guidelines for the older CF child or adult.

Nutritional therapy consists of:
- High calorie, high protein diet.
- Replacement of pancreatic digestive enzymes with all meals and snacks.
- Vitamin/mineral supplementation to maintain normal serum levels or prevent deficiency. Fat soluble vitamins in a water miscible form are generally prescribed.
- Liberal use of table salt to replace NaCl lost in sweat, especially during times of extremely hot weather, strenuous exercise, or febrile illness.

The diet for CF should be well balanced with emphasis on increased caloric and protein intake. A child or adult with CF will often need an intake of 150% of RDA for calories and 200% RDA for protein. The diet, however, should be individually adjusted to meet each patient's specific needs. Five to six meals and three snacks may be required to meet these goals. Some patients may experience a fat intolerance and may want to reduce their fat intake or limit the amount of fat within a specific meal, In general, a rigid fat restriction is avoided as fat can be a significant source of calories. Instead, additional pancreatic enzymes, or bile salts, are given to improve digestion.

Nutritional supplements are often used in addition to regular meals when a patient is having trouble gaining weight or maintaining adequate intake. At times, enteral feeding via nasal gastric tube or TPN is required to maintain adequate nutrition.

Infants with CF are usually placed on pre-digested formulas containing MCT oil. Solid foods are generally added to the infant's diet later than usual (5-6 months) and cereals should be given in reduced amounts because of the filling effect. Also, they are a less desirable source of calories and protein. Concentrating the formula or adding a glucose polymer supplement may be required to provide 24-calories per ounce formula for the infant who is not gaining weight. Infants with CF can be successfully breastfed, but must be monitored closely for weight gain.

As the CF patient population has grown older, more patients are being diagnosed with insulin-dependent diabetes. Nutritional goals for this populations are: even distribution of calories to coincide with insulin therapy, control of concentrated carbohydrates, and consistency in amount of food and timing of meals.

Adequacy
The diet can be adequate in all nutrients.

Professional References
1. Chase, HE, Long, MS, Lavin, MH. Cystic Fibrosis and malnutrition. J Pediatr 1979; 95:337.
2. Consensus Conferences Concepts in Care: Nutrition Assessment and Management in Cystic Fibrosis. CF Foundation 1992.
3. Creveling, S, Light, M, Gardner, P, Greene, L. Cystic Fibrosis, nutrition and the health care team. *Ped Nutr* 1994; 18(3).
4. Holliday, KE, Allen, JR, Waters, DL, *et al.* Growth of human milk-fed and formula-fed infants with cystic fibrosis. *J Pediatr* 1991; 118:77-79.
5. Moore, MC, Green, HL, Donald, WD, *et al.* Enteral tube feeding as adjunct therapy in malnourished patients with CF: A clinical study and literature review. *Am J Clin Nutr* 1986; 44:33-41.
6. Ramsey, B, Farrell, P, Penshcarz, P. Nutritional assessment and management in Cystic Fibrosis: Consensus conference. *Am J Clin Nutr* 1992; 55:108-116.
7. *Seminars in Pediatric Gastroenterology and Nutrition.* Cystic Fibrosis. Summer, 1993; vol 4:no 2.
8. Stark, L, Knapp, L, Bowen, A. Increasing calorie consumption in children with cystic fibrosis: Replication with 2 year follow-up. *J Appl Beh Analysis* 1993; 26:435-450.
9. Tomezsko, J, Stallings, V, Scanlin, T. Dietary intake of healthy children with cystic fibrosis compared with normal control children. *Pediatrics* 1992; 90:547-553.

Failure to Thrive

Description

The term Failure to Thrive (FTT) describes an infant or child whose weight is less than the fifth percentile on standard growth charts, or whose growth pattern has dropped more than two major percentile groups over a 3-6 month period. If the FTT becomes a chronic situation, the height and then head circumference begin to drop from the established curve.

Prolonged FTT leads to lasting deficits in growth and development, therefore early identification and intervention is essential.

Etiology

The etiology of FTT has been divided into organic and non-organic categories. However, current findings suggest that this classic division may be clinically inadequate and overly simplified. Most often FTT presents with some type of mixed etiology, rarely being either organic or non-organic.

Organic FTT may be a symptom of or secondarily result from pediatric diseases which may include: Genetic, congenital, and chromosomal abnormalities; gastrointestinal, cardiac, pulmonary, renal, and neurologic diseases; as well as other miscellaneous conditions which include: Chronic infection, intrauterine growth retardation, fetal alcohol syndrome and anemia.

Non-organic FTT is multifactorial in etiology. It typically includes one, or some combination, of these factors:

- **disordered feeding interactions** between parent and child resulting in inadequate intake and retention of calories. This frequently focuses on the mother as she is often the primary feeder. However, interactions with other feeders must be reviewed as well.
- **disordered non-feeding interactions** which primarily focuses on neglect of a child's emotional needs.
- **stressful social environment/dysfunctional family,** which may include poverty, poor parenting skills, marital stress, and/or chronic illness in immediate or related family members.
- **Individual temperament.** Quite often the child is perceived as picky or difficult, and frequently presents with inconsistent, strong-willed, or withdrawn behaviors, further complicating the parent-child interaction. Parental temperament may play into this to a little or great extent.

Incidence

Failure to Thrive presents in 80% of cases before the age of 18 months and accounts for 1-5% of all pediatric hospitalizations.

Diagnosis

History, physical examination, and review of growth history are the primary tools for diagnosis. Laboratory studies are then ordered based on signs or symptoms gained from the history and physical as an evaluation for organic cause for FTT. The growth failure is further defined by anthropometric measurements such as: weight for age, height for age, and weight to height ratio.

Given the prevalence of non-organic causes or contributions to FTT, a problem-oriented multidisciplinary approach that includes: Medical, nutritional, social and behavioral-interactional assessments should be part of the initial diagnostic work-up.

Nutritionist's Role in Diagnosis Nutrition History

Past history: breast vs. bottle fed, formula(s) and method of preparation, age at introduction to solids, eating skills development.

Present: 24 hour recall &/or a 3 day food record, daily eating pattern, food preferences, and use of vitamin/mineral or nutritional supplements.

Eating environment: identifying the primary feeder(s) and assessing their knowledge of nutrition, and determining whether a child typically eats alone or with others.

Assessment

Diet should be assessed for adequacy of calories, protein, calcium, iron, zinc, and general balance. Daily eating pattern should be assessed for these common problems seen in children of toddler age with FTT:

- excess caloric liquids, especially juice, in the diet. Juice intake greater than 4-8 oz./day and/or milk intake greater than 20 oz./day can result in a decrease in solid food intake, overall daily calories, and inadequate nutrient intake.
- continual nibbling of foods or sipping of liquids throughout the day, or continued nighttime feedings when the child is past 12 months of age, appears to interrupt a child's hunger pattern and result in decreased daily calories.
- Growth should be assessed by plotting past and current growth data on a standard growth chart and calculating ideal body weight (IBW) and weight/height ratio. (See Nutrition Assessment section for these calculations.)

The finding of low weight for age alone suggests acute malnutrition (wasting), while depressed height for age suggests chronic malnutrition (stunting). Children at highest risk are those for whom both weight for height and height for age are deficient, indicating acute malnutrition superimposed upon chronic.

Management of Failure to Thrive

The initial goals of treatment for Failure to Thrive are:
-medical stabilization
-nutritional rehabilitation
-social intervention and developmental stimulation

Nutritional Rehabilitation

The nutritional goal of therapy for all stages of FTT is catch-up growth which is 2-3 times the average rate of gain.

I. Estimating Energy, Protein, Vitamin and Mineral Needs

A. Estimating energy needs

Differing methods are cited for estimating energy needs for catch-up growth.

1. Energy needs(kcal/kg) = [RDA kcal/kg for weight age X IBW (kg)] ÷ [actual weight (kg)] where wt. age is the age at which present weight would be 50th%.
2. Energy needs (kcal/kg) = [120 cal/kg X median wt.(kg) for current ht] ÷ [actual weight (kg)]
3. Murray and Glassman cite that many children with FTT will not gain weight unless intakes are in excess of 150 cal/kg. They suggest catch-up energy needs begin at that level and be adjusted upward to achieve a weight gain of 30 gm/day for infants and 60-90 gm/day in young children. Which ever method is used, it is important to continually monitor weight and adjust calorie goals as necessary.

B. Estimating protein needs
Protein needs are estimated at 1.5-2 times the RDA for age. Quite often this is
2-2.5 grams protein/kg/day.

C. Estimating vitamin and mineral needs
Vitamin and mineral needs are based on the RDA for age. Deficiencies of vitamins and minerals, especially iron and zinc, are so common that unless a child is to begin a formula supplement, a routine part of nutritional rehabilitation is to begin a complete children's multivitamin that contains iron and zinc.

D. Special considerations
A severely malnourished child may be at risk for Refeeding Syndrome as rehabilitation is begun. This may require less than basal calories to begin with and advanced slowly until the child is metabolically stable.

II. Education of the parent/caregiver(s) for appropriate high calorie nutrition for the child.
This should include:
- encouraging high calorie, high protein foods. (See the High Calorie, High Protein suggestion sheet in this manual.) Some children will eat the amount of food needed to meet desired calorie intake, however, in many cases, use of a 24-30 cal/oz. supplement will be needed. Whole milk fortified with powdered milk or instant breakfast powder, pediatric 30 cal/oz. supplement, or concentrated infant formula (e.g. 24 or 27 cal/oz.) can be used. Besides nutrient composition, the family's budget and medical insurance should be considered when deciding on a supplement.
- encouraging a balanced diet. Children that consume excess caloric liquids should be limited to 4 oz. of juice/day and 16 oz. milk/day. Keep in mind, however, that calories and protein are the key to therapy, not a broad variety of foods.
- consistent daily eating pattern of 3 meals and 2-3 planned snacks, and discouraging continual nibbling of foods and sipping of liquids.
- daily multivitamin with iron and zinc.

III. Monitoring intake and tolerance of rehabilitation. Calorie Counts/Food Records may used both inpatient and outpatient. Accuracy of outpatient records will depend on the motivation of the feeder(s). Records may used for inpatient as well as outpatient though accuracy will depend on the motivation of feeder(s).

IV. Follow-up of patients with FTT is an essential part of management. Continued nutritional counseling including weight checks and periodic food record assessment, along with treatment for disordered feeding and non-feeding interactions, as well as social problems are often needed for an extended period of time. Frequent height and weight measurement provides the most important indicator of progress, ideally leading to a return to normal weight and height velocities over time.

Professional references

1. Hendricks KM, Walker WA: Manual of Pediatric Nutrition 2nd ed. B.C. Decker Inc.: Toronto/Philadelphia 1990; 68: 160-164.
2. Frank DA, Zeisel SH: Failure to Thrive. Pediatric Clinics of North America. Dec. 1988; 35(6): 1187-1206.
3. Peterson KE, Rathbun JM: Nutrition in Failure to Thrive as found in: Pediatric Nutrition in Theory and Practice. Grand RJ, Sutphen JL, Dietz WH (eds.)Butterworth: Stoneham. 1987 pp. 421, 627-637.
4. Frank DA et al: Failure to Thrive: Mystery, myth, and method. Contemporary
5. Pediatrics Feb. 1993 pp. 114-123.
   Bithoney WG et al: Failure to Thrive/Growth Deficiency. Pediatrics in Review. Dec. 1993; 13(12): 453-460.
6. Ekvall SW: Pediatric Nutrition in Chronic Diseases and Development Disorders. Oxford University Press: New York. 1993 183-188.
7. Rathbun JM, Peterson KE: Nutrition in Failure to Thrive as found in: Grand RJ, Sutphen JL, Dietz WH (eds.). Pediatric Nutrition. Boston: Butterworths. 1987.
8. Gomez F et al: Mortality in second and third degree malnutrition. J Trop Pediatr 1956; 2:77.
9. Waterlow JC: Some aspects of childhood malnutrition as a public health problem. BMJ 1974; 4:88.
10. Waterlow JC: Classification and definition of protein-calorie malnutrition. BMJ 1972; 3: 566.
11. Solomon SM, Kirby DF: The Refeeding Syndrome: A Review. JPEN 1990; 14(1):90
12. Smith MM, Lifshitz F: Excess Fruit Juice Consumption as a Contributing Factor in Nonorganic Failure to Thrive. Pediatrics March 1994; 93(3): 438.

High Calorie, High Protein Diet

The suggestions listed below are to give assistance in increasing the calories and protein in a child's diet. Foods high in sugar and fat do have calories which may be helpful for weight gain but they have "empty" calories (i.e. low nutrient density).

A good rule of thumb is to provide foods from all of the basic food groups first before adding high sugar/high fat foods or to combine fats and sweets with other nutritious foods.

- Eat more often (3 meals and 3-4 snacks)
- Offer whole milk with meals
- Use fortified milk (1 cup non-fat dry milk added to 1 quart whole milk) as a beverage or in cooking
- Use cream or non-dairy creamer in cooking
- Add additional margarine, cream cheese, sour cream, or cheese to potatoes, macaroni, rice, cooked cereal, vegetables, scrambled eggs, casseroles, etc.
- If appropriate for age, add dried fruits or chopped nuts to foods.
- Use bread or cracker coatings on meats, poultry, or fish
- Serve yogurt, graham crackers with peanut butter, or puddings as dessert
- Add non-fat dry milk to foods or drinks, up to 8 tablespoons/day
- Offer higher calorie starch choices such as: au gratin or scalloped potatoes, tater tots, pancakes, french toast or waffles (margarine or syrup can be added), muffins or banana bread, bagel with cream cheese
- High calorie supplements may be offered as a beverage. Available from grocery stores are Sport Shake and Instant Breakfast. Available from pharmacies are a variety of complete nutritional supplements. These are listed in the Enteral nutrition section. These supplements should be used with guidance from your child's dietitian, doctor, or nurse.
- For milk intolerant children try soy cheese, soy based ice cream, or tofu.

Snack suggestions

Limit sweets such as fruit-flavored drinks, pop, candy, cookies, gelatin, and popsicles. Sweet foods such as these can suppress the appetite and are low in nutrients. Try the following snacks, and see the recipes on the following page:

Cheese slices or cubes	Fruit yogurt as a snack itself
Pudding/custard	or as a dip for fruit
Cottage cheese with fruit	Yogurt-sicles (freeze yogurt
Muffins	in popsicle tray)
Banana, pumpkin or other	Cheese or peanut butter on
quick breads	bread or crackers
Sandwiches	Yogurt-juice drinks
Cereal Mix- see recipes	Commercial Eggnog

Special hints

- Make mealtime a relaxed time
- Eat family meals together so the child can observe others eating
- Have a quiet time to relax before eating
- Praise the child for eating well
- Avoid negative comments about foods disliked
- Space meals and snacks two to three hours apart
- Finger foods cut in different shapes may be appealing

High-Calorie, High-Protein Recipes
#1—Fortified Milk

1 cup nonfat dry milk powder	1 quart whole milk

Mix well and chill before using. Use this in place of regular milk for drinking and cooking. One cup provides 220 calories; 15 grams protein.

#2—Strawberry/Banana Yogurt Shake

1/2 cup strawberries	1/2 cup fortified milk
1/2 cup plain yogurt	1 tbsp. sugar
1/2 banana	

Combine ingredients in blender and blend until smooth, about 30 seconds. Pour into tall glass. Provides 330 calories; 17 grams protein.

#3—Chocolate Milk Shake

1/4 cup chocolate syrup	1-1/2 cups ice cream
1/2 cup nonfat milk powder	1/2 cup fortified milk

Combine ingredients in blender and blend until smooth. Makes approximately cups. One-half of this recipe, or approximately one cup, provides 415 calories; 15 grams protein.

#4—Sherbet Shake

1 cup sherbet	3/4 cup fortified milk

Blend ingredients in blender until smooth. Provides 400 calories; 14 grams protein.

#5—Cheese Cookies *

3/4 cup flour	2 tbsp. butter or margarine
2 tbsp. water	3 cups (1/2 pound) grated Cheddar cheese

Preheat oven to 400 degrees. Mix all ingredients, adding more water as needed to make a stiff dough. Roll dough into small (3/4 inch) balls. Place cheese balls on cookie sheet. Bake until lightly browned (10-15 minutes). Serve warm or cold. Makes about 24 cookies; One cookie provides 60 calories; 2.7 gms protein

#6—Peanut Butter Balls *

1/2 cup peanut butter	3 tbsp. dry milk powder
2 tsp. sugar or honey+	

Combine all ingredients and roll into balls. Store in refrigerator. Yields 8 one inch balls; Each provides 108 calories; 5.5 grams protein.

#7---Cereal Mix

10 cups of any combination of the following: any unsweetened cereal, pretzels, bite-size crackers, fish-shaped crackers, sesame sticks

6 tbsp. margarine   1 tbsp. Worcestershire sauce
2 tsp. garlic powder

Heat oven to 250 degrees. Melt margarine in 13" X 9" pan. Add Worcestershire sauce and garlic powder and mix. Add 10 cups of cereal/cracker mix and stir well to coat. Heat for 45 minutes, stirring every 15 minutes. Makes 10 cups. 1/2 cup provides 125 calories; 2 grams protein.

#8---Munch Mix

1/2 cup toasted coconut   1/2 cup raisins
1/2 cup sunflower seeds   1/2 cup chocolate chips
1 cup peanuts

Mix well and store in an airtight container. Cashews, walnuts, pecans, and soy nuts, as well as various dried fruits, may be combined for this high-calorie snack. One-half cup provides 490 calories; 13 grams protein.

#9---Granola

4 cups rolled oats	1/4 cup sesame seed
1/3 cup brown sugar	1/3 cup vegetable oil
1/2 cup wheat germ	1/4 cup honey+
1/2 cup coconut	1 tsp. vanilla

Heat oven to 350 degrees. Spread rolled oats in 13" X 9" X 2" baking pan. Heat in oven 10 minutes. Remove from oven; stir in sugar, wheat germ, coconut, and sesame seed. Mix oil, honey, and vanilla. Pour into pan and stir until dry ingredients are well coated. Bake 20 to 25 minutes, stirring mixture frequently. Cool. Stir until crumbly. Store in tightly covered container. Makes 6 cups. One cup provides 250 calories; 6 grams protein.

#10---Cream Cheese Fruit Spread

1-8 oz. container strawberry cream cheese
1-10 oz. jar marshmallow creme

Mix well. Refrigerate. 1/4 cup (4 Tbsp.) provides 186 kcals; 2.4 gram protein

#11---Bean and Cheese Dip

1-13 oz. can refried beans   1-12 oz. jar processed cheese spread

Mix and microwave until heated through, stopping frequently to stir. Serve with crackers, on tortillas, in tacos, or with tortilla chips. 1/4 cup provides: 110 kcals; 6.25 grams protein.

* recipe adapted from: Practical Strategies to Increase Energy Intake; Nutrition Focus 8(2) : March/April 1993
+ honey should not be given to children under 12 months of age

Galactosemia
Description
Galactosemia is an inherited metabolic disorder of carbohydrate metabolism. There are three known enzymes necessary in the conversion of galactose to glucose:
1. Galactokinase
2. Galactose-1-phosphate uridyltransferase (GALT)
3. Uridine diphosphate galactose-4-epimerase

While elevated levels of galactose in the blood can result from a deficiency of any of the above enzymes, it is a deficiency in the GALT enzyme that results in "classic" galactosemia, the most common and most severe form. Early symptoms include prolonged jaundice, hepatomegaly, vomiting, diarrhea, lethargy, irritability, feeding problems and growth retardation. E. Coli sepsis and shock are symptoms that can be fatal in the neonatal period if untreated. Mental retardation, cataracts and cirrhosis of the liver may occur in untreated patients. Symptoms may occur at birth but more often appear at the onset of milk feeding. Despite treatment, some older patients exhibit symptoms of developmental delay, ataxia, ovarian failure or growth failure.

There are now known to be at least nine mutations in the GALT cDNA with resultant varying amounts of galactose-1-p-transferase activity. Differential diagnosis is necessary via mutation analysis and by measurement of RBC galactose-1-p-transferase activity. Need for diet therapy in all variants is unclear but is generally initiated if GALT function is less than 25% or if RBC gal-1-phosphate is greater than 2 mg/dL

Screening
Screening for galactosemia is mandatory at birth in many states.

Treatment
A diet restricted in galactose should be initiated to maintain RBC galactose -1-phosphate in the 1 to 4 mg/dL range.

Galactose Free Diet
General Considerations
Galactose is derived from the hydrolysis of lactose into glucose and galactose. Therefore, the galactose free diet must eliminate all sources of lactose. Label reading is imperative as milk and milk derivatives are added to many foods. Foods containing milk, milk products, whey, casein, caseinates, lactalbumin, or lactoglobulin must be avoided. Hydrolyzed protein may be of milk protein origin and should be avoided. Lactose is also added to some medication, spices, chewing gum and artificial sweeteners. Check with a pharmacist or food manufacturer for clarification of ingredients.

Recent research has indicated that certain fruits and vegetables may contain some soluble galactose. It remains controversial as to whether or not a restriction of these foods is necessary. This most likely should be determined on an individual basis and would be dependent on blood galactose-1-phosphate levels.

Kosher or foods labeled 'parve' are generally lactose/galactose free but must be avoided if they contain caseinates.

Dietary restrictions should be continued for life.

Adequacy

This diet is nutritionally adequate if milk substitutes* are used. Adequate calcium, riboflavin and vitamin D intakes are often difficult to maintain in the older children who fail to consume adequate amounts of the milk substitute. Supplements of these nutrients are recommended.**

*Caution should be used when referring to milk substitutes as they may be confused with non-dairy cream substitutes. Examples of appropriate milk substitutes are Isomil, Prosobee, Nutramigen etc.

**Neo Cal Glucon, a calcium supplement, contains galactose and should not be prescribed.

Recommended Client Resources

A Lactose Free Cookbook
Parents of Galactosemic Children, Inc.
(see address below)
Living with Galactosemia--A Handbook for Families, Third Edition, 1993
Metabolism Clinic
James Whitcomb Riley Hospital for Children
Indiana University School of Medicine
Send $3.00 per copy to:
I.U.P.U.I. Bookstores
1830 West 16th Street
Indianapolis, IN 46202

Parents Guide to the Galactose Restricted Diet
Bureau of Public Health Nutrition
California State Department of Public Health
2151 Berkeley Way
Berkeley, CA 94704

Parents of Galactosemic Children--A Nationwide Organization
2871 Stage Coach Dr.
Valley Springs, CA 95252

Understanding Galactosemia: A Diet Guide
Lori Hartz, M.S. R.D.
Kimberly Pettis, R.D.
Sandy van Calcar, M.S. R.D.
August 1995
Biochemical Genetics Program
University of Wisconsin

References

1. Acosta PB, Yannicelli S: The Ross Metabolic Formula System Nutrition Support Protocols: Ross Labs, Columbus Ohio. 1993. 253-273.
2. Gross KC, Acosta PB: Fruits and vegetables are a source of galactose: Implications in planning the diets of patients with galactosemia. Journal of Inherited Metabolic Disorders 1991: 14:253-258.
3. Segal S: The challenge of galactosemia. International Pediatrics.1993: 8:125-132.
4. Waggoner DD, Buist N: Long-term complications in treated galactosemia: 175 US cases: International Pediatrics: 1993: 8-97-100.
5. Wenz E: Galactosemia in Pediatric Nutrition in Chronic Diseases and Developmental Disorders edited by Ekvall S: New York: Oxford Press: 1993:363-367.

Phenylketonuria

Description

Phenylketonuria (PKU) is an inherited metabolic disorder characterized by the inability to metabolize the amino acid phenylalanine to tyrosine. This defect is due to the absence or decreased activity of the liver enzyme phenylalanine hydroxylase. Phenylalanine and its' alternate metabolites accumulate in the blood, urine and other body tissues. Symptoms of untreated PKU are detectable between 3 to 6 months of age and include mental retardation, eczema, growth retardation, microcephaly, abnormal EEG with seizures, a musty odor and hyperkinesis.

Mandatory screening programs in most states have made it possible to detect PKU shortly after birth and initiate diet therapy before 3 weeks of age. Early diet therapy is necessary to prevent irreversible brain damage. The goal of the diet is to reduce the serum phenylalanine level to between 2 and 6 mg/dL (Normal=0.8 mg/dL).

Overview of Diet

Since phenylalanine is an essential amino acid necessary for normal growth and development, the diet of a patient with PKU must contain some phenylalanine. The amount of phenylalanine that is tolerated varies depending on enzyme activity, age and growth rate. Diets need to be calculated and monitored on an individual basis. In addition to phenylalanine, attention must be given to tyrosine, which becomes an essential amino acid, protein and calories. Requirements for these nutrients are assessed by frequent evaluation of serum phenylalanine and tyrosine levels, height and weight development, and analysis of actual dietary intake. An elevated serum phenylalanine usually indicates ingestion of too much phenylalanine secondary to over prescription, eating more than the prescribed amount, or misunderstanding of the diet. It may also be due to tissue catabolism secondary to acute infections or inadequate intake of phenylalanine, protein or calories. An inadequate intake of these nutrients will usually be accompanied by weight loss or failure to gain weight.

In order to restrict phenylalanine, high protein foods such as meat, dairy products, eggs, poultry, fish, nuts and legumes are eliminated from the diet. In order to provide adequate protein, especially the essential amino acids other than phenylalanine, semi-synthetic formulas have been developed (see enteral nutrition section). Some of these formulas contain small amounts of phenylalanine while others are phenylalanine-free. The protein to calorie ratio varies from formula to formula as does the concentration of vitamins and minerals. Without these products, it is not possible to maintain an adequate protein intake. Considerations for formula selection include nutrient needs and palatability.

Since the formula alone will not supply the amount of phenylalanine required by the patient, phenylalanine must be added to the diet in the form of food. Infants are given a specified amount of infant formula or breast milk that is mixed directly in their PKU formula. Breast feeding can be used as the supplement, however, it requires more careful monitoring. As the infant advances to solids, the amount of normal infant formula or breast milk gradually decreases and is replaced by a daily "allowance" of phenylalanine from foods. The allowance may be expressed in mg of phenylalanine or exchanges (1 exchange =15 mg of phenylalanine). Food lists have been developed for menu planning (see client resources). Since phenylalanine is a part of all protein, it is found in any food containing protein. The only "free" foods are pure sugars or fats. Special low protein foods such as pastas, cookies, bread and baking mixes have been developed to increase variety and are essential in meeting calorie needs.

Diet prescriptions for the volume of formula and phenylalanine allowance are determined on an individual basis by the dietitian and physician.

The following guidelines for nutrient requirements were developed from data collected by the PKU Collaborative Study, literature review, and through clinical experience at the University of Minnesota Metabolic Clinic to assist in planning PKU diets. They are merely guidelines and each patient should be carefully monitored and dietary changes made as necessary.

AGE	PHENYLALANINE mg/kg/day	PROTEIN* gm/kg/day	Energy kCal/kg/day
0-6 mo	25-60	3	110-120
6 mo-1 yr	25-40	2.5	110-105
1-3 yr	20-40	25 to 30 gm total	900-1800 total
4-6 yr	20-4015-35	30 to 40 gm total	1300-2300 total
7-10 yr	15-30	35 to 45 gm total	1650-3300 total
Females:			
11-14 yr	10-25	45 to 50 gm total	1500-3000 total
15-19 yr	10-20	45 to 50 gm total	1200-3000 total
Males:			
11-14 yr	10-25	55 to 60 gm total	2000-3700 total
15-19 yr	10-20	55 to 60 gm total	2100-3900 total

Recommendations for Pregnancy

Trimester and Age	PHE mg/day	Protein gm/day	KCal avg/day
Trimester 1:			
15-19 yrs	200-820	76	2500
19-24 yrs	180-800	74	2500
≥ 24 yrs	180-800	5.1-7.4 74	2500
Trimester 2:			
15-19 yrs	200-1000	76	2500
19-24 yrs	180-1000	74	2500
≥ 24 yrs	180-1000	5.1-7.4 74	2500
Trimester 3:			
15-19 yrs	330-1200	76	2500
19-24 yrs	310-1200	74	2500
≥ 24 yrs	310-1200	5.1-7.4 74	2500

*protein needs of individuals with PKU are recommended to be higher than normal. It is believed that when a formula is derived from casein hydrolysates or L-amino acids, as are PKU formulas, the nitrogen requirement increases.

Diet for Life

Discontinuing the diet therapy of PKU patients is a much debated issue. During the past fifteen years, metabolic clinics have been maintaining diet therapy during adolescence and young adulthood. Several reasons for this change in therapy are the unknown effects of elevated serum phenylalanine levels on normal intellectual and neurologic functioning and the more known harmful effects of elevated serum phenylalanine on the fetuses of pregnant PKU females.

Maintaining the diet for a longer period of time has led to the need for greater education programs that encourage the PKU patient to accept responsibility for his or her own diet therapy.

Client Resources

Food Value Lists and Cookbooks

1. Chef Lophe's PHE-Nominal Cookbook
   Barr, L, Trahms, C. 1988
   Child development and Mental Retardation Center
   U of Washington, Seattle, WA 98195

2. International PKU Recipe Book
   Barton, S. Portnoir, P. 1992
   Scientific Hospital Supplies Inc.
   1-800-365-7354

3. Low Protein Bread Machine Baking for PKU
   Schuett, V. 1993
   Plaid Printing, Seattle WA
   available from Dietary Specialties
   1-800-544-0099

4. Low Protein Cookery for Phenylketonuria
   Schuett, V. 1988
   U of Wisconsin Press
   608-262-8782

5. Low Protein Food List for PKU
   Schuett, V. 1995
   Available from Dietary Specialties
   1-800-544-0099

6. Phe for Three
   Evans, J, Prince, A, Huntington, K. 1992
   Nutrition Section
   Child Development and Rehab Center 0HSU
   PO Box 574
   Portland OR 97207

General Information

1. Education of Students with Phenylketonuria
   US Department of Health and Human Services
   NIH Publication #92-3318,1991

2. Living with PKU, 1989
   Mead Johnson publication #LB122-3-89
   Written by Inherited Metabolic Disease Clinic
   U of Colorado Health Science Center

3. National PKU News
   Schuett, V. editor
   6869 Woodlawn Ave. NE #116
   Seattle Washington 98115-5469

National Support Groups

1. Children's PKU Network
   8388 Vickers St. Suite 113
   San Diego, CA 92111
   619-233-3202

2. New England PKU Connection
   508-261-1291

Sources of Low Protein Foods

1. Dietary Specialties
   PO Box 227
   Rochester, NY 14601
   1-800-544-0099

2. Ener-G Foods, Inc.
   5960 1st Ave S.
   PO Box 84488
   Seattle, Washington 98124-5787
   1-800-3259788

3. Med-Diet, Inc.
   3050 Ranchview Lane
   Plymouth MN 55447
   1-800-633-3438

Professional References

1. Acosta PB, Austin V, Castiglioni L, Michals-Matalon K, Rohr F, Wenz E. Protocol for Nutrition Support of Maternal Phenylketonuria. Maternal PKU Collaborative Study. Los Angeles. 1992.
2. Acosta P, Yannicelli S. Phenylketonuria-Protocol 1. in Nutrition Support Protocols, The Ross Metabolic Formula System. 1-56. Ross Labs. Columbus, Ohio. 1993.
3. Azen et al. Intellectual Development in 12-Year-Old Children Treated for Phenylketonuria. AJDC. 1991. 145:35-39.
4. Hunt M, Berry H. Phenylketonuria. in Ekvall S (ed) Pediatric Nutrition in Chronic Diseases and Developmental Disorders. 327-334. Oxford University Press. NY. Oxford. 1993.
5. Koch R, Wenz E. Phenylketonuria. in Dietary Management of Metabolic Disorders. 10-16. Mead Johnson publication #L-B168-7-91. Evansville, IN. 1991.
6. Matalon K, Matalon R. Nutrition Support of Infants, Children and Adolescents with Phenylketonuria. Ross Metabolic Currents. Vol 2 No 2. 1989.
7. Medical Research Council Working Party on PKU. Phenylketonuria due to Phenylalanine Hydroxylase Deficiency: An Unfolding Story. BMJ. 309:115-119. 1993.
8. Recommendations in the Dietary Management of PKU: Report of the Medical Research Council Working Party on PKU London England. Archives of Disease in Childhood. 68:426-427. 1993
9. Yannicelli S, Davidson A, vanDoorninck W. Nutrition Support for the Late-Treated Adult with Phenylketonuria. Ross Metabolic Currents. vol 3 No 1. 1990.

Nutritional Management of Infants and Children with Renal Disease

The goal of nutritional management of infants and children with renal disease is to provide adequate nutrition to promote optimal growth and development while minimizing the metabolic imbalances caused by the disease process. These imbalances may include uremia, acidosis, serum calcium and phosphorus imbalances, hyperparathyroidism, hyperkalemia, hypertension, sodium and fluid retention and altered iron metabolism.

The success of nutritional therapy is often influenced by:
- patient's age
- patient's age at disease onset
- degree of renal function
- medical/pharmacological management
- psychosocial and economic issues.

Therapy needs to be individualized, dependent upon the patient's:
- age and development
- medical/pharmacological management
- degree of renal function
- if receiving dialysis, type of dialysis.

Nutritional Needs

Infants

Predialysis
If GFR > 15% = minimum RDA calories and protein for statural age.
If GFR < 15% = minimum RDA calories for statural age; protein = 1.5 - 1.6 gm/kg, or 9.12 kcal/cm and .15 gm protein/cm.

Hemodialysis
RDA calories and protein for statural age.

Continuous Cyclic Peritoneal Dialysis
RDA calories for statural age, and protein at 2.5 - 3 gm/kg.

Continuous Ambulatory Peritoneal Dialysis
RDA calories for statural age, and protein at 3 - 4 gm/kg.

Children and Adolescents

Predialysis
If GFR > 15% = minimum of RDA calories and protein for height and age.
If GFR < 15% = minimum of RDA for calories and maximum of RDA protein for height and age.

Hemodialysis
Minimum RDA for calories and RDA of protein for height and age.

CCPD and CAPD
Minimum RDA for calories, *consider glucose calories absorbed from dialysate*, and protein above RDA for height and age, usually .5 - 1 gm additional.

Restrict phosphorous, sodium, potassium, and fluid as necessary. Formulas of choice for infants with renal disease are low in renal solute load and phosphorous.

Supplement vitamins and minerals as needed. Dialysis patients will need to be supplemented with water soluble vitamins, B complex, C, and folic acid, due to dialysate losses. Active vitamin D and calcium supplements are generally prescribed. Aluminum containing phosphate binders may be prescribed, but usually are avoided, or used sparingly, to avoid secondary aluminum toxicity.

Because of inadequate intake, either because of poor appetite and/or fluid restrictions, it often becomes necessary to concentrate infant formulas, or to use high calorie low phosphorus supplements for the older child. Tube feeding may become necessary if there is marginal oral intake over a prolonged period.

References

1. *A Clinical Guide to Nutrition Care in End-Stage Renal Disease*. The American Dietetic Association, Renal Dietitian Dietetic Practice Group, 1987. Editors Gillit, Stover, Spinozzi.
2. Nelson, P, Stover, J. Principles of Nutritional Assessment and Management of the Child with ESRD In: Fine, RM, Gruskin, AB, eds. *End Stage Renal Disease in Children*. Philadelphia: WB Saunders, 1984:209-226.
3. Chantler, C. Nutrition Therapy in Children with Chronic Renal Failure. *Am J Clin Nutr* 1980; 33:1622.

Protein Controlled Diet Food Groups List

SPECIAL NOTES

Your physician has ordered this diet for you as an important part of your treatment. It is necessary to control both the **amount** and the **kind** of protein you eat. Protein from animal sources is of the best quality and will make up most of the protein in your diet. Adequate calorie intake is especially important. Be sure to eat **all** the foods on your diet.

Your total daily intake will include the following number of choices from each food group listed below.

	Food Group	Amount of Protein Provided
_____	Meat and Meat Substitute group	_____ grams of protein
_____	Milk and Milk Products group	_____ grams of protein
_____	Starch group	_____ grams of protein
_____	Fruit group	_____ grams of protein
_____	Vegetable group	_____ grams of protein
_____	Fat group	_____ grams of protein
_____	Sweets group	_____ grams of protein

MEATS AND SUBSTITUTES

Each of the following foods contains 7 grams of protein.
Choose _____ servings from this list each day. At least one of these servings should be an egg.

Lean beef, pork, veal, lamb	1 ounce
Fish (except clams and oysters)	1 ounce
Clams and oysters	2 ounces
Poultry	1 ounce
Egg	1 large
Cottage cheese	1/4 cup
Cheese	1 ounce

MILK AND MILK PRODUCTS

Each of the following foods contains 4 grams of protein.
Choose _____ servings from this list each day.

Cream, Half & Half	1/2 cup
Cream, heavy whipping	3/4 cup
Milk	1/2 cup
Ice cream, ice milk (hard)	2/3 cup
Ice milk, soft serve	1/2 cup
Pudding, cornstarch	1/2 cup
Sherbet	1-1/2 cups
Yogurt	1/2 cup

Protein-Controlled (continued)

STARCH GROUP

Each of the following foods contains approximately 2 grams of protein.
Choose _____ servings from this list each day.

Biscuit or muffin	1 small
Bread	1 slice
Doughnut (no nuts)	1
Hamburger or hot dog bun	1 small
Pancake	1 (3" diameter)
Sweetroll (no nuts)	1/2 average
Waffle, frozen	1 (4" x 4")
Waffle, homemade	1/2 (4" x 4")
Cereals*	
Cereal, hot	1/2 cup
Cereal, ready to serve	2/3 cup
Shredded Wheat	1 biscuit
Flour	2 tbsp.
Pasta	1/2 cup
Potato, white	1/2 cup
French fries	10
Potato chips	20
Rice	1/2 cup
Animal crackers	15
Graham crackers	4 small squares
Melba toast	4 oblong or 6 round
Round crackers	8
Popcorn	2-1/2 cups, popped
Saltines	8 small squares
Cake, plain	2" x 2" x 2" piece
Angel or sponge cake	1/18th of cake
Pound cake	1/4" slice
Cookies, assorted	4 cookies (2" diameter)
Gingersnaps	6 small
Vanilla wafers	10 small
Sugar wafers	5 small
Pie, fruit (double crust)	1/8 of an 8" pie
Candy	
Caramels	2 ounces
Milk chocolate	1 ounce
Chocolate covered mints	3 small
Soup, broth based (made with water)	1/2 cup

*Avoid bran, granola, and high-protein cereals.

Protein-Controlled (continued)

FRUIT GROUP

Each of the following foods contains approximately 0.5 grams of protein.
Choose _____ servings from this list each day.

Canned fruit	1/2 cup
Fresh fruit	1/2 cup or 1 medium
Fruit juices	
Apple, cranberry	1-1/2 cups
Grape, peach	1 cup
Apricot, grapefruit, lemon, lime,	
prune, pineapple, or pear	1/2 cup
Orange, tomato, vegetable juice cocktail	1/4 cup

VEGETABLE GROUP

Each of the following foods contains approximately 1 gram of protein.
Choose _____ servings from this list each day.

1/4 cup equals 1 serving	**1/2 cup equals 1 serving**
Asparagus	Bamboo shoots
Brussels sprouts	Beans, green or wax
Broccoli	Bean sprouts
Corn	Beets
Mixed vegetables	Cabbage, red or regular
Olives	Carrots
Spinach, cooked	Cauliflower
Sweet potatoes	Celery
	Eggplant
	Mushrooms
	Onions
	Parsnips
	Pumpkin
	Rutabaga
	Sauerkraut
	Squash, summer
	Squash, winter
	Tomatoes
	Turnips

In addition, the following vegetables contain negligible protein and may be taken in larger portions:

Cucumbers	Pickles
Green pepper	Radishes
Lettuce	Watercress

Avoid lima beans and peas.

Protein-Controlled (continued)

FATS AND OILS GROUP

Each of the following foods contains negligible protein and approximately 45 calories.
Choose at least _____ servings from this list each day.

Butter, margarine		1 tsp.
Oil, shortening		1 tsp.
Cream, sour		2 tbsp.
Dry cream substitute		2 tbsp.
Tartar sauce		2 tsp.
Liquid cream substitute:	Mocha Mix®, Farm Rich®	1/4 cup
	Poly Rich®	2 tbsp.
Nondairy whipped topping		2 tbsp.
Salad dressings (except blue cheese dressing)		1 tbsp.

SWEETS AND SPECIAL PRODUCTS

Each of the following foods contains negligible protein and approximately 100 calories.
Choose at least _____ servings from this list each day.

Koolaid, lemonade, limeade, carbonated beverages, and commercial fruit drinks	8 ounces
Candy	
Fondants	3 (40 per pound)
Gumdrops	7 large or 8 small
Jelly beans	20
Lollipops	1 medium
Chiquita Fruit and Juice Bars®	2 bars
Danish Dessert®	1/2 cup
Dole Fruit and Juice Bars®	1 bar
Fruit ice	1/2 cup
Popsicle®	1 twin bar
Sorbet	1/2 cup
Low-protein rusks	2
Low-protein pasta	2/3 cup, cooked
Low-protein cookies	2
Low-protein bread	1 slice
Low-protein gelled dessert	2/3 cup
Cranberry sauce or relish	2 tbsp.
Honey or syrup	2 tbsp.
Jam or jelly	2 tbsp.
Sugar, granulated or powdered	2 tbsp.
General Mills Fruit Roll Ups®	2 rolls
Polycase®	1/4 cup

Protein-Controlled (continued)

MISCELLANEOUS

The following items may be taken as desired:

Baking powder	Low protein baking mix
Baking soda	Mustard
Catsup	Pimiento
Chili sauce	Soy sauce
Cocoa powder	Steak sauce
Cornstarch	Tabasco sauce
Extracts	Tapioca
Flavorings	Vinegar
Herbs and spices	Wheat starch
Lemon juice	Worcestershire sauce
Lime juice	

Coffee, regular or decaffeinated
Tea, regular or herbal

The following foods contain excessive amounts of low-value protein and generally should not be used on your diet:

Dried peas, beans, lentils
Gelatin
Nuts and peanut butter

Protein Controlled Diet Counter List

SPECIAL NOTES

Your physician has ordered this diet for you as an important part of your treatment. It is necessary to control both the **amount** and the **kind** of protein you eat. Protein from animal sources is of the best quality and will make up most of the protein in your diet. Adequate calorie intake is especially important. Be sure to eat **all** the foods on your diet.

You should eat a total of _____ points from the following lists each day.

One point equals **1 gram** of protein.

DAIRY PRODUCTS

	Portion	Points
Milk		
skim, 1%, 2%, whole	4 oz.	4
buttermilk	4 oz.	4
condensed	2 oz.	6
evaporated skim	2 oz.	5
Ice cream	1/2 cup	3
Ice milk, soft serve	1/2 cup	4
Mocha Mix® Frozen Dessert	1 cup	2
Pudding	1/2 cup	4
Sherbet	3/4 cup	2
Yogurt, plain or fruit flavored	1/2 cup	4

FATS

Each of the following foods contains approximately 50 calories per serving.
At least _____ servings should be eaten each day.

	Portion	Points
Butter, margarine, oil, shortening	1 tsp.	0
Cream, Half & Half, whipping (light)	1 oz.	1
Cream, sour or heavy whipping	3 tbsp.	1
Dry cream substitute	3 tbsp.	1
Liquid cream substitute:		
Mocha Mix®, Farm Rich®	1 cup	1
Poly Rich®	1/2 cup	1
Mayonnaise	1 tbsp.	0
Nondairy whipped topping	2 tbsp.	0
Salad dressing (except blue cheese)	1 tbsp.	0
Blue cheese dressing	1 tbsp.	1
Tartar sauce	1 tbsp.	0

(continued)	Portion	Points
Apple	2 medium	1
Applesauce	2-1/2 cups	1
Apricots, canned	1/2 cup	1
Apricots, dried	1/4 cup	1
Banana	1/2 of 8" banana	1
Blackberries	1/2 cup	1
Blueberries	1 cup	1
Cantaloupe	1/2 of 5" melon	1
Cherries	1/2 cup	1
Dates	5 whole	1
Fruit cocktail	1 cup	1
Grapefruit, fresh	1/2 cup	1
Grapes	1 cup	1
Honeydew melon	1/6 of medium	1
Kiwi	1 medium	1
Lemon	1-1/2 medium	1
Lime	2 medium	1
Nectarine	1 medium	1
Orange	1 (2-1/2" diam.)	1
Peaches	1 (or 1 cup)	1
Pear, fresh	1 small	1
Pear, canned	2 cups	1
Pineapple	1 cup	1
Plum, fresh	2	1
Prunes	1/4 cup	1
Raisins	1/4 cup	1
Raspberries, red	2/3 cup	1
Rhubarb	1 cup	1
Strawberries	1 cup	1
Tangerine	2 medium	1
Watermelon	1 cup	1

Fruit Juices

	Portion	Points
Apple	40 oz.	1
Apricot nectar, lemon	8 oz.	1
Grape	20 oz.	1
Grapefruit, orange	6 oz.	1
Peach nectar, lime	12 oz.	1
Pear nectar	33 oz.	1
Pineapple	10 oz.	1
Prune, vegetable juice cocktail	5 oz.	1
Tomato	4 oz.	1

MEAT AND SUBSTITUTES

	Portion	Points
Egg	1 large	6
Meats		
Bacon	3 slices	5
Beef, pork, veal, lamb, poultry	1 oz.	7
Bologna	3 slices (10 per 8 oz.)	8
Canadian bacon	1 oz.	7
Luncheon meat	1 oz.	5
Pork sausage	1 oz. patty	5
Liver (beef, pork, chicken)	1 oz.	7
Wiener (no cereal added)	1 (10 per pound)	5
Fish, Seafood		
Clams	1 oz.	7
Saltwater (except flounder/sole)	1 oz.	6
Flounder/sole	1 oz.	7
Lobster	1 oz.	6
Oysters	1 oz.	4
Salmon	1 oz.	8
Sardines	4 medium	12
Scallops	1 oz.	7
Shrimp	1 oz.	6
Shrimp, canned	1 oz.	6
Tuna	1 oz. or 1/4 cup	8
Cheese		
American	1 oz.	6
Bleu or Roquefort	1 oz.	6
Brick, cheese food	1 oz.	6
Cheddar	1 oz.	7
Cottage cheese	1/4 cup	7
Cream cheese	1 oz.	2
Parmesan	1 oz.	10
Swiss	1 oz.	8
Cheese food spreads	1 oz.	5

	Portion	Points
Breads		
Bagel, water	1	6
Baking powder biscuit	1 (2" diam.)	2
Bread, white	1 slice	2
Bread, whole wheat	1 slice	3
English muffin	1/2	2
Hamburger or hot dog bun	1 small	3
Pita bread, round whole	1/2	2
Popover	1 average	4
Tortilla	1 (6" diam.)	3
Crackers		
Animal	15	2
Bread sticks	2 small	1
Graham crackers	2 squares	1
Matzoth	1 piece (6" diam.)	3
Melba toast	2 slices	1
Round crackers	4	1
Ry-Krisp®	2 triple crackers	1
Saltines	4 small squares	1
Soda	3 small squares	1
Zwieback toast	1	1
Cereals and Grains		
Barley	2 tbsp.	8
Cooked cereals		
Cream of rice	1 cup, cooked	2
Cream of wheat, Farina, Maltomeal ®	1/2 cup, cooked	2
Oatmeal, Ralston®	1/2 cup, cooked	3
Pettijohns	1/3 cup, cooked	2
Cold cereals		
Cocoa Puffs®, Puffed Rice®	1 cup	1
Cornflakes®, Puffed Wheat®, Rice Krispies®	1 cup	2
Cocoa Krispies®, Frosted Flakes®, Golden Grahams®	3/4 cup	1
Cheerios®, Raisin Bran®	1/2 cup	2
Shredded Wheat®	1 large biscuit	2
Flour, white	1 tbsp.	1
Macaroni, spaghetti	1/2 cup, cooked	2
Noodles	1/2 cup, cooked	3
Popcorn	2 cups, popped	2
Rice, white or brown	1/2 cup, cooked	2

STARCHES

(continued)		Portion	Points
Potatoes			
Baked, boiled		1 (2-1/2" diam.)	3
French fries		10 medium	2
Hashed browns		1/2 cup	2
Mashed		1/2 cup	2
Prepared Foods			
Brownie		1 piece (2"x2"x1")	2
Cake: angel food		1/12th of 9" cake	3
	pound	1" slice	2
Cookies:	chocolate chip	2 (2" diam.)	1
	cream filled	2 (2" diam.)	1
	gingersnaps	3	1
	shortbread	2	1
	sugar	2 medium	1
	vanilla wafers	5	1
Danish pastry, no nuts		1 small	3
Donut, cake or yeast		1 medium	2
Muffin, no nuts		1 average	3
Pancake		1 (4" diam.)	2
Pie, fruit		1/8 of 9" pie	2

SWEETS AND SPECIAL PRODUCTS

The food items listed below have approximately 100 calories per serving.
At least _____ servings should be eaten each day.

Beverages	Portion	Points
Cranberry juice cocktail	6 oz.	0
Fruit drinks, iced tea (sweetened),		
Koolaid®, lemonade, limeade, pop	8 oz.	0
Candy		
Candy corn	20 pieces	0
Gumdrops	28 small	0
Hard candy	5 small pieces	0
Jelly beans	20 pieces	0

SWEETS AND SPECIAL PRODUCTS

(continued)	Portion	Points
Candy		
Lifesavers®	12	0
Lollipop	1 medium	0
Marshmallows	5 large	0
Sugar mints, butter or party	1 oz. (14 pieces)	0
Fruit Desserts		
Chiquita Fruit and Juice Bars®	2 bars	0
Danish dessert	1/2 cup	0
Dole Fruit and Juice Bars®	1 bar	0
General Mills Fruit Roll Ups®	2 rolls	0
Popsicle® (approx. 3 oz.)	1 twin bar	0
Sorbet	1/2 cup	0
Low Protein Products		
Aproten® rusk	2	0
Low-protein bread	1 slice	0
Low-protein cookies	2	0
Low-protein pasta	2/3 cup, cooked	0
Low-protein gelled desserts	2/3 cup	0
Polycose®	1/4 cup	0
Sugars and Syrups		
Honey, syrup	2 tbsp.	0
Ice cream topping	2 tbsp.	0
Jam or jelly	2 tbsp.	0
Sugar (brown, granulated or powdered)	2 tbsp.	0

VEGETABLES

	Portion	Points
Asparagus	1/2 cup	2
Bamboo shoots	1/2 cup	1
Beans, green or wax	1/2 cup	1
Beans, lima	1/2 cup	5
Bean sprouts	1/2 cup	1
Beets 1/2 cup	1	
Beet greens	1/2 cup	2
Broccoli 1/2 cup	3	
Brussels sprouts	1/2 cup	3
Cabbage, raw	1 cup	1
Cabbage, cooked or red	1/2 cup	1
Carrots 1/2 cup	1	

VEGETABLES

(continued)	Portion	Points
Cauliflower	1/2 cup	1
Celery 1 cup	1	
Corn 1/2 cup	2	
Cucumber	1-1/2 cup, sliced	1
Eggplant 1 cup, diced	1	
Lettuce 1-1/2 cup	1	
Mushrooms	1/2 cup	1
Onion 1/2 cup	1	
Parsnips 1/2 cup	1	
Peas 1/4 cup	2	
Pepper, green	1 whole medium	1
Pumpkin 1/2 cup	1	
Radish 4 small	0	
Rutabaga	1/2 cup	1
Sauerkraut	1/2 cup	1
Spinach, raw	1/2 cup	1
Squash, summer	1/2 cup	1
Squash, winter	1/2 cup	1
Sweet potato	1/2 cup	2
Tomato 1/2 cup or 1 whole	1	
Turnip 1 cup	1	
Water chestnuts	1/2 cup	1

MISCELLANEOUS

The following may be eaten as desired:

Coffee
Cornstarch
Flavorings and extracts
Herbs and spices
Lemon juice, lime juice
Low protein baking mix
Pimiento
Tabasco sauce
Tapioca
Tea
Vinegar
Wheat starch

Ketogenic Diets
Description and Indications for Use

The Ketogenic Diet is a high fat, low carbohydrate and low protein diet developed in the 1920s as a treatment for intractable childhood seizures associated with epilepsy. The purpose of the diet is to induce and maintain a state of ketosis. Effective anti-convulsant drugs and the fact that the diet requires strict patient compliance may give the dietary approach a minor role in therapy. However, the Ketogenic Diet often is used in cases where other forms of treatment have failed or in cases of drug toxicity. It appears to be most effective in children under 10 years of age. It is used primarily to treat medically refractory atonic, amyoclonic and atypical absence seizures (Lennox-Gestaut Syndrome).

Withrow, 1990, summarized the effects of the Ketogenic Diet as follows: "Initiation of the diet results in several changes in blood biochemical parameters, the most important of which appears to be a rise in blood ketone bodies. After several days the system adapts in some way to use ketones as a partial fuel source. An anti-convulsant effect results and is maintained as long as the blood ketone bodies remain elevated

There are two ketogenic diets:
The standard high-fat diet based on conventional fats.
The medium chain triglyceride (MCT oil diet).

Nausea and vomiting is likely to occur if the diet is rapidly changed from a regular diet to a Ketogenic Diet. Therefore, if the patient is placed on the standard high-fat diet, the patient is given a diet containing 75 grams of carbohydrate on the first day, 50 grams on the second day, and the prescribed amount on the third or fourth day. As the carbohydrate level is reduced, the caloric level is kept constant by a corresponding increase in the fat intake. If nausea develops at any stage during the reduction of carbohydrates, small amounts of orange juice should be given, and further carbohydrate reduction held until nausea has subsided.

If the patient is started on an MCT oil diet regimen, Huttenlocher and Stephenson fast patients 24-48 hours before initiating the diet. This induces ketosis more rapidly. When the urine tests positive for ketones, Stephenson provides 10 cc of MCT oil on the first day and then gradually increases the MCT oil dose during the next 2 to 3 days, until the patient is receiving the prescribed amount of MCT oil.

The Ketogenic Diet is monitored by blood test to assure the level of the ketone d(-) ß-hydroxybutrate is maintained above 2 mM and, more easily, by daily testing for urinary ketones with the goal of moderate to high ketones.

It usually requires 5 to 10 days to adjust the calorie level of the diet to the child's requirements. If too many calories are prescribed, ketosis will not remain constant. Most children will lose weight during the first few days of the Ketogenic Diet. If weight loss continues, the calories provided will have to be increased. Hunger is a common complaint during the initial phase of the diet. However, if adequate calories are being provided, this usually subsides in a few days.

According to the studies by Dodson , there is a latency period of 10 to 21 days after initiation of a Ketogenic Diets before complete seizure control is achieved, and if the diet is not effective within three months, it will not work at all. If the diet is successful, it is recommended to continue the diet for two years and then gradually return to a regular diet.

Height and weight must be monitored closely and calories increased to support continued growth due to rigidly controlled energy intake which may compromise growth if the diet is maintained on a long-term basis.

If any medications are used that contain carbohydrate, i.e., cough drops, cough syrup, prescription pills or syrups including seizure medications, this carbohydrate must be calculated into the Ketogenic Diet plan that is prescribed.

Marked hyperlipidemia and increased incidence of uric acid renal stones have been observed in children on the standard high--fat diet. Transient abdominal pain, vomiting and diarrhea may occur using the MCT oil diet.

Nutritional Adequacy
The traditional high-fat diet is deficient in the B-complex vitamins, iron, calcium, and Vitamin D. The MCT oil diet is nutritionally inadequate, and must be supplemented with all vitamins and minerals.

1. Standard High-Fat Diet
The standard high fat diet is ordered as either a 3:1 or 4:1 ratio. The ratio specifies the ratio of the grams of fat (or ketogenic material) in the diet to the grams of non-fat (or non-ketogenic) material in the diet. Thus, in the 3:1 ketogenic diet, for every one gram of non-ketogenic material, there are 3 grams of ketogenic material. A gram scale is used for weighing foods.

Children under the age of five receive the 3:1 ratio diet, while those over age five are usually given the 4:1 diet. The calories of the 3:1 diet are 87% fat. The 4:1 diet is 90% fat.

Calculation
1. Determine calories/kg and calculate the total calories per day, following the RDA. Dodson recommends providing 75 kcal/kg of bodyweight initially.
2. Determine the protein/kg and calculate the total protein allowance per day. (One gram of protein/kg bodyweight is usually sufficient to maintain lean body mass.
3. In the 3:1 diet, one dietary unit = 31 calories since (3 grams fat x 9 calories/gram) + (1 gram nonfat x 4 calories/gram) = 31 calories. In the 4:1 diet, one dietary unit = 40 calories since (4 grams fat x 9 calories/gram) + (1 gram nonfat x 4 calories/gram) = 40 calories.
4. Divide total calories by 31 or 40 to equal the number of dietary units.
5. Number of dietary units x 3, or 4, = grams of fat in the diet.
6. Number of dietary units - grams of protein = grams of carbohydrate in the diet
7. Divide grams of carbohydrate, protein and fat by 3 to equal the amount per meal

Example of an 18 kg child on a 3:1 ratio diet:
70 calories/kg - 18 x 70 = 1260 calories/day.
1 gram protein/kg = 18 grams protein/day.
One dietary unit = 31 calories.
1260 divided by 31 = 40.6 dietary units.
40.6 x 3 = 121.8 grams of fat per day.
40.6 - 18 = 22.6 grams of carbohydrates per day.
121.8 divided by 3 = 40.6 grams of fat per meal.
18 divided by 3 = 6 grams of protein per meal.
22.6 divided by 3 = 7.5 grams of carbohydrate per meal.

2. MCT Oil Diet
This ketogenic diet is more palatable than the traditional high fat diet since larger amounts of protein and carbohydrate are allowed. The diabetic exchange lists and household measures may be used rather than a gram scale.

The MCT oil dose is divided into three (3) doses. Some experts suggest mixing the MCT oil with skim milk and serving it chilled. Others suggest including the MCT oil in recipes.

Calculations

Determine energy requirements according to age and weight. MCT oil at 7.7 kcal/ml provided 60% of the calories.

Determine protein as recommended for patient's age, approximately 10% of the calories.

Carbohydrate provided 18% of the calories.

Dietary fat provides 12% of the calories. this should include a source of linoleic acid such as corn or safflower oil to prevent essential fatty acid deficiency.

Example of a 15 kg child:

1400 calories. 60% of 1400 = 840 calories from MCT oil. 840 divided by 7.7 kcal/ml = 109 ml. 15 ml/tablespoons = 7 tablespoons + 1 teaspoon.

35 grams of protein.

63 grams of carbohydrate.

19 grams of fat.

Information for Ketogenic Diets

The lists of Foods to Avoid and Foods to Use as Desired can be used by both types of Ketogenic Diets.

Foods to Avoid

The following foods and products should be avoided because they contain measurable amounts of carbohydrate.

Sugar	Honey	Peas
Catsup	Ice creams	Pastries
Cake	Invert sugar	Preserves
Candy	Jam	Pies
Cereals	Jelly	Puddings
Chewing Gum	Lactose	Rolls
Cookies	Mannitol	Sherbet
Cough drops or cough syrup	Marmalade	Sorbitol
which contain sugar	Molasses	Sucrose
Dextrin	Muffins	Syrup
Dextrose	Pancakes	Waffles
Doughnuts		

Foods to Use as Desired

The following foods can be eaten as desired:

Artificial sweeteners:	Cucumbers
NutraSweet	Flavoring extracts, e.g., Vanilla, Mint, Almond
Aspartame	Unsweetened gelatin
Saccharin	Herbs and spices
but NOT Sorbitol	Lemon Juice
Artificially sweetened jams/jellies	Lime Juice
Artificially sweetened pop or	Low Calorie Salad Dressings Mustard
Kool-aid	Pepper
Broth, bouillon	Unsweetened Pickles
Celery	Radishes
Chives	Salt
Coffee	Tea
Cranberries without sugar	Vinegar

Food Units for Use with the Standard High-Fat Ketogenic Diet
Meat Units

One meat unit in the weight listed is equal to approximately 7 gm Protein and 5 gm Fat. The meat should be weighed after cooking and after bone, skin, and excess fat has been removed. Prepare by baking, broiling, or boiling. If fried foods are desired, part of the fat allowance may be used for frying the items.

	GRAMS		GRAMS
Meat (medium fat)		**Cheese**	
Beef, ham, lamb, pork, or veal	30	American, brick, cheddar,	30
Liver (add 1 fat unit, omit I vegetable unit)	30	Roquefort, Swiss, and processed cheese (omit 1 fat)	
Sausage, Pork (omit 2 fat units)	40	Cottage cheese, creamed	50
Beef, dried (add 1 fat unit)	20	(add 1 fat unit) (omit 1/2	
Bacon (omit 2 fat units)	25	vegetable unit)	
Cold cuts			
Bologna, luncheon meat, minced ham, liverwurst (all meat, no cereal)	45		
Salami (omit 1 fat unit)	30		
Frankfurters or wieners (all meat, not cereal) (omit 1 fat unit)	50		
Fowl		**Peanut Butter**	30
Chicken, duck, goose, or turkey	30	(omit 1 1/2 fat units) (omit 1/2 fruit unit)	
Fish		**Egg (one)**	50
Salmon or tuna, canned	30		
Sardines	35		
Shellfish			
Clams (add 1 fat unit) (omit 1 vegetable unit)	50		
Lobster (add 1 fat unit)	40		
Oysters (add 1 fat unit) (omit 1 vegetable unit)	70		
Scallops (add 1 fat unit)	50		
Shrimp (add 1 fat unit)	30		

Starch Units

One starch unit is equivalent to the weight listed and contains approximately 6 gm Carbohydrate and 1 gm Protein.

	GRAMS		GRAMS
White Bread	12	Mashed Potatoes	40
Corn (drained)	30	Potato chips (omit 1 fat)	12
Animal Crackers	8	Pretzels	7
Graham Cracker (plain)	8	Rice (cooked)	25
Saltines	8	40% Bran Flakes	8
Soda Crackers	8	Raisin Bran	8
Macaroni (cooked)	25	Cheerios	8
Egg Noodles (cooked)	25	Corn Flakes	7
Spaghetti (cooked)	25	Kix	7
Oatmeal (cooked)	60	Rice Krispies	7
Popcorn (popped)	8	Puffed Rice	7
Boiled Potatoes	40	Vanilla Wafers	8

Vegetable Units

One vegetable unit is equal to the weight listed and yield 3 gm Carbohydrate and 1 gm Protein.

	GRAMS		GRAMS
Asparagus	85	Mushrooms	100
Beans, green or wax	65	Okra	50
Beets	40	Onions	35
Broccoli	65	Green Peppers	60
Brussel Sprouts	45	Pumpkin	50
Cabbage, raw	55	Spinach	100
cooked	50	Summer Squash	100
Carrots, raw	30	Winter Squash	30
cooked	50	Tomatoes	70
Cauliflower	75	Tomato Puree	35
Eggplant	75	Tomato Juice	70
Kohlrabi	55	Vegetable Juice Cocktail	80

Fruit Units

One fruit unit is equivalent to the weight listed and provides 6 gm Carbohydrate. The Fruit may be raw, canned, cooked, dried, or frozen *without additional sugar.* If the fruit is canned or frozen, the label should state one of the following: no sugar added, juice packed, water packed, artificially sweetened, or unsweetened.

	GRAMS		GRAMS
Apple, fresh	40	Figs, canned	60
sauce	60	fresh	30
juice	60	Fruit Cocktail	60
Apricots, canned	60	Grapefruit, fresh, edible portion	60
fresh	60	juice	60
nectar	40	sections, canned	75
Banana, edible portion	30	Grapes, canned	40
Blackberries	50	fresh	40
Blueberries	40	juices, bottled	30
Boysenberries	60	juice, frozen	40
Cherries, canned	60	Lemon Juice	75
fresh	40	Lime Juice	65
Mango, fresh	35	Loganberries	50
Melon, edible portion:		Mandarin Oranges	100
Cantaloupe	100	Pineapple, canned	60
Honeydew	100	fresh, edible portion	40
Watermelon	100	juice	40
Nectarine, edible portion	40	Plums, canned, edible portion	60
Orange, fresh, edible portion	50	fresh, edible portion	40
Orange, juice	60	Prune Juice	30
Papaya	60	Raspberries	50
Peach, canned	60	Strawberries	75
fresh, edible portion	40	Tangerine, fresh, edible portion	50
nectar	40	juice	60

Fat Units

One fat unit is equivalent to the weight listed and provides 4 gm of Fat.

	GRAMS		GRAMS
Avocado (omit 50 grams of a vegetable)	30	Nuts:	
		Almonds, slivered	5
Butter or Margarine	5	Pecans, shelled	5
Cooking fats (shortening)	5	Walnuts, shelled	5
Mayonnaise	5	Oils, salad	5
		Olives, green or ripe	30

Whipping Cream Units

One whipping cream units equals 60 grams of whipping cream and equals 2 gm Carbohydrate, 1.5 gm Protein, and 19 gm Fat.

The whipping cream may be weighed before or after whipping, Water may be added to make the whipping cream more like milk.

Whipping cream must be at least 32% fat. Sixty grams of whipping cream may be exchanged for 1/2 vegetable unit and 5 fat units.

References

1. Berman, W. Medium chain triglyceride diet in the treatment of intractable childhood epilepsy. Dev Med Child Neurol 1978; 20:249.
2. Clark, BJ, House, FM. Medium chain triglyderide oil ketogenic diets in the treatment of childhood epilepsy. J Hum Nutr 1978;32:111.
3. Dodson, WE, Prensky, AL, DeVivo, DC, Goldring, S, Dodge, PR. Management of seizure disorders; selected aspects. J Pediatr 1976; 89:695.
4. Francis, D, Hamilton, MB, Coutts, J. Ketogenic diets. J Hum Nutr 1978; 32:212.
5. Gordon, N Medium chain triglycerides in a ketogenic diet. Dev Med Child Neurol 1977; 19:535.
6. Herzberg, GZ, Fivush, BA, Kinsman, SL, Gearhart, JP. Urolithiasis associated with the ketogenic diet. J Pediatr 1990; 117(5):743-5.
7. Huttenlocher, PR. Ketonemia and seizures: metabolic and anti-convulsant effects of two ketogenic diets in childhood epilepsy. Pediatr Res 1976; 10:536.
8. Huttenlocher, PR, Wilbourn, AJ, Signore, JM. Medium chain triglycerides as a therapy for intractable childhood epilepsy. Neurology 1971; 21:1097.
9. Keith, HM. Convulsive Disorders in Children. Litte, Brown and Co. Boston, 1963; 146-224.
10. Kinsman, SL, Vining, EP, Quaskey, SA, Mellits, D, Freeman, JH. Efficacy of the ketogenic diet for intractable seizure disorders: review of 58 cases. Epilepsia 1992; 33(6):1132-6.
11. Stephenson, JBP, House, F, Stromberg, P. Medium chain triglycerides in a ketogenic diet. Dev Med Child Neurol 1977; 10:696.
12. Wilder, RM. The effects of ketonemia on the course of epilepsy. Mayo Clin Proc 1921; 2:307-8.
13. Withrow, CD. The ketogenic diet: mechanism of anticonvulsant action. Adv Neurol 1980; 27:635.

Patient Resources

MINCEP® Epilepsy Care
Minnesota Comprehensive Epilepsy Program ™, P.A.
5775 Wayzata Boulevard
Phone: 612-525-2400
Fax:: 612-525-1560

Food Sensitivity

Description

Food sensitivity is the preferred term used to refer to all the adverse reactions to foods, both immunological and nonimmunological.

Food allergy

True food allergies are those reactions to foods that are mediated by the immune system and can be consistently reproduced. They are more common in early childhood; their incidence usually diminishes with age and they can be managed by totally eliminating the offending food from the diet. Foods such as soy, milk, wheat and egg produce food allergies that are frequently outgrown. Allergies produced by peanuts, nuts, fish, and shellfish are less commonly outgrown, and are the most frequently implicated in anaphylactic reactions.

Food intolerance

Food intolerance is the term preferred to describe nonimmunological reactions to foods. These reactions represent a diverse collection of mechanisms:

Gastrointestinal disorders (lactase deficiency, gluten enteropathy).
Inborn errors of metabolism (phenylketonuria, galactosemia).
Psychological/idiosyncratic reactions.
Noxious natural constituents (alkaloids in mushrooms, hemagglutinins in beans).
Reactions to pharmacological agents in foods (tyramine in cheddar cheese, wines; histamine in fermented foods).
Contaminants in foods (microorganisms such as aflatoxins in peanuts and grains).
Additives (sulfiting agents, tartrazine, and salicylates).

From this list, it is evident that nonimmunological reactions are the most common and account for the majority of the food sensitivities.

Incidence

The incidence of clinically significant food sensitivity is far less common than generally perceived. The incidence of true food allergy in children has been estimated to range from 0.3% to 7% in the United States. Subjective reporting, self-diagnosis, and a wide array of symptoms common with various other diseases make it more difficult to establish useful prevalence figures.

Symptoms

Symptoms fall into four major categories:
Gastrointestinal—nausea, vomiting, abdominal pain, diarrhea, malabsorption
Respiratory—rhinitis, wheezing, chronic cough, asthma, sinusitis, otitis media
Skin —urticaria (hives and welts), atopic dermatitis, rash, swelling of lips, mouth, tongue, face or throat
Behavioral—hyperactivity, attention problems, fatigue, anxiety, etc.
Systemic—anaphylaxis, failure to thrive

In addition to these symptoms, a variety of headaches (including migraine-type), urinary tract infections, arthritis, and Meniere's disease have been associated with food sensitivity.

Diagnosis

No single test can determine a conclusive diagnosis of food sensitivity. It is based on accumulated evidence, including the following:
History
Physical examination
Appropriate immunological tests
Trial elimination diet
Food challenge

A dietitian can provide valuable help during history taking and initial evaluation of nutritional status, and in planning an elimination diet by identifying the hidden sources of the suspected offending foods.

Treatment and management

Treatment and management is relatively simple compared to the complexity of the diagnosis. In most cases, identifying and avoiding the offending food is the most effective treatment. Severity of elimination depends on the tolerance level of the individual. Immunologically mediated food sensitivities require extensive precautions and careful management. A dietitian's help is needed in identifying hidden sources of allergens and in finding substitute foods. Also, some foods could be allergic in one form and not in another, while some foods may share their antigenic property with the other members of the same botanical family. Thorough scrutiny of food labels is necessary, and a food manufacturer's help should be solicited. A mild to moderate level of sensitivity may mean that a person may be able to tolerate small amounts of the offending food without a reaction. The challenge for a dietitian counselor lies not only in eliminating the offending food(s), but in meeting nutritional needs as well.

Many popular diets claim to alleviate symptoms of food sensitivity. Other treatments, such as drugs and oral desensitization, have not been very effective.

Adequacy

Depending on the foods eliminated, diets may be deficient in vitamins and minerals, according to the Recommended Dietary Allowances of the National Research Council.

Professional references

1. Taylor SL. Food allergies and sensitivities. J Am Dietetic Assoc 1986; 86:599-600.
2. Emerson JL, Johnson JL. Adverse reactions to foods—an overview. Food Technology in Australia 1985; 37(11):496-505.
3. Bock SA. Food sensitivity. Nutrition News 1984; 47(Oct.):9-11.
4. National Dairy Council. Food sensitivity. Dairy Council Digest 1983; 54(2):7-11.
5. Bock SA. Food allergy—a primer for people. Denver Colo.: A.J. Publishing, 1982.
6. Bahna SL. Factors determining development of allergy in infants. Allergy Proc (13(1) 1992.
7. Schwartz RH. Allergy, intolerance, and other adverse reactions to foods. Pediatric Annals 21:10, 1992.
8. Esteban MM. Adverse food reactions in childhood: concept, importance, and present problems. Journal of Pediatrics 121:5, 1992.
9. Sampson HA. Ig-E mediated food intolerance. J Allergy Clin Immun 81:3, 1988.
10. Food Hypersensitivity. In: Pediatric Nutrition Handbook. 3rd Ed. American Academy of Pediatrics. Elk Grove Village, IL 1993.
11. Dobler ML. Food Allergies. The American Dietetic Association. Chicago, IL 1991.

Soy or Legume Sensitivity

Soybeans are classified as a legume. Other foods in the legume family are navy, kidney, string, and pinto beans; black-eyed and green peas; chick peas; lentils; carob; licorice; and peanuts. Sensitivity to peanuts is the most common, but soybean sensitivity is prevalent, too. Sensitivity to one legume can often occur in association with sensitivity to another legume. **All labels on foods must be read for products or ingredients containing soy:** Vegetable protein, Soy protein isolate, Lecithin, Soy flour, VPC (vegetable protein concentrate), HVP (hydrolyzed vegetable protein), TVP (textured vegetable protein), Soy vegetable oil, Soybeans.

The composition of any food product may be changed without notice. Read every label and contact manufacturer when in doubt about an ingredient listed.

FOOD GROUP	FOODS TO AVOID
Breads/Starches	Breads, crackers, cereals, cakes, rolls, or pastries containing soy oil or flour. Processed and so-called "natural" cereals (ready-to-eat or cooked). Pasta made with soy flour or oil. Foods fried in soy oil, such as potato chips, cheese curls, or corn chips.
Vegetables	Soybean sprouts, vegetables prepared with soy sauce.
Fruit	None
Meat & Substitutes	Sausages or luncheon meats made with soy additives; commercially prepared meats in which soy is used as a meat extender (e.g., HVP, TVP). Soybeans are sometimes roasted and used instead of nuts. Some cheese substitutes contain soy. Soy cheese, Tofu.
Milk	None, except milk substitutes that contain soy. Non-dairy creamer.
Soups & Combination Foods	Soy is used in many canned soups, commercial entrees, and combination foods.
Desserts & Sweets	Baked goods, such as cakes, cookies, pastries containing soy flour. Soy products may be used in some ice creams. Hard candies, nut candies, fudge, and caramels made with soy flour. Lecithin is used in candies, especially in chocolate.
Fats & Oils	Soybean oil, margarine or vegetable shortening. Some salad dressings and mayonnaise.
Beverages	Soy-based milk substitutes and formulas, coffee substitutes made with soy.
Condiments/Miscellaneous	Commercial vegetarian products, foods fried in soy oil, Worcestershire and steak sauces may contain soy, fermented soybean pastes, miso, and natto.

Adapted from: Bronson-Adatto C, ed. Food sensitivity—a resource including recipes (food sensitivity series). Chicago: American Dietetic Association, 1985. Used with permission.

Wheat Sensitivity

Wheat is an allergen because it is capable of initiating an immunological reaction. Most often the gluten, a protein found in wheat, is the cause of food sensitivity; but that is due to food intolerance, a reaction not mediated by the immune system. In both instances, one should be aware that products labeled "wheat free" may or may not be gluten free. Strict adherence to a wheat-free diet presents a tremendous challenge.

Foods to avoid

- Ingredients such as modified food starch, wheat-based emulsifiers and stabilizers, hydrolyzed vegetable proteins.
- Malt or cereal extracts.
- All types of wheat or wheat-based flours: all-purpose, pastry, cake, bread, gluten and graham flours
- Wheat containing products such as: semolina, graham, bran and farina

NOTE: For more information about foods to use and avoid, refer to the Gluten-Restricted Diet in this manual.

All wheat and products made from wheat are eliminated from the diet. **All labels on foods must be read for products containing:** any wheat flour (cake, whole wheat, graham, bread, gluten, all-purpose), wheat germ, bran, farina, bread crumbs, crackers meal, or flour used as a thickening agent.

The composition of any food product may be changed without notice.

FOOD GROUP	FOODS TO AVOID
Breads/Starches	Bread or bread crumbs made from wheat flour. Wheat crackers. Matzos. Doughnuts, muffins, rolls, dumplings, biscuits, pancakes, french toast. All wheat-based pasta, bread and cracker stuffing. Multigrain breads containing wheat. Ready-to-serve or cooked cereals containing wheat. Rice or potato products thickened with wheat flour or starch.
Vegetables	Any breaded or prepared with wheat flour.
Fruit	None, except strained fruits with wheat cereal added.
Meat & Substitutes	Sausage products or luncheon meats containing wheat as a filler. Floured or breaded meats, fish, or poultry.
Milk	None
Soups & Combination Foods	Soups or convenience foods containing wheat-based pasta or thickened with wheat flour or starch.
Desserts & Sweets	All products made with wheat flour: cake, cookies, pie, pastries, ice cream cones. Commercial ice cream, sherbet. Frosting. Prepared mixes. Packaged puddings.
Fats & Oils	Commercially prepared salad dressings, thickened with wheat flour. Commercial or other gravies made with wheat flour.
Beverages	Beer, whiskey, wheat-based grain drinks (e.g., Postum)

FOOD GROUP	FOODS TO AVOID
Condiments/Miscellaneous	Sauces thickened with wheat flour. Pretzels. Some seasoning blends. Many commercial candies contain wheat products-ask manufacturer. Some brands of yeast. Soy sauce.

Adapted from: Bronson-Adatto C, ed. Food sensitivity—a resource including recipes (food sensitivity series).Chicago: American Dietetic Association, 1985. Used with permission.

Egg Sensitivity

Eggs are a commonly used food that may cause food sensitivity reactions. Persons with egg sensitivity may find it relatively easy to eliminate visible eggs, but may not be aware of the variety of food products that contain eggs. **All labels on foods must be read for products containing:** eggs, egg powder, dried egg, powdered egg whites, or albumin.

The composition of any food product may be changed without notice.

FOOD GROUP	FOODS TO AVOID
Breads/Starches	Any containing eggs or crust, glazed with egg. Pancakes, waffles, french toast, doughnuts, muffins, zwieback, soda crackers, pretzels. Egg noodles or pasta, including vermicelli, macaroni, and spaghetti. Baking mixes, fritter batter, batter-fried foods.
Vegetables	Any prepared with sauces or breading that contain eggs in any form.
Fruit	None
Meat & Substitutes	Eggs in any form, including egg powders or commercial egg substitutes. Souffles, breaded meats, fish, and poultry, meatballs, meat loaf, croquettes, some sausages.
Milk	Cocomalt, eggnog, malted beverages.
Soups & Combination Foods	Broth, consomme, bouillon clarified with egg. Mock turtle and egg noodle soups. Prepared entrees or combination foods that contain eggs in any form.
Desserts & Sweets	Cakes, cookies, cream-filled pies, meringues, custard, puddings, ice cream, sherbet. Chocolate candies with cream or fondant fillings, marshmallow candy, commercial divinity, fudge, and cake icings. (Many candies are brushed with egg white.) Dessert powders. Frozen dairy desserts containing the fat substitute Simplesse.
Fats & Oils	Commercial salad dressings and mayonnaise, unless egg-free.
Beverages	Root beer (egg may be used as a foaming agent), wine or coffee (if clarified with egg). Some malted cocoa drinks.
Condiments/Miscellaneous	Cream sauces made with eggs, such as Hollandaise, tartar sauce, marshmallow sauce. Baking powder that contains egg white or albumin.

Adapted from: Bronson-Adatto C, ed. **Food sensitivity—a resource including recipes (food sensitivity series). Chicago: American Dietetic Association, 1985. Used with permission.**

Milk Sensitivity

Milk sensitivity is most common and frequent among infants and young children. It is an immunological reaction and may be caused by one of the many proteins found in cow's milk. Some individuals react to the lactose content in milk, which is a condition described as lactose intolerance.

Refer to the Cow's milk protein-free diet or the Lactose-Free or Low lactose diets in this manual.

Professional references (for milk and wheat sensitivity)

1. Bronson-Adatto C, ed. Food sensitivity—a resource including recipes (food sensitivity series). Chicago: American Dietetic Assoc., 1985. Used with permission.
2. Dobler ML. Food Allergies-a resource including recipes. Chicago: American Dietetic Association. 1991.

Cow's Milk Protein Sensitivity

All milk and milk products are eliminated from the diet. **All labels on foods must be read for products containing milk or milk products:** instant non-fat dry milk powder, milk solids, butter, whey, curd, margarine, casein, casein hydrolysate, ice cream, cheese, lactose. The composition of any food product may be changed without notice.

FOOD GROUP	FOODS TO AVOID
Bread/Starches	Any made with milk or milk products: doughnuts, pancakes, waffles, hot breads, biscuits, crackers, some rolls, rusk, zwieback. Any potatoes, rice or pasta prepared with milk or milk products.
Vegetables	Any prepared or creamed with milk or milk products.
Fruit	None
Meat & Substitutes	Cheese, cottage cheese, sausage products or luncheon meats that contain milk products as fillers. Breaded or creamed meats, fish, or poultry. Eggs or egg substitutes prepared with milk.
Milk	All cow's milk, nonfat dry milk, evaporated milk, condensed milk, yogurt. Milk-based infant formulas. Cocoa containing or prepared with milk. Non-dairy creamers containing caseinate.
Soups & Combination Foods	Cream soups. All soups prepared with milk or milk products.
Desserts & Sweets	Any prepared with ingredients not allowed. Commercial cakes, cookies, pies, puddings, ice cream, sherbet. Prepared baking mixes. Frozen dairy desserts containing the fat substitute Simplesse.
Fats & Oils	Butter, cream, margarines containing milk solids. Salad dressings and mayonnaise with ingredients not allowed.
Beverages	Milk beverages as eggnog, cocoa, milkshakes, malts.

FOOD GROUP	FOODS TO AVOID
Condiments/Miscellaneous	Milk chocolate. Cream sauce. Au gratin dishes. Curd, whey. Foods fried in butter or batter. Imitation chocolate chips.

Adapted from: Bronson-Adatto C, ed. Food sensitivity—a resource including recipes (food sensitivity series). Chicago: American Dietetic Association, 1985. Used with permission.

Client resources for the food-sensitive individual

1. The Food Allergy Network. 4744 Holly Avenue, Fairfax, VA 22030-5647. (703) 691-3179.
2. Hartsook, E. Gluten Intolerance Group Cookbook, 2nd ed. PO Box 23053 Seattle, WA 98102-0353, 1990.
3. Wood, M. Coping with the gluten-free diet. Springfield, IL: Charles C. Thomas, 1982.
4. Zukin, J. Dairy-Free Cookbook. Rocklin, CA: Prima Publishing and Communications. 1989.
5. Gluten Intolerance Group of North America (GIG), PO Box 23053 Broadway Station, Seattle, WA 98102-0353, (206) 325-6980.
6. Allergy Kitchen Series (3 volumes). Allergy Publications, PO Box 640, Menlo Park, CA 94026.
7. Kidder B. The Milk-Free Kitchen. New York, NY:Henry Holt and Co. 1991.
8. Special Recipes and Allergy Aids, General Mills Consumer Center, White Plains, NY 10625.
9. Recipes Using Rice Flour, The Rice council of America, 3917 Richmond Avenue. PO Box 22802, Houston, TX 77027.
10. Yoder ER. Allergy-Free Cooking. Reading, MA: Addison-Wesley Publishing Co., 1987.
11. Celiac Sprue Association, CSA Pantry Collection #1,2, & 3, 1990. PO Box 31700, Omaha, NE 68131-0700.
12. Food Allergy News Cookbook. The Food Allergy Network. 4744 Holly Avenue, Fairfax, VA 22030-5647. (703) 691-3179.
13. Dobler ML. Food Allergies. Chicago: American Dietetic Association 1991.
14. Dobler ML. Gluten Intolerance. Chicago: American Dietetic Association 1991.
15. Beaudette T. Adverse Reactions to Food Chicago: American Dietetic Association 1991.
16. Ener-G Foods, Inc. 5960 1st Avenue South. Seattle, WA 98124-5787, (800) 331-5222.

Elimination Diet
Description
This diet should be followed only while the patient is under a physician's guidance. It is used to aid in identifying the patient's food allergy; therefore, it should be used only for a short period. Foods should be added at intervals of 4 to 5 days according to the physician's directions.

Indications for use
The diet should be followed in the presence of an undefined food allergy or allergies that appear to be related to dietary factors.

Adequacy
The Elimination Diet is inadequate in many nutrients, according to the Recommended Dietary Allowances of the National Research Council. It is recommended for short-term use only, and a vitamin and mineral supplement appropriate for the age of the patient is recommended.

Using the elimination diet
This diet should be followed for a short period and only under a physician's guidance. Its purpose is to discover which foods cause an allergic reaction.

FOOD GROUP	ALLOWED/RECOMMENDED	AVOID/USE SPARINGLY
Breads/Starches	Puffed rice, rice flakes, Rice Krispies®, tapioca	All others
Potatoes/Pasta/Rice	Rice, sweet potato	All others
Vegetables	Asparagus, beets, carrots, lettuce	All others
Fruit or Juices	Apricot, cranberries, peach, pear, pineapple	All others
Meat & Substitutes	Lamb and chicken	All others, including cheese
Milk	None are allowed	All milk and milk products are omitted
Soups & Combination Foods	Only those made with allowed ingredients	All others
Desserts & Sweets	Allowed fruits. Desserts made with allowed ingredients. Cane or beet sugar, honey.	All others
Fats & Oils	Margarine made without milk., non-soybean oils and shortenings, olive oil	All others

FOOD GROUP	ALLOWED/RECOMMENDED	AVOID/USE SPARINGLY
Beverages	Bubble-UP® (a carbonated, dye-free beverage)	All others, including coffee, tea, and colored beverages
Condiments/Miscellaneous	White vinegar, salt	All others, including pepper, spices, chewing gum. Medications that are not specifically ordered.

Gluten Sensitivity

Description

Gluten is the water-insoluble protein found in many grains. Each individual grain has a characteristic gluten composed of several protein fractions. Present in wheat, rye, oats, and barley, alpha-gliadin is a gluten fraction that produces intestinal injury when ingested by susceptible individuals. Other foods may contain gluten (for example, corn or rice), but these glutens are well tolerated.

The toxic glutens have a devastating effect on the small bowel. The intestinal mucosa assume a flat appearance, due to the disappearance of the villi and the thickening of the surface. This results in decreased absorptive surface area and an immature cell population, with diminished enzyme activities and transport capabilities. The damaged mucosa is incapable of normal function, and there is subsequent malabsorption of major nutrients.

Biopsy of the small intestine is usually required for a positive diagnosis of gluten sensitivity. Dietary treatment consists of eliminating foods and food ingredients from wheat, oats, rye, and barley. When these are excluded completely from the diet, most patients regain function of the small intestine.

Strict compliance is important even during symptom-free periods—the patient must realize that this is a lifelong diet. During the initial stages of treatment, some people will also need to restrict lactose, due to a decrease in lactase activity as a result of damage to the brush border of the small intestine.

Indications for use

Celiac disease/nontropical sprue/gluten-sensitive enteropathy
Dermatitis herpetiformis

Adequacy

The Gluten-Controlled Diet is nutritionally adequate according to the Recommended Dietary Allowances of the National Research Council when alternate grains are used.

Professional references

1. American Dietetic Association. Gluten restricted, gliadin free diet. In: Handbook of clinical dietetics. New Haven: Yale University Press, 1980: C 23 - C 27.
2. Bronson-Adatto C, ed. Gluten intolerance—a resource including recipes (food sensitivity series). Chicago: American Dietetic Association, 1985.
3. Dobler ML. Gluten Intolerance. Chicago: American Dietetic Association. 1991.
4. Hartsook EL. Gluten-restricted, gliadin-free diet instruction. Seattle, Wash.: Gluten Intolerance Group of North America, 1987.
5. Kasarda D. The relationship of wheat protein to celiac disease. Cereal Foods World 1978; 240.
6. Shils ME, Olson JA, Shike M. Celiac Disease. In: Modern Nutrition in Health and Disease 8th ed. Lea & Febiger: Philadelphia 1994.

Gluten-Free Diet

Gluten from wheat, rye, oat, and barley protein interferes with the absorption of food in individuals with gluten sensitivity. It is important to read all labels, as gluten may have been added as an incidental ingredient. **Words to check for on the label include:** flour, starch, modified food starch, cereal, thickening, fillers, emulsifiers, and hydrolyzed vegetable protein. A "Gluten-Controlled Diet Product Ingredient List" is available from your dietitian.

If you are not sure whether an ingredient contains gluten, be sure to check with the manufacturer. Also, note that some manufacturers may change ingredients without notice. **Always read labels.**

The following is a strict Gluten-Free Diet. Since flour and cereal products are quite often used in the preparation of foods, it is important to be aware of the methods of preparation used as well as the foods themselves. This is especially true when you are dining out.

FOOD GROUP	ALLOWED/RECOMMENDED	AVOID/USE SPARINGLY
Breads/Starches *4 servings or more**	Only those prepared from arrowroot, corn, potato, rice, and soybean flours. Low-gluten wheat starch, if tolerated muffins, pancakes, Buckwheat(-)	All bread, rolls, etc., made from wheat, rye, oats and/or barley. Commercial gluten bread, commercially prepared for biscuits, cornbread, waffles, etc
Crackers	Rice wafers(*), pure cornmeal tortillas, popcorn, some crackers and chips(*)	All others containing wheat, rye, oats and/or barley
Cereals	Hot cereals made from cornmeal, Cream of Rice®, cold cereals such as puffed rice, Kellogg's Sugar Pops®, Post's Fruity & Chocolate Pebbles®, Van Brode's®, corn flakes and crisp rice, Featherweight's® corn flakes, General Mills'® Cocoa Puffs®	All wheat, rye, and/or oat cereals; wheat germ, barley, oatmeal, bran, graham, malt, bulgar, millet(-), spelt. NOTE: Cereals containing malt as a flavoring may be used only with physician's approval.
Potatoes/Pasta/Rice	White or sweet potatoes, yams, hominy, rice or wild rice, special gluten-free pasta, some oriental rice noodles or bean noodles.	Regular noodles, spaghetti, macaroni, most packaged rice mixes(*)

Flours and thickening agents Notes
(A) Good thickening agent
(B) Good when combined with other flours
(C) Best combined with milk and eggs in baked products
(D) Best in grainy-textured products
(E) Produces drier product than other flours do
(F) Produces moister product than other flours do
(G) Adds distinct flavor to product, use in moderation
	Arrowroot starch (A)
	Corn bran (B)
	Corn flour (B,C,D)
	Corn germ (B)
	Cornmeal (B,C,D)
	Corn starch (A)
	Potato flour (B,C,E)
	Potato starch flour (B,C,E)
	Rice bran (B)
	Rice flours:
	  Plain, brown (B,C,D,E)
	  Sweet (A,B,C,F)
	Rice polish (B,C,G)
	Soy flour (B,C,G)
	Tapioca starch (A)
		Wheat starch (manufacturer states that it contains gluten)
		
		All flours containing wheat, rye, oats, and/or barley

FOOD GROUP	ALLOWED/RECOMMENDED	AVOID/USE SPARINGLY
Vegetables *3 servings or more**	Most plain, fresh, frozen, or canned vegetables	Creamed vegetables(*), vegetables canned in sauces(*). Any prepared with wheat, rye, oats, or barley
Fruit *3 servings or more**	All fresh, frozen, canned, or dried fruits(*). Fruit juices.	Thickened or prepared fruits, some pie fillings(*)
Meat & Substitutes *2 servings or more** *(4 to 6 oz. Total per day)*	Meat, fish, poultry, or eggs prepared without added wheat, rye, oats, or barley, luncheon meat(*), stabilizers; frankfurters(*), and pure meat . All aged cheese, processed cheese products(*), cottage cheese(+), cream cheese(+), dried beans and peas, lentils	Any meat or meat alternate containing wheat, rye, oats, barley, or gluten stabilizers. Bread-containing products such as Swiss steak, croquettes, and meatloaf. Tuna, canned in vegetable broth(*), turkey with HVP injected as part of the basting, any cheese product containing oat gum as an ingredient
Milk *2 cups or the equivalent*	Milk, yogurt made with allowed ingredients(*)	Commercial chocolate milk which may have cereal added(*), malted milk
Soups & Combination Foods	Homemade broth and soups made with allowed ingredients, some canned or frozen soups are allowed(*). Combination or prepared foods that do not contain gluten(*). Read labels.	All soups containing wheat, rye, oat, or barley flours. Bouillon and bouillon cubes that contain hydrolyzed vegetable protein (HVP). Combination or prepared foods that do contain gluten(*).
Desserts & Sweets **In moderation**	Custard, junket, homemade puddings from cornstarch, rice, and tapioca, some pudding mixes(*). Gelatin desserts, ices, and sherbet(*). Cake, cookies, ices, and sherbet(*). Cake, cookies, and other desserts prepared with allowed flours. Some commercial ice creams(*).	Cakes, cookies, doughnuts, pastries, etc., prepared with wheat, rye, oat, and/or barley flour. Some commercial ice creams(*). Ice cream flavors which contain cookies, crumbs, or cheesecake(*); ice cream cones. All commercially prepared mixes for cakes, cookies, and other desserts(*); bread pudding, puddings thickened with flour
Sweets **In moderation**	Sugar, honey, syrup(*), molasses, jelly, jam, plain hard candy, marshmallows, gumdrops(*), homemade candies free from wheat rye, oats, or barley. Coconut	Commercial candies containing wheat, rye, oats, or barley(*). Almond Roca is dusted with wheat flours. Chocolate-coated nuts, which are often rolled in flour.

FOOD GROUP	ALLOWED/RECOMMENDED	AVOID/USE SPARINGLY
Fats & Oils **In moderation**	Butter, margarine, vegetable oil, sour cream(+), whipping cream, shortening, lard, cream, mayonnaise(*). Some commercial salad dressings(*). Peanut butter	Some commercial salad dressings(*).
Beverages	Coffee (regular or decaffeinated), tea, herbal tea (read label to be sure that no wheat flour has been added). Carbonated beverages, some root beers(*).	Cereal beverages such as Postum®, or Ovaltine®, beer, ale, malted milk, some root beers. Whiskey, vodka, gin.
Condiments/Miscellaneous	Salt, pepper, herbs, spices, extracts, food colorings, cider, rice and wine vinegar, bicarbonate of soda, baking powder, Chun King® soy sauce, nuts, coconut, chocolate, and pure cocoa powder. Olives, pickles(#), catsup(#), and mustard(#). Heinz white vinegar.	Some curry powder(*), some dry seasoning mixes(*), some gravy extracts(*), some meat sauces(*), some catsup(*), some prepared mustard(*), horseradish(*), some soy sauce(*), chip dips(*), some chewing gum(*), distilled white vinegar(#). MSG. Yeast extract (contains barley). Caramel color (may contain malt)

(*) Check labels and investigate any questionable ingredients. Also see the "Product Ingredient List," available from your dietitian.

(#) Distilled white vinegar uses grain as a starting material. A very small amount of protein may be carried over into the distillate during large-scale distillation processes. For this reason, it is advisable to use cider or wine vinegar in food preparation such as making salad dressing and pickles and in cooking. Commercially prepared pickles, catsup, mustard, mayonnaise, steak sauce, and other condiments are usually made with distilled grain vinegar; however, the maximum amount of gluten present in such products via the vinegar is insignificant. Moderate use of the above-mentioned commercial condiments may be allowed. In extreme gluten sensitivities, however, they should be avoided.

(-) Additional research is needed before this product can be recommended.

(+) Check vegetable gum used.

* These amounts indicate the **minimum** number of servings needed from the basic food groups to provide a variety of nutrients essential to good health. The word "maximum" is used if amounts of certain foods eaten must be controlled. Combination foods may count as full or partial servings from the food groups. Dark green, leafy, or orange vegetables are recommended 3 or 4 times weekly to provide vitamin A. A good source of vitamin C is recommended daily. Potatoes may be included as a serving of vegetables.

Note: Brand names are used for clarification only, and do not constitute an endorsement. Also, ingredients may be changed by the manufacturer without notice. **Always read labels.**

Source: Adapted from: Hartsook EL. Gluten-restricted, gliadin-free diet instruction. Seattle, Wash.: Gluten Intolerance Group of North America, PO Box 23053, Seattle, Wash. 98102-0353, 1987. Used with permission.

Gluten-Free Diet

SAMPLE MEAL PLAN*

Breakfast	Noon Meal	Evening Meal
Fruit and/or Juice	Meat or Substitute	Meat or Substitute
Cereal (from allowed grains)	Gluten-free bread	Potato or Rice
Toast (from allowed grains)	Vegetable and/or salad	Salad with dressing and/or
Margarine or butter	Margarine or butter	soup
Jam or jelly	Fruit or dessert	Gluten-free bread
Milk	Beverage	Margarine or Butter
Vegetable	Milk	Fruit or Dessert
		Beverage

SAMPLE MENU*

Breakfast	Noon Meal	Evening Meal
Orange Juice	Chicken salad sandwich (with	Roast beef
Banana	gluten-free bread and mayonnaise)	Baked potato/margarine
Rice or corn cereal	Sliced tomatoes	Lettuce salad with gluten-free
Toast (gluten-free bread)	Broccoli	dressing
Margarine	Margarine	Gluten-free bread
Jam	Apple	Margarine
Coffee/tea	Custard	Coffee/tea
Milk	Coffee/tea	Milk

* These meal plans are provided as samples; your daily meal plans will vary.

References you may find helpful

The following additional information is available from your dietitian:

- Gluten-Restricted Diet Product Ingredient List
- Selected Additives that are Gluten-Free
- Refer to: Client Resources for the Food Sensitive Individual in this manual

Gluten-Controlled Diet

Always check the source of the following ingredients before eating any product containing them. When writing the manufacturer, request information on the specific starting material(s) used in the ingredient. For example, when "modified food starch" is listed on the label, ask for the specific type of starch used--potato starch, tapioca starch, etc. Use only those products that are made from allowed sources.

Ingredient	Allowed	Omitted
Hydrolyzed vegetable protein (HVP), texturized vegetable protein (TVP), or hydrolyzed plant protein (HPP)	Soy, Corn	Mixtures of wheat with corn or soy
Flour or cereal products	Rice flour, corn flour; corn meal; potato flour, soy flour	Wheat, rye; oats; barley
Vegetable protein	Soy, corn	Wheat, rye; oats; barley
Malt or malt flavoring	Those derived from corn	Those derived from barley, barley malt syrup
Starch	When listed as such on a U.S. manufacturer's ingredient list, can only be **cornstarch**	
Modified starch or modified food starch	Arrowroot; corn; potato; tapioca, waxy maize, maize	Wheat starch
Vegetable gum	Carob bean; locust bean; cellulose gum; guar gum; gum arabic; bum acacia; bum tragacanth; xanthan gum	Oat gum
Soy sauce, soy sauce solids	Those that do not contain wheat	Those that contain wheat
Mono- and di-glycerides	Those using a gluten-/gliadin-free carrier	Those which use a wheat starch carrier

Source: Hartsook EL. Gluten-restricted diet instruction. Seattle, Wash.: Gluten Intolerance Group North America (PO Box 23053, Seattle, Wash. 98102-0353), 1987. Used with permission.

Selected additives that are gluten free

Adipic Acid
Ascorbic acid
BHA/BHT
Beta Carotene
Biotin

Calcium phosphate
Calcium chloride
Calcium pantothenate
Carboxymethylcellulose
Carrageenan
Citric acid
Corn sweetener
Corn syrup solids

Demineralized whey
Dextrimaltose
Dextrose--dextrins
Dioctyl sodium sulfosuccinate

Extracts

Folic acid--folacin
Fructose
Fumaric acid

GUMS: Acacia; arabic; carob;
       Bean; cellulose; guar,
       Locust beans; tragacanth;
       xanthan

Invent sugar

Lactic acid
Lactose
Lecithin

Magnesium hydroxide
Malic acid
Mannitol
Microcrystalline cellulose
Monosodium glutamate (MSG)

Niacin--niacinamide

Polyglycerol
Polysorbate 60 and 80
Potassium citrate
Potassium iodide
Propylene glycol monostearate
Propylgallate
Pyridoxine hydrochloride

Riboflavin

Sodium acid pyraphosphate
Sodium ascorbate
Sodium benzoate
Sodium caseinate
Sodium citrate
Sodium hexametaphosphate
Sodium nitrate
Sodium silico aluminate
Sucrose
Sorbitol
Sulfosuccinate

Tartaric acid
Thiamine hydrochloride
Tri-calcium phosphate

Vanillin
Vitamins and minerals

Note: The above is not an exhaustive list.

Source: Hartsook EL. Gluten-restricted, gliadin-free diet instruction. Seattle, Wash.: Gluten Intolerance Group of North America (PO Box 23053)

Client resources

1. CELIAC SPRUE ASSOCIATION/UNITED STATES OF AMERICA, INC. (CSA/USA)
   P.O. Box 31700
   Omaha, NE 68131-0700
   402-558-0600

2. MIDWEST GLUTEN INTOLERANCE GROUP (MGIG)
   For membership information contact:
   Sandy Carroll
   8201 158th Ln. NW
   Ramsey, MN 55303

3. MEDICATIONS (prescription and over-the-counter drugs)
   All medications have fillers/dispersing agents added to them that are usually lactose or corn starch. Wheat starch may also be used. Before you take any medication, you should check with the manufacturer to make sure the product is free of gluten/gliadin. When you call or write to them, you will need to tell the drug company the lot number of the product.
   Questions for a pharmacist 1-900-903-7847. There is a charge per minute.

4. GLUTEN FREE PANTRY
   P.O. Box 881
   Glastonbury, CT 06033
   203-633-3826

5. THE REALLY GREAT FOOD CO.
   P.O. Box 319
   Malverne, NY 11565

6. DIETARY SPECIALTIES
   P.O. Box 227
   Rochester, NY 14601-0227

7. ENER-G-FOODS, INC.
   P.O. Box 84487
   Seattle, WA 98124-5787

Gluten-Controlled Diet

Always check the source of the following ingredients before eating any product containing them. When writing the manufacturer, request information on the specific starting material(s) used in the ingredient. For example, when "modified food starch" is listed on the label, ask for the specific type of starch used—potato starch, tapioca starch, etc. Use only those products that are made from allowed sources.

INGREDIENT	ALLOWED/RECOMMENDED	OMITTED
Hydrolyzed vegetable protein (HVP), texturized vegetable protein (TVP), or hydrolyzed plant protein (HPP)	Soy, corn	Mixtures of wheat with corn or soya
Flour or cereal products	Rice flour, corn flour, corn meal, potato flour, soy flour	Wheat, rye, oats, barley
Vegetable protein	Soy, corn	Wheat, rye, oats, barley
Malt or malt flavoring	Those derived from corn	Those derived from barley, barley malt
Starch	When listed as such on a U.S. manufacturer's ingredient list, can only be **cornstarch**	
Modified starch or modified food starch	Arrowroot, corn, potato, tapioca, waxy maize, maize	Wheat starch
Vegetable gum	Carob bean, locust bean, cellulose gum, guar gum, gum arabic, gum acacia, gum tragacanth, xanthan gum	Oat gum
Soy sauce, soy sauce solids	Those that do not contain wheat	Those that contain wheat
Mono- and diglycerides	Those using a gluten/gliadin-free carrier.	Those which use a wheat starch carrier

Medications (prescription and over-the-counter drugs)

All medications have fillers/dispersing agents added to them that are usually lactose or corn starch. Wheat starch may also be used. Before you take any medication, you should check with the manufacturer to make sure the product is free of gluten/gliadin. When you call or write to the drug company, you will need to know the lot number of the product.

SOURCE: Hartsook EL. Gluten-restricted, gliadin-free diet instruction. Seattle, Wash.: Gluten Intolerance Group of North America (PO Box 23053, Seattle, Wash. 98102-0353), 1987. Used with permission.

Tyramine- and Dopamine-Controlled Diet
Description

This diet identifies foods high in tyramine, either naturally or through aging (a process that increases tyramine content by protein breakdown), and/or foods high in dopamine. Both need to be limited while a person is using a monoamine oxidase inhibitor, and for two weeks after discontinuing the drug.

Tyramine and dopamine are monoamines. Monoamines cause constriction of blood vessels and abnormal elevation of blood pressure. Normally, these amines are harmless because of an enzyme, monoamine oxidase (MAO), which efficiently and rapidly detoxifies them. The MAO-Inhibitor (MAO-I) class of drugs decreases this effect. Therefore, ingestion of foods high in tyramine in the presence of an MAO-I drug can result in a hypertensive crisis.

The severity of the crisis depends on several factors:
1. The amount of tyramine consumed:
   - 6 mg can produce mild elevation in blood pressure
   - 10 mg may show a marked elevation
   - 25 mg can result in a severe hypertensive crisis
2. The rapidity of gastric emptying
3. The type of MAO-I (tranylcypromine, trade name Parnate, is most likely to cause a hypertensive reaction)
4. The duration of MAO-I treatment:
   - Reactions are less severe during the first few weeks of treatment
5. The size of the dose
6. The interval between the dose and the ingestion of tyramine-containing food
   - Greater risk if ingestion of a high-tyramine food closely follows the MAO-I dose

Indications for use

The Tyramine- and Dopamine-Controlled Diet is indicated whenever one of the following monoamine oxidase inhibitors (MAO-I) is prescribed:

Generic name	Trademark
furazolidone	Furoxone (Norwich-Eaton)
isocarboxazid	Marplan (Roche)
pargyline hydrochloride	Eutonyl (Abbott)
pargyline hydrochloride and methylclothiazine	Eutron (Abbott)
phenelzine sulfate	Nardil (Parke-Davis)
procarbazine	Matulane (Roche)
tranylcypromine sulfate	Parnate (Smith, Kline and French)

Adequacy

Diets restricted in tyramine and dopamine are nutritionally adequate, according to the Recommended Dietary Allowances of the National Research Council.

Professional references

1. Walker JI, Davidson MB, Zung WK. Patient compliance with MAO inhibitor therapy. J Clin Psychiatry 1984; 45(7, Sec. 2):78-80.

2. McCabe BJ, Tsuang MT. Dietary considerations in MAO inhibitor regimens. J Clin Psychiatry 1982; 43(5):178-81.

3. Maxwell MB. Re-examining the dietary restrictions with procarbazine (on MAO-I). Cancer Nursing 1980; (Dec.):451-7.

4. Sullivan EA, Schulman KI. Diet and monoamine oxidase inhibitors: a re-examination. Can J Psychiatry 1984; 29:707-11.

5. Davidson J, Zung WK, Walker JI. Practical aspects of MAO inhibitor therapy. J Clin Psychiatry 1984; 45(7,Sec. 2):81-4.

6. McCabe BJ. Dietary tyramine and other pressor amines in MAO-I regimens: a review. J Am Dietetic Assoc 1986; 86(8):1059-64.

7. Moneret-Vautron DA. Biogenic amines. Bibl Nutr Dieta Basel Karger, 48:66-71, 1991.

Tyramine- and Dopamine-Restricted Diet
Special notes

This diet should be followed while taking any monoamine oxidase inhibitor (MAO-I) drug, and for two weeks after discontinuing the drug. Consuming any food high in tyramine or dopamine while taking an MAO-I drug may cause elevated blood pressure. Symptoms can include pounding headache, choking sensations, racing heart, and neck stiffness. Symptoms will usually occur within two hours after eating.

FOOD GROUP	ALLOWED/RECOMMENDED	AVOID/USE SPARINGLY
Breads/Starches *4 servings or more**	Any except those listed to avoid.	Bread or crackers containing aged cheese.
Vegetables *2 servings or more**	Any except those listed to avoid.	Any spoiled vegetable. Pods of broad green beans**, including fava beans and Italian green beans. Sauerkraut.
Fruit *2 servings or more**	Any except those listed to avoid.	Banana peel; any spoiled fruit.
Meat & Substitutes *2 servings or more** *(4 to 6 oz. Total per day)*	Fresh poultry, meat, fish, or eggs. Tofu, cottage cheese, cream cheese, processed cheese and American cheese.	Spoiled or aged protein foods. Pickled herring. Cheese aged six (6) months or longer. (Limit these to 4 oz. Per day).
Milk *2 cups or the equivalent**	Any except those listed to avoid.	Any spoiled milk or milk product.
Soups & Combination Foods	Any except those listed to avoid.	Any that have become spoiled or putrid. Any that contain pods of broad beans or excessive amounts of cheese.
Desserts & Sweets *In moderation*	Any except those listed to avoid.	Desserts that contain excessive amounts of cheeses.
Fats & Oils *In moderation*	All are allowed.	None are omitted.
Beverages	Beverages are allowed; however, limit the following to the amounts shown: Coffee, tea-4 to 5 cups per day*** Spirits-1 to 2 oz. Per day Wines – 8 oz. Per day Beer-12 to 24 oz. Per day	Alcohol, coffee, or tea in excess of limits. Limit caffeine-containing carbonated beverages to fewer than ten servings per day.
Condiments/Miscellaneous	Any except those listed to avoid.	Brewer's yeast, marmite. Any food that has become spoiled or putrid

* These amounts indicate the minimum number of servings needed from the basic food groups to provide a variety of nutrients essential to good health. The word "maximum" or "limit" is used if amounts of certain foods eaten must be controlled. Combination foods may count as full or partial servings from the food groups. Dark green, leafy, or orange vegetables are recommended 3 or 4 times weekly to provide vitamin A. A good source of vitamin C is recommended daily. Potatoes may be included as a serving of vegetables.

** Contains dopamine, another amine that can cause elevated blood pressure.

*** Caffeine in large amounts may cause hypertension and cardiac arrhythmias in persons taking an MAO-I.

Tyramine Levels in Average Portions

Tyramine levels vary with samples, methods of analysis, and methods of food storage. Although not precise, the following values serve as a guide to relative levels of tyramine in some common foods.

Extremely High Levels—greater than 100 mg per average serving
- Pickled herring, 3 oz.   259 mg
- Stilton cheese, 2 oz.   124

Very High Levels—50 to 100 mg per average serving
- Cheddar cheese, 2 oz.   88 mg
- Camembert cheese, 2 oz.   76
- Boursault cheese, 2 oz. 64
- Emmenthaler cheese, 2 oz.   57

High Levels—20 to 50 mg per average serving
- Yeast extract, 1 tsp.   35 mg
- Brick cheese, 2 oz.   30
- Roquefort cheese, 2 oz. 30
- Herring, salted and dried, 2 oz. 27
- Mozzarella cheese, 2 oz.   23

Moderate Levels—5 to 20 mg per average serving
- Blue cheese, 2 oz.   15 mg
- Romano cheese, 2 oz.   14
- Chianti wine, 8 oz.   6

Low Levels—1 to 5 mg per average serving
- Meat extract, 1 tsp.   5 mg
- Beer, 12 oz.   3
- Processed cheese, 2 oz. 2
- Avocado, 3-1/2 oz.   1
- Orange, 2-1/2 in. diameter   1

Minimal Levels—less than 1 mg per serving
- Cream cheese   Yeast
- Cottage cheese Unfermented soy sauce
- Yogurt Fruits, including bananas
- Champagne   Distilled spirits—vodka, whiskey, etc.

Only the pods of broad beans are restricted because of their dopamine content. No other foods known to date have been identified as being high in dopamine.

Lactose-Controlled Diets
Description

Lactose is a carbohydrate that is found primarily in milk and milk products, as well as in foods with added milk or whey. In order to be used by the body, lactose must be hydrolyzed into galactose and glucose by the enzyme lactase. Lactose intolerance occurs when there is a deficiency of this enzyme.

If the small intestine contains insufficient lactase activity to hydrolyze an ingested load of lactose, the unabsorbed lactose remains in the intestine and acts osmotically to draw water into the area. This may cause symptoms of nausea, bloating, and cramping. Later, when the lactose and water enter the colon, the lactose is metabolized by bacteria, producing carbon dioxide, hydrogen, and organic acids. The patient can experience additional bloating and cramping, plus gas and diarrhea.

Classifications of lactase deficiency

Congenital lactase deficiency: A rare, inborn error of metabolism in which infants develop severe diarrhea when fed breast milk or a milk-based formula.

Primary lactase deficiency: The most common type, characterized by a gradual decrease in lactase activity. It occurs after weaning.

Secondary lactase deficiency: Occurs following injury to the small intestinal mucosa as a result of diseases such as celiac disease, nontropical sprue, infectious gastroenteritis, malnutrition, parasites, or inflammatory bowel disease. It can also occur after treatment with antibiotics or cancer drugs or as a result of surgery.

Tolerance to lactose varies widely, and each person must determine how much milk can be consumed without developing symptoms. Drinking smaller portions of milk throughout the day may be beneficial. Some studies suggest that slowing gastric emptying may help increase tolerance of milk products. This may be accomplished by:

- Consuming milk or milk products with a meal rather than alone
- Using milk with a higher fat content
- Drinking chocolate milk instead of unflavored milk
- There are several dairy products that may be tolerated better than milk by some people:
- Cheese (especially aged cheese) has lactose content is much lower than in milk.
- Yogurt contains bacterial lactase, which is active in the intestinal tract and helps digest the lactose.

The use of cultured dairy products such as buttermilk, cottage cheese, and sweet acidophilus milk for lactase-deficient individuals is controversial. Lactose-hydrolyzed milk (Lact-Aid®) contains 40 to 90 percent less lactose than milk. This product decreases symptoms of milk intolerance.

Indications for use

Lactose-Free Diet

1. Congenital lactase deficiency
2. Galactosemia
3. Initial treatment stages of some gastrointestinal diseases

Low-Lactose Diet

1. Primary lactase deficiency
2. Secondary lactase deficiency

There is no clear-cut dividing point between the two diets. As stated previously, there is much variance in patients' tolerance to lactose. A person may start out with a strict Lactose-Free Diet and eventually may be able to tolerate small amounts of lactose. Conversely, some people's symptoms may not respond to the Low-Lactose Diet, and they may need to follow the Lactose-Free Diet.

Adequacy

These diets may be deficient in calcium, riboflavin, and vitamin D, according to the Recommended Dietary Allowances of the National Research Council. Depending on individual tolerances and the use of milk substitutes, milk, or other dairy products, these recommendations may be met.

Professional references

1. American Dietetic Association. Lactose free diet. In: Handbook of clinical dietetics. New Haven, Conn.: Yale University Press, 1980:D13-10.
2. Bayless TM, Rosenberg IH, Walker WA. When to suspect lactose intolerance. Patient Care 1987; (Sept. 30):136-47.
3. Martini MC, Smith DE, Savaiano DA. Lactose digestion from flavored and frozen yogurt, ice milk, and ice cream by lactase-deficient persons. Am J Clin Nutr 1987; 46:636-40.
4. Bayless TM, Paige DM, eds. Lactose digestion: clinical and nutritional implications. Baltimore, Maryland, and London: Johns Hopkins University Press, 1981.
5. Bronson-Adatto C, ed. Lactose intolerance—a resource including recipes. Chicago: American Dietetic Association, 1985.
6. National Dairy Council. Cultured and culture-containing dairy foods. Dairy Council Digest 1984; 55(3).
7. National Dairy Council. Nutritional implications of lactose and lactase activity. Dairy Council Digest 1985; 56(5).
8. Newcomer AD, McGill DB. Clinical consequences of lactase deficiency. Clinical Nutrition 1984; 3 (Manual of Clinical Nutrition Supplement):53-8.
9. Savaiano DA, Abov El Anovar A, Smith DE, Levitt MD. Lactose malabsorption from yogurt, pasteurized yogurt, sweet acidophilus milk and cultured milk in lactase-deficient individuals. Amer J Clin Nutr 1984; 40:1219-23.
10. Skinner S, Martens RA. The milk sugar dilemma: living with lactose intolerance. East Lansing, Mich.: Medi-ed Press, 1987.

Lactose- (and Galactose-) Free Diet
Special notes

Lactose and galactose are carbohydrates. The major food source is dairy products. Reading food labels is important. Many products add lactose, even when they are not made from milk. Look for the following words: whey, milk solids, dry milk solids, nonfat dry milk powder. Typical sources of lactose other than dairy products include breads, candies, cold cuts, prepared and processed foods, and commercial sauces and gravies.

Lactalbumin, lactic acid, and lactate do not contain lactose and do not have to be eliminated.

All foods must be prepared without milk, cream, or other dairy foods.

A vitamin/mineral supplement may be necessary. Consult your physician or dietitian.

Lactose also is found in many prescription and over-the-counter medications.

Soy milk and lactose-free supplements may be used as an alternative to milk.

In order to make this diet galactose free, the following foods must also be omitted. Do this only upon the recommendation of your physician or dietitian.

Organ meats	Lima beans
Dried beans	Peas
Sugar beets	Soybeans
Lentils	

FOOD GROUP	ALLOWED/RECOMMENDED	AVOID/USE SPARINGLY
Breads/Starches *4 servings or more**	Breads and rolls made without milk. French, Vienna, or Italian bread.	Breads and rolls that contain milk. Prepared mixes such as muffins, biscuits, waffles, pancakes. Sweet rolls, donuts, French toast (if made with milk or lactose).
Crackers	Soda crackers, graham crackers. Any crackers prepared without lactose.	Zwieback crackers, corn curls, or any that contain lactose.
Cereals	Cooked or dry cereals prepared without lactose (read labels).	Cooked or dry cereals prepared with lactose (read labels).
Potatoes/Pasta/Rice	Instant potatoes, frozen French fries, Any prepared without milk or lactose. Popcorn.	Escalloped or au gratin potatoes.
Vegetables *2 servings or more**	Fresh, frozen, and canned vegetables.	Creamed or breaded vegetables. Vegetables in a cheese sauce or with lactose-containing margarines.
Fruit *2 servings or more**	All fresh, canned, or frozen fruits that are not processed with lactose	Any canned or frozen fruits processed with lactose.
Meat and Substitutes *2 servings or more**	Plain beef, chicken, fish, turkey, lamb, veal, pork, or ham. Kosher prepared meat products. Strained or junior meats that do not contain milk. Eggs, soy meat substitutes, nuts. Soy cheese. Tofu.	Scrambled eggs, omelets, souffles that contain milk. Creamed or breaded meat, fish, or fowl. Sausage products such as wieners, liver sausage, or cold cuts that contain milk solids. Cheese, cottage cheese, or cheese spreads.

FOOD GROUP	ALLOWED/RECOMMENDED	AVOID/USE SPARINGLY
Milk[**] *(See Beverages for milk substitutes. See Desserts for ice cream and frozen desserts.)*	None.	Milk (whole, 2%, skim, or chocolate). Evaporated, powdered, or condensed milk; yogurt; buttermilk; malted milk; sweet acidophilus milk.
Soups & Combination Foods	Bouillon, broth, vegetable soups, clear soups, consomme. Homemade soups made with allowed ingredients. Combination or prepared foods that do not contain milk or milk products (read labels).	Cream soups, chowders, commercially prepared soups containing lactose. Macaroni and cheese, pizza. Combination or prepared foods that contain milk or milk products.
Desserts & Sweets *In moderation*	Water and fruit ices; gelatin; angel food cake. Homemade cookies, pies, or frozen cakes made from allowed ingredients. Pudding (if made with water or a milk substitute). Lactose-free tofu desserts. Sugar, honey, corn syrup, jam, jelly; marmalade; molasses (beet sugar); Pure sugar candy, marshmallows.	Ice cream, ice milk, sherbet, custard, pudding, yogurt. Commercial cake and cookie mixes. Desserts that contain chocolate. Pie crust made with milk-containing margarine; reduced calorie desserts made with a sugar substitute that contains lactose. Toffee, peppermint, butterscotch, chocolage, caramels. Frozen dairy desserts containing the fat substitute Simplesse.
Fats & Oils *In moderation*	Butter (as tolerated-contains very small amounts of lactose). Margarines and dressings that do not contain milk. Vegetable oils, shortening, Miracle Whip®, mayonnaise, nondairy cream and whipped toppings without lactose or milk solids added (examples, Coffee Rich®, Borden's Cremora®, Carnation Coffeemate®, Rich's Whipped Topping®, PolyRich®.	Margarines and salad dressings containing cream, cream cheese; peanut butter with added milk solids, sour cream, chip dips made with sour cream.
Beverages	Carbonated drinks; tea; coffee and freeze-dried coffee; some instant coffees (check labels). Fruit drinks; fruit and vegetable juice; Postum®, Milk substitutes, such as soy milk and lactose-free supplements, and soy formulas. (Refer to the Enteral nutrition section for listing.)	Ovaltine®, hot chocolate. Some cocoas; some instant coffees; instant iced teas; powdered fruit drinks (read labels). Diet carbonated beverages that contain a lactose carrier.
Condiments/Miscellaneous	Soy sauce, carob powder, olives, gravy made with water, baker's cocoa, pickles, pure seasonings and spices, wine, pure monosodium glutamate, catsup, mustard.	Some chewing gums, chocolate, some cocoas. Dietetic preparations (read labels), Certain antibiotics and vitamin/mineral preparations. Spice blends if they contain milk products. MSG extender. Artificial sweeteners that contain lactose. Some nondairy creamers (read labels).

* These amounts indicate the minimum number of servings needed from the basic food groups to provide a variety of nutrients essential to good health. A maximum amount is listed if intake of certain foods must be controlled. Combination foods may count as full or partial servings from the food groups. Dark green, leafy, or orange vegetables are recommended 3 or 4 times weekly to provide vitamin A. A good source of vitamin C is recommended daily. Potatoes may be included as a serving of vegetables.

** The Lactose-Free Diet will be deficient in the Milk/Milk Product Group servings.

A sample meal plan for the Lactose-Free Diet is available from your dietitian.

Ingredients in any product may be changed by manufacturers. Always read labels.

Additional consumer information, available from your dietitian, includes
- Substitutions for Lactose-Containing Ingredients
- Consumer Resources (publications) and Alternative Products
- Lactose Content of Various Foods

Reference
1. Skinner S, Martens RA. The milk sugar dilemma: living with lactose intolerance. East Lansing, Mich.: Medied Press, 1987. Used with permission.

Low-Lactose Diet
Special notes

Lactose is a carbohydrate. The major food source is dairy products. Reading food labels is important. Many products contain lactose, even when they are not made from milk. Look for the following words: whey, milk solids, dry milk solids, nonfat dry milk powder, lactose.

Foods processed with minor amounts of milk or milk products may be used as tolerated. The quantity of lactose or milk tolerated varies from one individual to another. Drinking one-fourth to one-half cup of milk at four separate times should be tried, rather than drinking one cup all at once. Taking milk or dairy products with a meal is recommended. Two percent or whole milk may work better than skim milk, and heating milk may also be of some benefit.

Many types of cheese are low in lactose, and aged cheeses are better tolerated in many individuals. A fermented dairy product, such as yogurt, seems to produce fewer symptoms, even though the lactose content is similar to that in milk.

Lactose-hydrolyzed milk, soy milk, and lactose-free nutritional supplements may be used as an alternative to milk.

In some individuals, chocolate milk may be better tolerated than whole milk.

A vitamin/mineral supplement may be necessary. Consult your physician or dietitian.

If the Low-Lactose Diet does not alleviate symptoms, refer to the Lactose-Free Diet.

NOTE: The foods in the Avoid/Use Sparingly column below contain lactose, but may be tolerated by some individuals. Refer to the above "Special Notes" for ideas about how to include them in your diet.

FOOD GROUP	ALLOWED/RECOMMENDED	AVOID/USE SPARINGLY
Breads/Starches *4 servings or more**	All.	None.
Crackers:	All.	None.
Cereals:	All.	None.
Potatoes/Pasta/Rice	All.	Those prepared with milk or milk products, such as au gratin or escalloped potatoes.
Vegetables *2 servings or more**	All.	Those prepared with milk or milk products.
Fruit *2 servings or more**	All.	None.
Meat & Meat Substitutes *2 servings or more** *(4 to 6 oz. Total per day)*	All meat, eggs, poultry, fish, peanut butter. Parmesan, monterey, Swiss. Dry cottage cheese. Nuts.	American processed cheese, Aged cheese such as cheese spreads, imitation blue, brick, cheddar, Edam, Gouda, cheese food, creamed cottage cheese, curd cheese.
Milk* * *2 cups or the equivalent**	Yogurt (as tolerated). Choose a brand of yogurt that contains "active" or "live" cultures. Lactose-reduced milk as tolerated, acidophilus milk***. Cocoa	Milk (whole, 2%, skim). Evaporated, powdered, condensed milk; malted milk; buttermilk***; sweet mixes. Frozen yogurt.
Soups & Combination Foods	Broth, bouillon, consomme. Homemade soups made from allowed ingredients. Combination foods that do not contain milk or milk products (read labels).	Cream soups, commercial soups containing milk or milk products. Combination foods that contain milk or milk products.

FOOD GROUP	ALLOWED/RECOMMENDED	AVOID/USE SPARINGLY
Desserts & Sweets *In moderation*	Fruit ice, gelatin, cakes, cookies or pastries. Lactose-free tofu desserts. Sugar, honey, corn syrup, jam, jelly, marshmallows, pure sugar candy, molasses. Chocolate and cream candy; caramel within tolerated limits.	Ice cream, ice milk, sherbet, pudding, custard.
Fats & Oils *In moderation*	Butter, margarine, lard, oil, shortening, nondairy cream substitutes, salad dressings.	Cream, sour cream, cream cheese (small amounts may be tolerated).
Beverages	Coffee, tea, fruit and vegetable juices, carbonated drinks. Milk substitutes, infant soy formulas, lactose-free supplements.	None except those mentioned under the Milk category.
Condiments/Miscellaneous	Spices, herbs, condiments, olives, unsweetened cocoa, vinegar, pickles.	White sauces, cocoa mixes.

* These amounts indicate the minimum number of servings needed from the basic food groups to provide a variety of nutrients essential to good health. A maximum amount is listed if intake of certain foods must be controlled. Combination foods may count as full or partial servings from the food groups. Dark green, leafy, or orange vegetables are recommended 3 or 4 times weekly to provide vitamin A. A good source of vitamin C is recommended daily. Potatoes may be included as a serving of vegetables.

** The Low-Lactose Diet will be deficient in the Milk/Milk Product Group servings unless 2 c. yogurt, or lactose-reduced milk or lactose-free supplement can be included.

*** Some individuals may be able to tolerate these products.

Additional consumer information, available from your dietitian, includes
- Sample Meal Pattern for the Low-Lactose Diet
- Substitutions for Lactose-Containing Ingredients
- Consumer Resources (publications) and Alternative Products
- Lactose- (and Galactose-) Free Diet

Reference

1. Skinner S, Martens RA. The milk sugar dilemma: living with lactose intolerance. East Lansing, Mich.: Medi-ed Press, 1987. Used with permission.

Lactose-Controlled Diets
Sample Meal Plans

Lactose- (and galactose-) free diet

SAMPLE MEAL PLAN*

Breakfast	Noon Meal	Evening Meal
Fruit and/or juice	Meat or substitute	Meat or substitute
Cereal	Bread or substitute	Potato or substitute
Nondairy creamer	Vegetable	Salad with dressing or soup
or milk substitute	Nondairy margarine or butter	Vegetable
Toast	Fruit or dessert without milk	Bread
Nondairy margarine or butter	Beverage	Nondairy margarine or butter
Beverage		Fruit or dessert without milk
		Beverage

SAMPLE MENU*

Breakfast	Noon Meal	Evening Meal
Orange juice	Chicken breast	Roast beef
Banana	Rice	Baked potato
Bran flakes	Green beans	Butter or milk-free margarine
Vienna bread (toasted)	Fresh melon	Broccoli
Butter or milk-free margarine	Coffee or tea	Lettuce salad with vinegar and oil
Coffee or tea	Non-dairy creamer	dressing
Non-dairy creamer		Angel food cake
		Coffee or tea
		Non-dairy creamer

Low-lactose diet

SAMPLE MENU*

Breakfast	Noon Meal	Evening Meal
Orange juice	Chicken breast	Roast beef
Banana	Rice	Baked potato
Bran flakes	Green beans	Broccoli
Toast	Fresh melon	Lettuce salad with Thousand
Margarine or butter	1 c. yogurt with active cultures	Island or French dressing
Coffee or tea	Coffee or tea	Bread with margarine or butter
		Oatmeal raisin cookie or cake
		Coffee or tea
	Snack	
	1-1/2 oz. Aged cheddar cheese	
	Crackers	

* Lactose-controlled diets will be deficient in the Milk/Milk Product Group servings unless 2 c. yogurt, lactose-reduced milk or lactose-free supplement can be included.

Additional consumer information, available from your dietitian, includes
- Substitutions for lactose-containing ingredients
- Consumer information (publications) available and alternative products

Substitutions for Lactose-Containing Ingredients
Lactose-Controlled Diets

In place of:	Use:
Cream, Half & Half (10-12% butterfat) 1 cup	1½ tbsp. Butter or milk-free margarine plus about 7/8 cup milk substitute OR ½ cup liquid non-dairy creamer plus ½ cup milk substitute
Cream, coffee (at least 20% butterfat) 1 cup	3 tbsp. Butter or milk-free margarine plus about 7/8 cup milk substitute
Cream, whipping, heavy (26-40% butterfat) 1 cup	1/3 cup butter or milk-free margarine plus about ¾ cup milk substitute (This substitution cannot be used for whipping.)
Cream, sour 1 cup	3 tbsp. Butter or milk-free margarine plus 7/8 cup buttermilk or yogurt. (Use buttermilk or yogurt only as tolerated).
Milk, whole 1 cup	1 cup soy milk or LactAid* or 1 cup coconut milk or 1 cup almond milk or 1 cup fruit juice or 1 cup potato water (The choice depends on the recipe and resulting flavor.) OR USE 1 cup lactose-free supplement and decrease sugar in recipe or ½ cup liquid non-dairy creamer plus ½ cup water or 1 cup water plus 1½ tsp. Butter or milk-free margarine.
Milk, Skim 1 cup	¼ cup liquid non-dairy creamer plus ¾ cup water

* Brand names are used for clarification only and do not constitute an endorsement.

Adapted from: Skinner S, Martens RA. The milk sugar dilemma: living with lactose intolerance. East Lansing, Mich.: Medi-ed Press, 1987. Used with permission.

Client Resources
Lactose-Controlled Diets

1. American Dietetic Association. Lactose intolerance (a resource including recipes). American Dietetic Association, 208 South LaSalle Street, Suite 1100, Chicago, IL 60604-1003.
2. Skinner, Sherlyn and Martens, Richard. The milk sugar dilemma: living with lactose intolerance. Medi-ed Press, 1987. (Available from Medi-ed Press, P.O. Box 957, East Lansing, MI 48823.)
3. LactAid"—samples and literature available. LactAid", P.O. Box 111, Pleasantville, NJ 08232.
4. Cooking with Isomil" (milk-free recipes). Ross Laboratories, 625 Cleveland Avenue, Columbus, OH 43216.
5. Meals without milk. Mead Johnson & Co., 2400 West Pennsylvania Street, Evansville, IN 47721-0001.
6. Zukin, Jane. Milk-free diet cookbook: cooking for the lactose intolerant. Sterling Publishing Co., Inc., New York, NY.
7. Byerly's (grocery stores). Special foods for special people—lactose-free diet. This shopping guide can be obtained from the home economist or the store manager at all Byerly's locations.
8. National Dairy Council. Getting along without milk—for people with lactose intolerance. Rosemount, Ill.: National Dairy Council, 1987. (Available from National Dairy Council, Rosemount, Ill., 60018-4233.)

Alternative products
LactAid® (lactase enzyme)

Available in liquid form to add to milk and in tablet form to be taken before consuming lactose-containing foods. LactAid® pretreated milk, cottage cheese, American processed cheese food, and ice cream are also available in some stores.

Soy milk

Various companies provide this product. It must be fortified with calcium in order to be nutritionally equivalent to milk. It is important to study the labels to determine how closely the nutrient content resembles that of milk.

Nondairy creamers

Check the labels; some have lactose added.

Special Considerations for High Risk Neonates

High risk infants include low birth weight (≤ 2500 grams), premature (≤ 37 weeks), small for gestational age (SGA) or intrauterine growth retarded infants. Preterm infants of a weight appropriate for gestational age have increased calorie needs compared to a full term infant. Provision of adequate calories is essential to prevent starvation, hypoglycemia and promote optimal growth of approximately 20-30 grams per day. Generally an intake of 120 kcal/kg/day enterally or 90-100 kcal/kg/day parenterally will meet these needs. Growth retarded or SGA infants have experienced insufficient calorie and nutrient intake for proper intrauterine growth. These infants may need a minimum of 120 kcal/kg/day enterally and up to 140-150 kcal/kg/day to catch up.

Proper distribution of protein, carbohydrate and fat helps assure a tolerable renal solute and gastrointestinal osmotic load. Due to the limited gastric capacity to handle the volume necessary to meet calorie needs, occasionally the standard 67 kcal/100 ml (20 kcal/oz.) formula must be concentrated to 81 kcal/100 ml (24 kcal/oz) or 91 kcal/100 ml (27 kcal/oz). Concentrated formulas may be needed for infants with cardiac or lung disease requiring fluid restriction. Concentration should be gradually increased to allow the gastrointestinal system time to accommodate to the increased osmolality. Fluid intake and output as well as urine osmolarity need to be monitored with increased formula concentrations. Normally a fluid intake of 100-150 ml/kg/day will maintain the infant. The range may vary from 100-200 ml/kg/day. Influences such as phototherapy, gastrointestinal losses, skin and lung losses and use of radiant warmers demand close monitoring. It is important to note that the actual fluid requirements depend on individual needs and must be calculated as such.

Protein needs also exceed those of a normal full term infant. An intake of 3-4 gms/kg/day orally is recommended. These amino acids are known to be essential for premature infants: histidine, cystine, taurine, and tyrosine. These needs will be met with the recommended intake of fortified human milk or premature infant formula. Parental amino acids should be limited to 2.5-3.0 gms/kg/day.

Carbohydrate generally poses no problem to the high risk infant. Although lactase reaches peak activity at nine months gestation, these infants generally tolerate the lactose in infant formulas and human milk. Formulas designed for premature infants have a reduced lactose content which is replaced in part by glucose polymers.

Fat is more likely to be malabsorbed by a preterm infant because of diminished bile acid pools and increased bile acid secretion. Medium chain triglycerides are tolerated better than long chain triglycerides and compose a large portion of the fats in premature infant formulas. In parenteral solutions lipids will provide essential fatty acids and are quite helpful as a calorie source. They should be limited to 2-3 gms/kg/day.

Other nutrients which most authors feel deserve careful consideration include sodium, calcium, phosphorus, vitamin E, vitamin D, and iron.

Recommended readings

1. Green HL, Hambridge KM, Schandler R, et al. Guidelines for the use of vitamins, trace elements, calcium, magnesium, and phosphorus in infants and children receiving total parenteral nutrition. *Amer. J. Clin. Nutr.* 1988; 48:1324-1342.

2. Keiner JA. *Parenteral Nutrition.* In: Walker WA, et al editors. Pediatric gastrointestinal disease volume two. Philadelphia, PA: B.C. Decker; 1991: 1645-1675.

3. Tsang RC and Nichols B (eds): Nutrition during Infancy. Hanley and Belfus Inc., Philadelphia, PA, 1988.

4. Tsang RC, Lucas A, Ricardo U, and Zlotkins (eds): Nutritional needs of the preterm infant. Williams and Wilkins, Baltimore, MD, 1993.

5. Groh-Wargo S, Thompson M, and Hovasi Cox J (eds): Nutritional care for high-risk newborns. Precept Press Inc., Chicago, IL, 1994.

6. Van Aerde J. Nutrition and metabolism in the high-risk neonate. In: Fanaroff AA and Martin RJ, (eds). *Neonatal-Perinatal Medicine Diseases of the Fetus and Infant.* St. Louis, MO, Mosby Year Book 1991:478-526.

7.. Rose J, Gibbons K, Carlson S, and Koo W. Nutrient needs of the preterm infant. *Nutrition in Clinical Practice* 1993; 8:226-232.

8. Gremse DA and Balistreri WF. Neonatal cholestasis. In: Lebenthal E, ed. Textbook of gastroenterology and nutrition in infancy, second edition. New York: Raven Press Ltd. 1989:909-948.

9. American Academy of Pediatrics, Committee on Nutrition. Nutritional needs of low-birth-weight infants. *Pediatrics* 1985; 75:976-986.

Nutritional Intervention for Diarrhea
Definition

Diarrhea is characterized by an increased volume (>20 gm/kg/day) and fluidity of stool, and an increase in frequency of bowel movements relative to the usual pattern for a particular child. It can be accompanied by an excessive intestinal loss of fluid and electrolytes. Diarrhea is usually termed either acute or chronic.

Acute diarrhea
Etiology

Acute diarrhea can be caused by infectious agents (viral, bacterial, or parasitic), antibiotics, food allergy or intolerance, inflammatory bowel disorders, or extraintes-tinal infections (e.g. otitis media, pneumonia or urinary tract infection). It may last a few days to a week.

Treatment

The goals of treatment are:
- Rehydration Therapy—to correct existing fluid and electrolyte deficits with an oral electrolyte solution (OES). See Enteral Nutrition section for listing or intravenous fluids, if needed.
- Therapy for ongoing loss—to replace ongoing fluid and electrolyte losses from stooling and/or vomiting with OES.
- Maintenance Therapy—to supply normal daily fluid needs with low salt fluids, such as breast milk, the usual milk-based feeds, and water.
- Antimicrobial therapy—as indicated.

Children with no signs of dehydration can be treated at home by the caregiver with increased fluids and continuation of the regular feeding and diet. Dilution of formula or milk is unnecessary. Continued feeding results in improved nutrition during and after recovery without prolonging the diarrhea illness.

Children with mild to moderate dehydration should receive OES over a 4-6 hour period or until rehydrated. Breast feeding should continue alternated with feedings of OES. Formula fed infants should be given OES. Maintenance therapy may begin when the existing fluid deficit has been corrected. Ongoing losses should be replaced with OES. The child's usual feedings and a carbohydrate rich diet should be resumed. If the diarrhea significantly worsens with milk-based formula, the formula may be diluted to half strength for 24 hours.

Children with severe dehydration should be treated with an intravenous electrolyte solution. An OES should be given as soon as they are able to drink on their own. Once the child is rehydrated, maintenance therapy should continue as described above.

Chronic Diarrhea
Definition

Stool output of >20 gm/kg/day for more than two to three weeks is considered chronic diarrhea.

Intractable Diarrhea of Infancy (IDI) is a syndrome not a disease. It is seen in infants three months of age or less and is associated with severe diarrhea that does not respond to usual treatment for diarrhea. Many conditions can initiate the syndrome. Control or irradication of the condition is necessary to relieve IDI. Nutritional treatment consists of fluid and electrolyte replacement and initiating some form of parenteral nutrition, elemental infant formula, or a combination or both.

Chronic Nonspecific Diarrhea (CNSD), also known as Irritable Bowel Syndrome of children, refers to children less than 3 years of age who do not show significant malabsorption. Two factors have been associated with CNSD: very low fat diets and large intake of liquids. Maintaining fat calories in the diet at 35 percent to 40 percent has been found in some infants to control diarrhea. Similarly, restricting the volume of common liquids such as: fruit juice, sports drinks, soda, and sugared fruit drinks to appropriate amounts for age has been found to relieve diarrhea in some children. Other conditions resulting in CNSD are cystic fibrosis, gluten sensitive enteropathy, milk intolerance and other food sensitivities are addressed in other portions of this manual.

References

1. Richards L, Claeson M, Pierce N: Management of acute diarrhea in children: lessons learned. Pediatr Infect Dis J 1993, 12: 5-9.
2. Brown KH: Dietary Management of Acute Childhood Diarrhea: Optimal timing of feeding and appropriate use of milks and mixed diets. J Peds April 1991. 118(4:2):S92.
3. Lifshitz F et al: Refeeding of infants with acute diarrheal disease. J Peds April 1991 118 (4:2): S99.
4. Ellett ML, Fitzgerald JF, Winchester M: Dietary Management of Chronic Diarrhea in Children. Society of Gastroenterology Nurses and Associate. Feb. 1993: 170.
5. Pediatric Nutrition Handbook. 3rd ed. American Academy of Pediatrics: Elk Grove Village, IL 1993.

Attention Deficit Hyperactivity Disorder (ADHD)
Description
Attention Deficit Hyperactivity Disorder, ADHD, is a neurologic disorder affecting 3-5% of school age children. The clinical diagnosis has specific criteria, i.e. inattention, impulsivity, hyperactivity, short attention span, an onset before 7 years of age and a duration of at least six months. Diagnosis should be made by a multidisciplinary team of trained health professionals. This disorder is more prevalent in boys than girls. Approximately one third of all ADHD children outgrow the disorder by puberty, another third by 19-20 years of age and the remaining may have problems as adults.

Nutrition related theories
In years past, diet was thought to contribute to the behavior of a child with ADHD. Dr. Benjamin Feingold, an allergist, introduced a diet avoiding the intake of natural salicylates, BHA, BHT, and artificial colors and flavors to treat children with ADHD. Early results appeared favorable, but controlled studies later have not supported the Feingold hypothesis. However, 5-10% of children may benefit from such a diet.

Sugar (sucrose) was thought to contribute to hyperactivity in children. However controlled studies have failed to demonstrate negative behavior after sucrose consumption.

Megavitamins have been used to treat hyperactivity. Controlled studies have not indicated by a benefit from megavitamin therapy. (1) Toxicity from overdosing of vitamins can occur, especially from the fat soluble vitamins.

Other considerations
Medications are sometimes used in treating ADHD. These drugs may cause anorexia, poor appetite, and possibly endocrine abnormalities leading to decrease in weight gain and physical growth.

Routine nutrition assessment may be recommended more frequently for children on medications. A normal balanced diet for age is recommended.

Professional references
6. Feucht S: Nutrition and Attention Deficit Hyperactivity Disorder. Nutrition Focus. 1990; 6(1): 1-4.
7. Lucas B: Diet and Behavior In: Pipes P. Nutrition in Infancy and Childhood. 4th ed. 1989; 387-401.
8. Queen P, Lang C: Handbook of Pediatric Nutrition. Aspen Publishers. 1993; 162
9. Silver LB: Attention-Deficit Hyperactivity Disorder- A Clinical Guide to Diagnosis and Treatment. American Psychiatric Press Inc. 1992; 133.
10. Pediatric Nutrition Handbook. 3rd Ed. American Academy of Pediatrics. 1993; 331.

Nutrition and Cocaine Abuse

In the past several years, cocaine drug abuse has been on the rise. Cocaine abuse during pregnancy has been associated with significant perinatal morbidity and mortality. There has also been more attention and study on how cocaine affects pregnancy and the developing embryo and fetus.

Prenatal Effects of Cocaine

Cocaine affects the central nervous system as a stimulant. It may subsequently cause vasoconstriction, tachycardia, and an abrupt rise in blood pressure. In pregnancy, vasoconstriction can affect the placenta causing a decrease in blood flow to the fetus and an increase in uterine contractions. There is an increased chance of premature labor, placental abruption, placenta previa, spontaneous abortions, and meconium staining of the amniotic fluid.

In utero, cocaine easily crosses the placenta. The fetus converts cocaine to norcocaine, a water-soluble substance, which is more potent than cocaine. It is excreted into the amniotic fluid, which the fetus takes as nourishment. Exposure to norcocaine can cause intrauterine growth retardation and lead to significant impairment in neonatal neurobehavioral capabilities.

Cocaine-Exposed Infants

Cocaine-exposed babies face numerous obstacles from physical to neurobehavioral problems, including feeding problems. These infants tend to be shorter, of lower birth weight, and have smaller head circumferences. There is an increased risk of genitourinary malformations, congenital cardiac anomalies, and in some infants an increased incidence of neural tube defects and ileal atresia secondary to intrauterine bowel infarction. In addition, cocaine-exposed babies have a tenfold increase in Sudden Infant Death Syndrome (SIDS), over the general population.

Upon birth, some cocaine-exposed infants exhibit symptoms of neonatal drug withdrawal. Some of these characteristics are irritability, hypersensitivity, and jittery behavior. Formal neurobehavioral evaluations at three days of age with the Brazelton Neonatal Behavioral Assessment Scale have revealed that such infants are largely unable to respond to the human voice and face, deficient in the ability to interact with others, and highly labile emotionally, responding poorly to attempts at comforting. Some cocaine-exposed infants go into a deep sleep for long periods of time to shut themselves off from outside stimulation. This type of situation makes it difficult to feed and care for the child. Bonding between the mother or caretaker to the infant is hindered, and abuse or neglect has been reported.

Feeding Suggestions/Comforting Techniques

The literature reports that cocaine can be passed via breast milk to the infant. Therefore, breast feeding is contraindicated in mothers who continue to use cocaine after delivery. A suitable formula should be substituted for the breast milk.

Due to hypersensitivity to the environment, a variety of parenting and soothing techniques need to be implemented to allow for a successful feeding session.

Feeding:
- Small, frequent feedings of formula or breast milk unexposed to cocaine.
- Burp frequently.
- Proper positioning: A sitting position seems to be more effective.
- Feed slowly.
- Support chin and cheeks if baby is sucking poorly.

Comforting:

- Quiet/secure environment.
- Dim lighting, soft music.
- Speak softly, rock gently, avoid bouncing.
- Wrap the baby tightly with arms folded against its chest.
- Hold the baby close to your body.

Cocaine-exposed babies are 40 times more likely to suffer delays in motor development as infants not exposed to drugs before birth. By four months of age, these children tend to be stiff and rigid, and have difficulties bringing their hands together and relaxing their fists. It would be helpful to consult a physical and/or occupational therapist about feeding difficulties as the child grows and develops.

Presently, there is very little information available on the long-term development of cocaine-exposed infants. However, these children should be considered in a high-risk category for developmental and learning disabilities. Close follow-up by the dietitian, including growth monitoring and feeding observations, will help identify nutritional problems and appropriate interventions, planned in conjunction with other health care providers.

Professional References

1. Bays, J, The care of alcohol and drug affected infants. *Pediatric Annals* 1992; 21(8):489.
2. Brody, JE, Cocaine: Litany of fetal risks grows. *New York Times*, Sept. 6, 1988; 19-23.
3. Chasnoff, I, Perinatal effects of cocaine. *Contemporary OB/GYN* 1987; 29(5):163-179.
4. Chasnoff, I, Lewis, D, Squires, L. Cocaine intoxication in a breast-fed infant. *Pediatrics* 1987; 80(6):836-838.
5. Neerhof, M, MacGregor, S, Retzky, S, Sullivan, T. cocaine abuse during pregnancy: Peripartum prevalence and perinatal outcome. *Amer J Obstet Gynecol* 1989;161(3):633-638.

Nutrition and Fetal Alcohol Syndrome

Fetal Alcohol Syndrome (FAS) is classified as those birth defects caused by maternal alcohol ingestion during pregnancy. The severity of damage to the fetus from alcohol appears to depend on the amount consumed and the stage of the pregnancy when it is consumed. The greatest damage appears during the first trimester when cell growth is occurring. alcohol may impair placental transfer of nutrients, such as amino acids, glucose, folate, and zinc to the fetus. In the United States, one out of every 750 newborns - or 5,000 babies per year - has FAS. It is the third most frequent cause of mental retardation in the United States. Children born with milder forms of FAS are classified as Fetal Alcohol Effects (FAE).

There are several distinct physical and mental abnormalities of FAS. They are listed below:

Prenatal:
- Intrauterine growth retardation (IUGR).

Postnatal:
- Decreased adipose tissue.
- Growth deficiency in height, weight, and head circumference.

Characteristic facial features:
- Microcephaly - abnormally small head.
- Micrognathia - unusual smallness of the jaw.
- Microphthalmia - abnormally small eyes and short opening between the eyelids.
- Underdeveloped philtrum, thin upper lip, and flatter mid-face.

Central nervous system:
- Neurological abnormalities - poor coordination, hypotonia, seizures, poor APGAR scores.
- Intellectual impairment - small brains, mental retardation.
- Behavioral problems - developmentally delayed, extreme nervousness, irritability, and hyperactivity.

Other:
- Cardiac anomalies, hemangiomas, eye and ear anomalies.

Growth and Nutrition

A child with FAS has several physical and developmental disabilities which may lead to serious feeding problems during preschool years. Infants with FAS tend to have a weak suck, tire easily when fed, and subsequently have poor intake. These babies may also demonstrate increased distractibility and hypersensitivity to oral feedings. Nasogastric feedings and/or gastrostomy feedings may be necessary to provide adequate nutrition. Significant delays in oral feeding development may occur.

As the child grows older, behavior problems associated with FAS may impair nutritional intake. Among these manifestations are fine motor problems, such as poor finger articulation; delay in establishing hand dominance; and weak grasp with delayed gross motor development. Oral feeding skills should be assessed by an Occupational or Speech Therapist. Growth and development of FAS infants and children should be monitored frequently.

References

1. Alpert, J, Zuckerman, B. Alcohol use during pregnancy: What is the risk? *Pediatric Review* 1991; 12(12):375-381.

2. Caruso, K, TenBensel, R. Fetal Alcohol Syndrome and fetal alcohol effects. The University of Minnesota experience. *Minnesota Medicine* 1993; 76(4):25-29.

3. Dedam, R, McFarlane, C, Hennessy, K. A dangerous lack of understanding. *The Canadian Nurse* 1993; 89(6):29-31.

4. Erickson, KE. Fetal Alcohol Syndrome: The health professional's role. Nutrition Update for Health Professionals March, 1984. St. Paul-Ramsey County Nutrition Program, 555 Cedar Street, St. Paul, Minnesota 55101.

5. Fetal Alcohol Syndrome. Public Health Education Information Sheet, March of Dimes Birth Defects Foundation National Headquarters, Community Services Department, 1275 Mamaroneck Avenue, White Plains, New York 10605. February 1985.

6. Fisher, DE, Karl, PI. Maternal ethanol use and selective malnutrition. *Recent Dev Alcohol*; 1988;6:277-289.

7. Preventing Fetal Alcohol Effects: A Practical Guide for Ob/Gyn Physicians and Nurses. US Department of Health and Human Services, DHHS Pub No (ADM) 81-1163, Superintendent of Documents, US Government Printing Office, Washington, DC 20402.

Client Information

1. "For Your Baby's Sake, Don't Drink" 15 pg booklet and 4 pg pamphlet, Governor's Citizens Advisory Council on Alcoholism, Division of Alcoholism, 160 N LaSalle St, Rm 1500, Chicago, IL 60601.

2. "Before You Drink, Think..." 4 pg pamphlet, and "Drugs, Alcohol, Tobacco Abuse during Pregnancy" pamphlet, March of Dimes. Contact the local chapter.

3. "Drinking and Dreams Don't Mix." Healthy Mothers, Healthy Babies, National Health Information Clearinghouse, PO Box 47, Washington, DC 20044.

Nutrition and Acquired Immune Deficiency Syndrome (AIDS)

Introduction

AIDS (Acquired Immune Deficiency Syndrome) has been reported in the pediatric population since 1983. AIDS is caused by the HIV (Human Immunodeficiency Virus). The body's health is defended by the white blood cells called lymphocytes. This process is hindered by AIDS by breaking down the body's immune system. When HIV enters the body, it infects special T cells, where the virus grows. The virus kills these cells slowly. As more and more of the T cells die, the body's ability to fight infection weakens.

A person with HIV infection may remain healthy for many years. Persons are said to have AIDS when they are sick with illnesses and infections that can occur with HIV.

Even before HIV causes AIDS, it can cause health problems. Maintaining optimal nutrition in the patient with AIDS is necessary to deter the consequences of malnutrition and its effects in the disease process. Good nutrition may help maintain weight, promote growth, prevent nutrient deficiencies, decrease the incidence and severity of infection, and improve the quality of life. Several nutrients such as sodium, potassium, iron, magnesium, phosphorus, sulfur and zinc are lost. Electrolyte problems such as fluid overload and anemia are common.

HIV Transmission in Babies and Children

HIV can be passed to a baby during pregnancy or delivery. An HIV-infected woman's chances of having a baby with HIV are one in four for each pregnancy. HIV can also be contracted through contact with blood or body fluids. Bathing, kissing, feeding and playing with your child are not risky and do not cause the spread of HIV. In the past some babies and children became infected through blood transfusions. Today the blood from all donors is screened for the virus and infection is unlikely..

Nutritional Disorders in AIDS/HIV

Over 95% of children with HIV infection will develop clinically significant malnutrition before death. 25-50% of infants with vertically transmitted HIV infection may be smaller and remain smaller for gestational age. With progression of HIV disease, the growth retardation becomes more profound and evolves into a wasting state.

Etiology of Nutritional Disorders

- Progression of HIV infection
- Concurrent infections (CMV, PCP, hepatitis, etc.)
- Oral, esophageal and small intestine infection (Candida, HSV)
- CNS involvement (appetite suppression, chewing and swallowing problems)
- Nausea and Vomiting (gastritis, medications, pancreatitis, etc.)
- Gastrointestinal disease/Malabsorption/Diarrhea
- Hypermetabolic State - increase in REE (fevers, infections)

Assessment and Management of Nutritional Disorders

Normal Growth and Weight

First year:	12 cm/year	7 kg/year
4-10 years:	5-6 cm/year	2-3 kg/year

Growth Measurements:
- Weight and height for age and weight for height
- Head Circumference to age 3 or further if appropriate
- Weight less than 5th percentile and not following the curve
- Weight loss that crosses two percentile lines
- Weight loss of 10% of baseline
- Weight/Height ratio of less than 5 percent

Laboratory Data:
- Albumin, Prealbumin
- Transferrin
- TIBC
- BUN
- Creatinine
- Hemoglobin
- SGOT, SGPT
- Nitrogen Balance studies
- Electrolytes, glucose, calcium

Estimating Energy Needs:
- RDA tables
- Bentler and Stannish formula for catch-up growth
- Metabolic Cart

NOTE: Some children may require as many as 200 kcal/kg and up to 4 grams protein/kg

Eating Problems:
- Diarrhea
- Nausea and Vomiting
- Mouth Ulcers/Dry Mouth
- Weight Loss
- Anorexia

Diarrhea
- Replace lost fluids.
- Replace lost potassium. Eat more bananas, potatoes, fish and meat.
- Don't skip meals.
- Eat small amounts often.
- Some foods may control diarrhea (bananas, white rice, applesauce, toast, macaroni, Jell-O, mashed potatoes, yogurt)
- Avoid fatty, greasy, spicy and crunchy fiber foods.
- Elemental feedings.
- Lactose restriction.
- Antidiarrheal medication.

Nausea and Vomiting
- Don't skip meals.
- Eat often and in small amounts if needed.
- Salty foods may be better tolerated than very sweet foods.
- Avoid greasy, fried foods.
- Take medications as directed.

Mouth Ulcers/Dry Mouth
- Consult physician to rule out and treat candidiasis (thrush).
- Use soft, cool foods. Avoid very hot foods.
- Blenderize foods if needed.
- Drink mild beverages like apple juice.
- Suck on hard candies
- Use moist foods.
- Serve high-calorie, high-protein beverages.
- Drink liquid through a straw.
- Use canned fruits or fruits without skins or seeds.

Weight Loss
- Eat more frequently.
- Eat high calorie, high protein foods (see High Calorie, High Protein Diet)
- Add extra fat if tolerated.
- Add cheese, meat, dried fruits to increase calories in foods.

Anorexia
- Choose favorite foods. Variety is not as essential as calorie intake.
- Eat often and slowly.
- Consume liquids after eating to avoid filling the stomach.
- Increase calories and protein by adding nonfat dry milk powder when possible.
- Offer finger foods and bite-sized pieces.
- Involve the child in food choices and self-feeding.
- Megestrol Acetate (Megace) may be used as an appetite stimulant.

Oral Refeeding with Formula/Supplements
1. Standard 20 kcal/oz formula
2. High calorie, high density formula (24 and 27 kcal/oz); 30 kcal/oz for older children
3. Supplement formulas with MCT oil (7.7 kcal/ml)- Microlipid; corn oil (8.0 kcal/ml)-be sure to shake bottle as it will rise to the top; Polycose (1 tsp = 8 kcal)
4. Semi-elemental or elemental formula (Alimentum or Pregestimil) may be required.
5. Nutritional Supplements (See Enteral Formula listings)

NOTE: Check renal function on formulas exceeding 24 calories/ounce.

Tube Feeding and Parenteral Nutrition

When severe malnutrition or inadequate oral intake occurs, enteral or parenteral nutrition may be necessary to supplement or replace oral feeding. If enteral, a continuous 12 hour infusion pump should be utilized. If parenteral nutrition, refer to Total Parenteral Nutrition section for guidelines. TPN should be short-term in order that enteral feedings may be resumed to stimulate normal immunologic and physiologic function. Risks of catheter infection and long-term complications associated with TPN should be carefully considered in a patient with an already compromised immune system.

References

1. Bahl, SM, Hickson, JF. Nutritional Care for HIV-Positive Persons: A Manual for Individuals and their Caregivers (Modern Nutrition). CRC Pr, 1995.
2. Bell, SJ. Positive Nutrition for HIV Infection and AIDS: A Medically Sound Take Charge Plan to Maintain. Chronimed, 1996.
3. Foshee, WS. A Manual for the Management of HIV Infections in Infants, Children and Adolescents. Medical College of Georgia, 1996.
4. Sherman, C, Raucher, B, Epstein, J, Berger, M. Quality Food and Nutrition Services for AIDS Patients. Aspen Pub, 1990.
5. Wilkes, CM. Cancer and HIV Clinical Nutrition Pocket Guide. Jones & Bartlett Pub, 1995.

Websites

6. HIVpositive.com A comprehensive resource for HIV/AIDS
7. http://www.nih.gov/ National Institutes of Health
8. http://www.eatright.org American Dietetic Association
9. http://www.medscape.com Medscape
10. http://www.gen.emory.edu/MEDWEB/medweb.html An enormous site which offers links to other health care-related sites

Resources

11. National AIDS Hotline 1-800-342-AIDS
12. National Pediatric HIV Resource Center 1-800-362-0071
13. Pediatric AIDS Coalition 1-800-336-5475
14. American Dietetic Association 1-800-336-1655

Nutritional Concerns for the Oncology Patient
General Considerations

The nutritional status of the pediatric cancer patient is a major concern to health care professionals. The side effects of cancer and cancer therapy (radiotherapy, chemotherapy, and surgery) can include any one or a number of problems, most of which are nutritionally related. In general, either (1) the child's desire or ability to eat or; (2) the physiologic machinery for nutrient digestion, absorption, and metabolism, or both, are affected. Since these side effects vary in type and intensity from one child to another and from one day to the next, successful nutrition regimes will also vary. The primary goals of nutritional therapy for the pediatric cancer patient are to prevent or manage cachexia, a common problem of the oncology patient, and to promote normal pediatric growth patterns.

Cachexia is a term used to describe the state of malnutrition, wasting, and debility. It is characterized by a loss of body weight, adipose tissue, visceral protein, and skeletal muscle. The degree of cachexia that an oncology patient may experience is related to nutritional intake, diagnosis, and cancer treatment. Cachexia may be caused by anorexia, metabolic abnormalities, or reduced caloric intake. These causes may be disease- or treatment-related.

Calorie and protein requirements, in addition to those of vitamin and minerals, may be increased as a result of the disease or its therapy. Therefore, high-calorie, high-protein diets are usually chosen for children with cancer (refer to the High-calorie, High-protein diet). A multi-vitamin and mineral supplement may also be recommended for these patients. Monitoring the child's growth patterns and serum biochemical values are appropriate methods for assessment of adequate dietary intake.

Special Considerations

Enteral tube feedings may be used for patients with continued, suboptimal oral intake. Nausea, vomiting, diarrhea, or tumor involvement of the gastrointestinal tract may prevent the use of enteral feedings. Tube placement into the duodenum or jejunum may be appropriate for patients experiencing nausea and vomiting. A night feeding often works well for patients to supplement inadequate oral intake during the day. For those patients who are not candidates for enteral feedings, parenteral nutrition may be indicated. The major benefits of any form of nutritional support are possible increased tolerance to oncology treatment and decreased morbidity, improved quality of life, and improvement or maintenance of nutritional status.

A Parent's Guide for Young People with Cancer

Good nutrition is an important part of your child's treatment. In general, your child's normal diet should be continued during cancer treatment unless your physician gives you a special one. A few diet hints are listed below:

1. Build meals around your child's favorite foods. Variety is not as important as intake.
2. Small, frequent meals and snacks are attractive to most children. You can freeze portions of a favorite dish and serve them when desired.
3. Smaller bites and frequent sips of water, milk, or other unsweetened drinks will make chewing and swallowing easier.
4. Avoid empty calorie foods. Such items (e.g., soft drinks, chips, candy) reduce your child's appetite without providing nutrients. By contrast, milkshakes, yogurt, fruit, juices, or instant breakfasts provide extra calories and protein.
5. Some types of chemotherapy may temporarily alter your child's sense of taste. Well-seasoned foods such as spaghetti, tacos, and pizza may seem especially good at times. Sometimes adding extra salt or sugar, or using less, may make foods taste better. However, because of fluid retention, patients on cortisone drugs should limit salt in their diets.

6. A decrease in appetite is common to some types of chemotherapy. But this must be countered with an increase in fluid intake beginning a few days before the chemotherapy and continuing for a few days after it.
7. If appetite is poor, the addition of a single multivitamin (one without folic acid, if your child is taking methotrexate) per day may be advisable. Be sure to ask your doctor before beginning vitamin supplements.
8. If your child is taking oral medication at home, the time of day that medication is given may be critical. Some are best given in the morning, some at midday, some on a full stomach, etc. Be sure to ask your doctor when and how medications should be administered.

Material taken from "Young People with Cancer: A Handbook for Parents". Published by the National Cancer Institute. NIH Publication No. 92-2378, Revised March 1988, Reprinted October 1991.

Side Effects of Cancer and of Cancer Treatment
Decreased Food Intake

Anorexia, often accompanied by weight loss, is frequently seen as a presenting symptom of cancer as well as a side effect of treatment. Guidelines for each patient must be individualized and will include some of the following suggestions:

- Consider eating as a treatment regimen. Eat often and when appetite is best; generally this is in the morning.
- Keep food easily accessible.
- Use high-calorie, high-protein foods a meals or for snacks. Take snacks long enough before the next meal so that they do not interfere with appetite.

Early satiety is the state of being hungry at the beginning of a meal and then feeling full after a few bites. Suggestions to increase intake despite early satiety include the following:

- Eating calorie-dense foods (to pack the maximum amount of calories into a small amount of foods)
- Possibly limiting high-fat foods, which delay gastric emptying, may ease the feeling of fullness; however, it is difficult to consume adequate calories when fat intake is limited
- Avoiding gas-producing foods
- Consuming small, frequent meals
- Eating slowly
- Adding skim milk powder to foods-it will affect flavor minimally and will increase calorie and protein levels without increasing volume
- Drinking liquids between meals; this decreases the volume of the stomach at meal times

Nausea and Vomiting

Nausea and vomiting are common side effects experienced by patients receiving chemotherapy and/or radiation therapy. These symptoms usually occur directly after treatment. Duration and severity vary widely among patients. Action to take for symptom alleviation include:

- Providing education to explain the symptoms-stressing the reasons for eating may increase the patient's acceptance of side effects. A positive outlook can increase the patient's sense of well-being.
- Offering generally well-tolerated foods following chemotherapy and radiation therapy such as soda, juice, soup and crackers, Jell-O®, and sherbet
- Reducing offensive food odors

- Scheduling meals and treatments carefully
- Using antiemetics (see list, page 407)

Mouth and Throat Problems

Stomatitis, or mouth ulceration.

Mucositis occurs when the oral mucous membranes are irritated by chemotherapy agents that act on rapidly dividing cells. Radiation therapy in the head and neck area can result in mouth soreness. As a result of avoiding many foods and sometimes whole food groups, vitamin and mineral deficiencies may result.

Xerostomia, or dry mouth, often occurs with radiation to the head and neck, resulting in injury of salivary glands as a part of the course of treatment. Dental hygiene becomes more critical when the protective effects of the saliva are absent.

To help with xerostomia, mucositis, or stomatitis:

- Limit highly acidic and spicy foods, such as (but not limited to) orange juice, grapefruit juice, tomatoes and tomato sauces, such as Mexican and some Italian foods.
- Avoid rough, coarse-textured foods. Well-tolerated foods include bland entrees such as macaroni and cheese, egg dishes, creamed turkey or chicken dishes, custards, eggnogs, ice cream, Jell-O®, milk and milk shakes, nectars, puddings, popsicles.
- Drink liquids with meals to add moistness to dry mouth.
- Use extra gravy, butter, or margarine to moisten food.
- Dip foods in liquids before eating them.
- Serve foods lukewarm rather than hot or cold.
- Avoid alcohol.
- Use a straw-it may make drinking easier.
- Use viscous Xylocaine, baking soda mouthwashes, corn syrup rinses (per doctor's or nurse's recommendation). This may help relieve pain and discomfort.

Odor and Taste Changes

These changes are common and often transient.

Meat Aversions

These suggestions may improve intake:
- Serve poultry and fish, meat mixed into casseroles, marinated meats or cold sliced meats.
- Serve cold, high-protein entrees such as meat and egg salads, sandwiches, cottage cheese, or deviled eggs.
- When a high salt threshold occurs, try ham, sausage, bacon, corned beef, and marinated or pickled meats.
- Serve hot egg entrees as high-quality protein.
- Serve cold, high-protein snacks such as nuts, peanut butter, gelatin with cottage cheese, yogurt, and bean dips and chips.
- Serve cold, high-protein desserts with fruit: pudding and pudding pops, custards, and milkshakes. Ice cream also contains some protein.

Bitterness aversions often occur along with meat aversions; coffee and chocolate may become unpalatable for the patient.

Increased sour threshold. When this occurs, offer tart fruit juices, pickled foods, and marinated fish, meats, and vegetables.

Increased sweet threshold. The taste threshold for sweets may rise, and it is easy to add more sugar to foods. For maximum nutritional value, concentrate on sweets such as pudding, custards, shakes, and fruit juices.

Sweet aversion is fairly common. Decrease sugar in recipes and buy fruit packed in water, juice, or light syrup. Serve tart fruits such as grapefruit.

Esophageal Reflux

This may occur during chemotherapy and/or radiation treatment.

Constipation

Chemotherapeutic agents, pain medication, inactivity, and limited food and fluid intake are causes of constipation for cancer patients. Constipation can also result when cancerous tumors interfere with normal bowel function. Increasing the intake of dietary fiber and fluid, as well as engaging in any feasible activities, will improve gastric mobility. Medications to ease constipation are available; an individualized treatment plan must be developed.

Diarrhea

The treatment of diarrhea must be specifically aimed at its cause(s). Therefore, it should be highly individualized and minimally restrictive. Causes of diarrhea are many, and include cancer therapies and the disease itself. There are no general guidelines for treating diarrhea; treatment must be chosen carefully, considering individual differences and verification of clinical disorders.

Changes in Serum Calcium Levels and Use of Calcium-Restricted Diets for Cancer Patients

The most common cause of hypercalcemia in hospitalized patients is malignancy. Other types of tumors commonly associated with hypercalcemia include hematologic cancers, such as myeloma, lymphosarcoma, Burkitt's lymphoma, and T-cell lymphoma; solid tumors with bone metastasis, such as lung and pancreatic tumors; and solid tumors without metastasis, such as lung, kidney, pancreatic, breast, and ovarian tumors.

Limiting the intake of calcium in the diet is not indicated for most patients with hypercalcemia of cancer, as these patients exhibit a low absorption of calcium because of a decrease in the levels of the hormones that facilitate calcium absorption. Only in conditions, such as sarcoidosis and vitamin D intoxication, where increased absorption of calcium is important in the pathogenesis of hypercalcemia can it be expected that dietary limitation of calcium will be of value. In most cases, the increased serum calcium of cancer occurs from bone resorption. Therefore, dietary restriction can be only of marginal value, and may contribute to even higher serum calcium levels by limiting the intake of phosphorus. Drugs are the most effective means of reducing high serum calcium levels in cancer patients.

```
┌─────────────────────────────────────────────────────────────────────┐
│                  Antiemetic and Orexigenic Agents                     │
│                                                                       │
│  Antiemetics  (very effective)                                        │
│                    Benadryl®        (diphenhydramine)                 │
│                    Compazine®       (prochlorperazine)                │
│                    Decadron®        (dexamethasone)                   │
│                    Marinol®         (cannabinoid)                     │
│                    Reglan®          (metoclopramide)                  │
│                    Zofran®          (ondansetron)  used in combination with │
│                                     dexamethasone and Kytril (granisetron) │
│                                                                       │
│                    Orexigenics      (appetite stimulants)             │
│  Corticosteroids                                                      │
│                    Hydrazine Sulfate                                  │
│                    Megace®          (megestrol acetate)-weight gain with │
│                                     increased protein stores          │
│                    Periactin®       (cyproheptadine)                  │
│                    Tetrahydrocannabbinol                              │
└─────────────────────────────────────────────────────────────────────┘
```

Professional References

1. Sachinder SH, et al, Hypercalcemia crisis due to unsuspected parathyroid in a patient with advanced breast cancer. American Surgeon 1984; 50:230-2.
2. Mundy GR, et al. The hypercalcemia of cancer. New England J Med 1984; 310(6): 1718-27.
3. Wilkkensar R. Treatment of hypercalcemia associated with malignancy. British Med J 1984; 74:475-80.
4. Stewart A. Therapy of malignancy-associated hypercalcemia. Am J Med 1983; 74:475-80.
5. Schneider AB, Sherwood LM. Calcium homeostasis and the pathogenesis and management of hypercalcemic disorders. Metabolism 1974; 23(10:975-1007).
6. American Dietetic Association. Handbook of clinical dietetics. New Haven, Conn.: Yale University Press, 1981: H18.
7. Stedman TL, Stedman's medical dictionary. Baltimore, MD.: Williams and Wilkins, 1984:892.
8. American Dietetic Association, Manual of Clinical Nutrition. Chicago, IL.: The American Dietetic Association, 1988.
9. Bloch, AS. Nutrition and Cancer: The Paradox. Ross Dietetic Currents, Vol 23, No. 2, 1996.

Client Resources

1. American Cancer Society. A nationwide, community-based voluntary health organization dedicated to eliminating cancer as a major health problem. Many publications are available.
    http://www.cancer.org
    Toll Free: 800-ACS-2345

2. American Cancer Society – Minnesota affiliate
    3316 W. 66th Street
    Minneapolis, MN 55435
    http://www.mn.cancer.org
    Toll Free: 800-ACS-2345

3. CancerNet from the National Cancer Institute. This is a World Wide Web resource which is constantly updated and provides valuable information for health care professionals on cancer as well as information on care, screening, and prevention.
    http://wwwicic.nci.nih.gov
    Toll Free: 800-800-4-CANCER

4. Nutrition Quackery Information
    http://www.quackwatch.com

5. Alternative Therapies – Recommended by National Council Against Health Fraud.
    http://www.ncahf.org

6   Leukemia Society of America – Information about leukemia, lymphoma, multiple myeloma and Hodgkin's disease. For the number of the local office, check your telephone directory.
    Home Office 600 Third Avenue
    New York, NY 10016
    http://www.leukemia.org
    Toll Free: 800-955-4LSA

7   Eating Hints for Cancer Patients
    National Institutes of Health
    National Cancer Institute
    NIH Publication No. 95-2079, July 1995.

8   Haller, J. What to Eat When You Don't Feel Like Eating, Lancelot Press Ltd. June 1994. Phone:902-684-9129, FAX: 902-684-3685.

NOTE: These are just a few of the many resources for persons living with cancer.

ADOLESCENT NUTRITION

Nutritional Considerations During Adolescence
General Description

Adolescence can be thought of as a time of transition from one stage in the life cycle (childhood) to the next (adulthood). There is an alteration in the lifestyle, self-concept, physical growth and nutritional needs. No single physical, psychological, intellectual, scholastic, legal or chronological criterion can adequately describe this complex phenomenon known as adolescence. The beginning of adolescence can be characterized by the onset of puberty and a psychological acceptance and reaction to these developmental changes. The end of adolescence is marked by preparedness for an opportunity to assume an adult role in society.

Adolescence is marked by a period of rapid growth in both males and females, commonly termed "growth spurt." Growth spurt is not only linear, but includes the increase in size of all organ systems of the body. The adolescent will gain about 20% of adult height and 50% of adult weight during pubertal growth. Females enter growth spurt 1 1/2 to 2 years sooner than males. Males acquire a greater percent of lean body mass (LBM) while body fat accumulates to a greater degree in females. The rapid growth and development of this time period has profound nutritional implications, and requirements for all nutrients increase.

Adolescents seem to be particularly influenced by bizarre unbalanced diets that are the current fad. They have a tendency to skip meals, do a lot of snacking, enjoy fast food, and diet to lose weight. Teens have many concerns related to the shape and size of their bodies, the condition of their skin, their sexual development, and social acceptance by their peers. They are beginning to experience and seek independence from family and desire freedom in making decisions. These factors, as well as use of alcohol and/or drugs, complicate the nutrient needs of this age group.

Nutritional status of adolescents as a group has been described as generally good. However, some studies have observed low dietary intakes and marginal or sub-clinical deficiencies of iron, calcium, riboflavin, and vitamins A and C. Female adolescents don't meet the recommended goal servings from the dairy and meat groups. Seventy-one percent of male teens eat meals out—comprising 35% of total energy intake (33% is from fast food). The following factors appear to limitations of fast food meals:

- Calcium, riboflavin and vitamin D are low unless a dairy product is ordered.
- Folate and fiber is low
- Fat, sodium, and energy are high in these meals.

Fast foods can contribute nutrients to diets of teens, but will not meet all of their nutritional needs.

Nutrient Requirements

There are no true guidelines for nutrient requirements for adolescents. Present RDA's are extrapolations from recommendations for children and adults. However, recommendations for nutrient intake are generally related to rate and timing of growth spurt. Evaluation of nutrient needs should be done on an individual basis, taking into account additional stresses due to increased involvement in sports, skipping meals, snacking between meals, and/or adherence to current dietary fads.

Estimated kilocalorie and nutrient requirements for adolescents have been based on physiological changes related to growth spurt. The adolescent's age, sex, stage of puberty, and current growth parameters must be taken into consideration. Caloric requirements and intake for males increase to age 16 years, when a maximum intake is achieved paralleling accelerated growth. After this time, the caloric intake decreases. In females the increase in caloric intake reaches a peak at 12 years, then declines by about 18 years, at which time it plateaus. The adequacy of energy intake can be assessed by evaluating growth and body composition.

Methods by which energy requirements can be estimated are:

a. RDA kilocalories, Adolescents. See Appendix.
b. Mayo Clinic Food Nomogram.
c. Harris and Benedict's Basal Energy Expenditure.
d. Height estimations, based on kcal/cm, applied as follows:

Age		Kcal/cm of Height	
Male		Mid Range	Range
	11 - 14	17.2	14.8 - 20.7
	15 - 18	15.9	13.2 - 21.0
	19 - 22	16.4	14.9 - 17.7
Female			
	11 - 14	14.0	11.1 - 17.6
	15 - 18	12.9	7.9 - 17.5
	19 - 22	12.9	11.0 - 14.6

e. FAO/WHO requirements as given in the following table:

Energy Requirements of Adolescents by Age in Years

Age in Years	Kcal/Kg/day	
	Male	Female
10	74	68
11	71	62
12	67	57
13	61	52
14	56	50
15	53	48
16	51	45
17	50	43
18	49	42
19	47	40

Protein Requirements for adolescents have been estimated at about 12 to 16 percent of total energy intake. The RDA for protein for adolescents is 44-56 grams/day. The requirement for protein is determined by the amount required for maintenance plus that needed for the formation of new tissue, which during adolescence may represent a substantial part of the total nitrogen needs. Caloric and/or protein deficits at peak growth periods may comprise deposition of LBM.

Methods by which protein requirements can be estimated are:

a. RDA for protein for adolescents. See Appendix.
b. Height Index:

	Ages	Gm/cm height
Males		
	11 - 14	.29
	15 - 22	.32
Females		
	11 - 14	.29
	15 - 18	.28
	19 - 22	.27

Calcium Requirements during adolescence are not firmly established. Needs depend on growth velocity, bone structure and size, and absorption rate. Forty-five percent of total bone growth occurs during adolescence. The largest gains in bone weight occur in females between ages 10 and 14 years and in males between 12 and 16 years. The RDA for calcium, has been established at 1200 mg per day for 11 to 18 year-old males and females.

Iron Requirements increase during adolescence and are directly related to rapid growth most obviously reflected in increase in blood volume and muscle mass. Iron absorption is known to become more efficient during periods of increased need and, hence, efficiency of iron absorption increases during a growth spurt. Iron deficiency anemias in adolescence can usually be explained on the basis of depletion of marginal stores by increased demand. Iron requirements for both males and females 11-18 years has been established at 18 mg/day. For females the increased need is related to menstrual losses as well as growth, and in males to increases in tissue mass plus the rise in hemoglobin levels.

Trace Elements, such as zinc, magnesium, copper and manganese, have been found to be marginally inadequate in the diets of teens. Depressed zinc plasma levels in the adolescent are thought to be due, in addition to marginal intake, to increased zinc requirements during periods of rapid growth of new skeletal and muscle tissue. Zinc requirements for both males and females 11 to 18 years old is 15 mg/day.

Nutritional Assessment

Nutritional assessment of the adolescent should include:

Dietary:

Food frequency determinations
Exclusion of food groups
Habits and eating patterns
Snacks
24-hour recall
Socio-economic status
Vitamin supplementation
Dietary additives
Special food beliefs
Who does food preparation

Medical:	History of previous diseases History of food allergies Family history
Anthropometric:	Height Weight Weight/height ratio Recent weight gain or loss Arm circumference and skinfold thickness are desirable, but not required.
Physical Activity and Exercise Patterns:	Physical Education at school Sports TV watching Computer time

Growth Grids

Height and weight can be plotted on growth grids for comparison. Early maturation of either sex will appear to deviate from previously followed percentiles for a year or so because most growth grids are based on chronological rather than developmental age, with the growth spurt of many adolescents out of phase with each other.

Growth charts are helpful to assess any deviations from previous growth patterns; however, they do not allow for accurate weight-for-height assessments. The Body Mass Index (BMI) allows for assessment of weight-for-height ratios in adolescents. Guidelines for using the BMI assessment are as follows:

Determine the BMI by one of the following methods:
1) Calculate the BMI using the formula, Weight in kg divided by height in meters ^{2}.
2) Use a BMI chart.
3) Use the BMI to evaluate the weight-to-height ratio
4) Refer to Table 1 (page 415) to determine weight-for height percentile.
   a) By gender, find the patient's age in the far left column.
   b) Read across the row to find the value corresponding the patient's BMI.
   c) Read up for the percentile.
5) Interpretation of percentile.
   a) = 95%ile indicates overweight.
   b) = 85%ile indicates risk for overweight.
   c) =15%ile indicates risk for low weight for height.
   d) = 5%ile indicates low weight for height. **Evaluate for eating disorder.**

Counseling Adolescents About Nutrition

Counseling adolescents can be a challenge. Changes in food behaviors that are considered desirable by nutritionists may not appeal to the target group who will make their own decisions.

It is important to stress to teens that healthy eating will aid them in accomplishing their goals, rather than telling them to eat certain foods because the foods are "good for them." Teens often doubt that nutrition is important because they are not experiencing any consequences from poor food habits and choices. Since food is only one aspect of their busy lives, it only receives a fraction of their attention. Many times what they need, and will eat, is unavailable to them at the places and times when they do eat. However, adolescents get hungry, like to eat, want energy and vigor, and the means to compete and excel in whatever they do. Some may have good habits from childhood that carry over to the teen years. Behavioral changes are most successfully achieved when related to physical development and sports performance.

Studies indicate that as much as 28% of caloric intake for teens is in the form of between meal snacks. Thus, snacks can be used to advantage in contributing significantly to nutrient intake. Snack choices should emphasize the daily requirements for protein, vitamins, and minerals, as well as energy. Snacks of choice should include: sandwiches, hamburgers, pizza, fruit, yogurt, milk, and raw vegetables. Teens can be encouraged to make decisions about snacks and snack foods by considering the following points:
1. Are the extra calories needed?
2. Does the snack count for more than calories, that is, will it supply protein, vitamins and/or minerals, as well as calories?

The following are suggestions for counseling adolescents:

1. Be aware of their developmental stage--physical, social, and emotional.
2. Show genuine interest; establish good rapport.
3. Give the teen credits for their nutrition knowledge base.
4. Provide the teen with an opportunity to talk and ask questions.
5. Be flexible; allow the teen to accept or reject an idea while talking about it.
6. Do not take sides in generation gap arguments.
7. Set realistic, short-term goals.
8. Give positive reinforcement.
9. Be patient; do not force issues.
10. Establish priorities and honestly express the importance of each goal.
11. Be a good role model; it can be the best teacher.
12. Remember that good nutrition is a long-term goal, not meal-by-meal.
13. Stress that no one food is perfect; recommend variety and moderation.
14. Support the teen in acceptance of self, rather than a dream image.
15. Emphasize the value of mixed foods common in the teen diet, such as pizza, lasagna, tacos, and cheeseburgers.

References:

1. Adolescent Health Survey Report. 4-H Development, Minnesota Extension Service, University of Minnesota 1989.
2. Barnes, HV. Physical growth and development during puberty. Med Clin North Am 1975:59:1305.
3. Brasel, JA. Factors that affect nutritional requirements in adolescents. Curr Concepts Nutr 1977; 5:53.
4. Brookman, RP. Adolescent nutrition. Med Clin North Am 1975;59:1473.
5. Brow, RT. Assessing adolescent development. Pediatr Ann 1978;7:587.
6. Dwyer, JT. Great Expectations: Overview of Adolescent Nutrition for the Year 2000 and Beyond. Adolescent Medicine 1992;3(3):377-390.
7. Hendricks, KM, Walker, WA. Manual of Pediatric Nutrition, 2nd ed. BC Decker Inc 1990.
8. Hines, JH, Williams, HD. Guidelines for Overweight in Adolescent Preventive Services: Recommendations from an Expert Committee. Am J Clin Nutr 1994;59:306-316.
9. Mahan, LK, Rees, JM. Nutrition in Adolescence. CV Mosby Co 1984.
10. Pediatric Nutrition Handbook. Adolescent Nutrition. American Academy of Pediatrics. 3rd ed. 1993.
11. Pembertom, CM, et al. Mayo Clinic Diet Manual, 6th ed. BC Decker Inc 1988.
12. Pipes, PL, Lucas, B, Rees, JM. Nutrition in Infancy and Childhood, 4th ed. CV Mosby Co 1989.
13. Read, MH, Harvey-Webster, M, Usinger-Lesquereux, J. Adolescent Compliance with Dietary Guidelines. Health and Education Implications. Adolescence 1988;23(91), Fall. Libra Publishers Inc.
14. Shen, JTY. The Clinical Practice of Adolescent Medicine. Appleton-Century-Crofts 1980. Pp 183-195.
15. Shils, M, Young, V. Modern Nutrition in Health and Disease 7th Ed, Lea & Febiger 1988. Pp 969-981.
16. The state of adolescent health in Minnesota. Minnesota Youth Health Survey, Adolescent Health Program, Department of Pediatrics, University of Minnesota, Minnesota Department of Health, Feb 1989.
17. VanOss, EM. The effect of nutrition education on the snack food choices of young teens. Plan B paper, Graduate School, University of Minnesota, 1980.
18. Williams, SR, Worthington-Roberts, BS. Nutrition Through the Life Cycle. Mosby Year Book, Inc. 1992. Pp 284-340.
19. USDA. Continuing Survey of Food Intakes by Individuals. 1994-96.

Table 1. Reference Data on %iles of Body Mass Index (wgt/hgt^2) for Adolescents

Percentiles

	5th	15th	50th	85th	95th
MALES - Age, Years					
10	14.42	15.15	16.72	19.60	22.60
11	14.83	15.59	17.28	20.35	23.73
12	15.24	16.06	17.87	21.12	24.89
13	15.73	16.62	18.53	21.93	25.93
14	16.18	17.20	19.22	22.77	26.93
15	16.59	17.76	19.92	23.63	27.76
16	17.01	18.32	20.63	24.45	28.53
17	17.31	18.68	21.12	25.28	29.32
18	17.54	18.89	21.45	25.92	30.02
19	17.80	19.20	21.86	26.36	30.66
FEMALES - Age, years					
10	14.23	15.09	17.00	20.19	23.20
11	14.60	15.53	17.67	21.18	24.59
12	14.98	15.98	18.35	22.17	25.95
13	15.36	16.43	18.95	23.08	27.07
14	15.67	16.79	19.32	23.88	27.97
15	16.01	17.16	19.69	24.29	28.51
16	16.37	17.54	20.09	24.74	29.10
17	16.59	17.81	20.36	25.23	29.72
18	16.71	17.99	20.57	25.56	30.22
19	16.87	18.20	20.80	25.85	30.72

Values = 85th percentile indicate risk for overweight, and those =95th percentiles indicate overweight. Values =15th percentile indicate risk for low weight for height and those =5th percentile indicate low weight for height. *Based on smoothed percentiles from NHANES I.*
Adapted from Must, A., Dallal, GE, Dietz, WH. Am Jour Clin Nutr 1991.

Nutritional Considerations for Adolescent Athletes

Nutritional Needs
Adolescent athletes have the same basic nutritional needs as less active adolescents. A well-balanced diet will support athletic training and competition and promote normal growth and development.

Adolescent athletes are generally receptive to the teaching of nutritional guidelines. This is due to a strong desire to increase sports efficiency as well as increased body awareness. However, this also leaves them vulnerable to sports nutrition myths and misinformation. It is important to have coaching and training staff that are knowledgeable in nutrition, to introduce good nutritional standards through sports.

Calories
Adolescent athletes require adequate calories to support basal metabolism, activity, and growth. Since the energy needs of training and competition are high and the growth rate during adolescence is rapid, caloric needs may be great. Insufficient calories may lead to sub-optimal sports performance and growth impairment. Excess calories, on the other hand, results in unnecessary fat deposition and an increased workload to the heart.

In determining an individual's caloric needs consider body size, level of training, type of sport, and rate of growth. The distribution of calories should follow the recommendations for the general public, that is, 15% of calories from protein, 30% from fat, and 55% from carbohydrates.

Fuel for Energy
Muscles use primarily carbohydrate and fat for fuel. During vigorous exercise, carbohydrate is the main energy source. This carbohydrate fuel is stored in the muscles and liver as glycogen. When glycogen stores are depleted, fatigue comes on rapidly and work performance decreases. Therefore, the amount of glycogen stored is one factor that determines the athlete's ability to sustain prolonged, vigorous exercise.

For submaximal work of long duration, fat is the primary fuel source. The endurance trained athlete becomes more efficient at using fat and can spare glycogen.

Carbohydrate
Carbohydrate is the most efficient and readily available source of food energy. Since carbohydrate cannot be stored in significant amounts, the active person needs an adequate amount at regular intervals. Diets containing less than 40% of the calories from carbohydrate lead to a steady decrease in glycogen stores with successive days of training. Athletes training exhaustively on successive days or competing in prolonged endurance events may benefit from diets with more than 70% of the calories coming from carbohydrate.

Protein
Many coaches and athletes believe that high protein diets increase muscle mass and improve performance. Contrary to this belief, the only way to increase muscle mass is with muscle training and increased calories in a balanced diet. The increased caloric intake of athletes will adequately provide the moderate increase in protein that is required. Thus, use of high protein intakes or amino acids or protein supplements (>20% of total calories) is contraindicated. Diets high in protein can actually impair performance. Consuming excessive protein may induce dehydration, loss of appetite, or diarrhea -- all conditions that will hinder performance -- and may put stress on the kidneys. Athletes who eat protein in the place of carbohydrate are using a less efficient and more expensive fuel for energy.

416

In addition to requiring protein for normal growth and development, adolescent athletes need protein to restore nitrogen lost through heavy sweating, to replace tissue lost through trauma, proteinuria, hemoglobinuria, or myoglobinuria, and for increased lean body mass due to training. This additional protein need is easily met by the high calorie diets consumed by adolescent athletes. Special foods and supplementary protein are unnecessary. (See Appendix for the RDA of protein for adolescents.)

Fat

Since fat can be stored by the body in almost unlimited amounts, there is no reason to increase the amount of fat in the athlete's diet. In general, most adolescents could benefit from a decrease in their total fat intake and an increase in their intake of complex carbohydrates. This is compatible with the athlete's need for a high carbohydrate diet.

Vitamins and Minerals

There is no conclusive evidence to support claims that vitamin supplements improve physical performance. The athlete has an increased need for B vitamins due to an increased caloric intake, but this need can be met by a balanced diet.

The iron status of adolescent athletes deserves special attention for several reasons. First of all, iron requirements are high for menstruating girls and rapidly growing adolescent males and females. Secondly, the iron intake of adolescents is often marginally adequate or deficient. This is more prevalent in adolescent females eating less protein. Thirdly, many athletes have abnormally low iron stores. Even when hemoglobin is normal, low iron stores may lead to a decrease in strength and endurance and to easy fatigue.

Considering these factors, iron status should be monitored in adolescent athletes. Occasionally, an iron supplement will be needed to correct a deficiency or maintain balance.

Calcium in the adolescent's diet should be addressed as well since recent surveys of teenage eating habits indicate carbonated beverages are often substituted for milk, thereby decreasing calcium intake. Education about the importance of calcium intake should stress dietary sources.

Indication for supplementation: A single daily multiple vitamin and mineral tablet may be called for, and is generally not harmful. However, megadosages of any vitamin or mineral may be harmful, and should be strongly discouraged.

Fluids and Electrolytes

During exercise, water is rapidly lost through sweat. Inadequate replacement of water can have serious consequences for athletes. With as little as a 2-3% decrease in body weight due to dehydration, physical performance is impaired. More severe dehydration can lead to heat exhaustion and even death.

Thirst is not always a good indicator of fluid needs. Drinking fluids to satisfy thirst usually replaces only 60-70% of water lost. Therefore, athletes may have to force fluids. The best way to monitor dehydration is by frequent body weight measurements. Ideally, the athlete should drink enough fluid to maintain pre-exercise weight. Each pound of weight lost during exercise should be replaced by one pint of liquid.

Some basic recommendations for fluid replacement are:

- Volume – 8-16 oz. of fluid prior to the exercise event is suggested. During exercise, 5-8 oz. should be consumed every 15 minutes and fluid replacement should continue after the event.
- Temperature – cold fluids are preferable. They empty from the stomach rapidly, so they
- are readily available to the body.
- Type of Fluid – in most cases plain water is the best fluid replacement. Commercial drinks containing glucose and electrolytes should be diluted with water and used sparingly. They should not contain greater than 2.5% sugar. Soft drinks and fruit juices contain 5-10% sugar and should be diluted. Drinks high in sugar are high in osmolarity and are likely to delay gastric emptying and may cause cramping, nausea, vomiting, and dehydration.

Special Considerations

Food Fads and Health Foods

There is no one food or group of foods that improves physical performance. Fad diets and "magical" health foods should be discouraged. Diets severely restricting the variety of foods eaten are incompatible with good health, adequate growth, and optimum athletic performance.

Vegetarian Diet

A vegetarian diet can support the nutritional needs of an adolescent athlete. The same basic nutritional guidelines for all vegetarians hold true. The vegetarian athlete needs to be aware of consuming adequate calories, protein, iron, calcium, zinc, and vitamin B-12.

Fiber

Dietary fiber is an important part of good nutrition for most people. Athletes are no exception. Prior to a weigh-in or a competitive event, however, athletes may want to decrease their fiber intake. Fiber retains fluid in the gut which increases body weight and creates a feeling of heaviness.

Precompetition Meal

The best precompetition meal is well tolerated and familiar. Encourage athletes not to experiment with food intake prior to an event. There is no magic in the precompetition meal that will help athletes win. The key is in training-not the meal-before the event. Liquid meals are not better, but may be preferred by athletes who suffer from nausea, vomiting and abdominal cramps due to nervous tension.

General guidelines for the precompetition meal are:

Timing	• 3-5 hours prior to the start of an event (this avoids retention of undigested food in the GI tract)
Quantity	• relatively light, about 500 calories
Composition	• high in carbohydrates, low in concentrated sugars • low in fiber and fat • unrestricted in fluid • moderate in salt (highly salted foods cause water retention and thirst)

Carbohydrate Loading

Carbohydrate loading is a technique used to increase glycogen in muscles with the aim of increasing endurance and improving performance. It should be used only for endurance events that last more than 90 minutes consisting of strenuous exercise such as marathon or triathlon training or events. The traditional method of carbohydrate loading should not be used by children and adolescents.

The traditional method requires six days of dietary manipulation. Over 2-3 days muscles are depleted of glycogen by exercising them to exhaustion and consuming a high-protein, low-carbohydrate diet. During this phase athletes often experience fatigue, irritability and general discomfort. Then for three days immediately prior to the competitive event, glycogen stores are increased two to three times above normal. This is accomplished by light training and consuming a high-carbohydrate diet.

A less stressful form of carbohydrate loading is recommended for athletes competing in prolonged endurance events. With this method the depletion phase is eliminated. A normal diet is consumed until three days prior to the event, when the athlete decreases the amount and intensity of exercise and consumes a high-carbohydrate diet. Muscles are not supersaturated with glycogen, but the available glycogen stores are filled to capacity. Since training alone increases glycogen stores, "filled to capacity" will be above normal for the highly trained athlete.

Traditional carbohydrate loading has been criticized for possibly having adverse effects on the cardiovascular system and muscle fibers. Opponents of this method also claim that it impairs performance by increasing body weight and causing muscle stiffness. This is due to the increased body water accompanying increased glycogen.

Weight Management

Reaching and maintaining ideal weight often improves athletic performance. For the adolescent athlete ideal weight will change as he or she grows and matures. For all athletes, ideal weight is influenced by percentage of body fat. An appropriate amount of body fat aids in strength, endurance, and speed for any sport.

The average 15-16 year-old boy has 14-16% of his body weight as fat. The average teenage girl has 20-26% of her body weight as fat. A body fat percentage of less than about 18% for an adolescent girl may result in amenorrhea.

An athlete should allow adequate time for either losing or gaining weight. Sudden increases or decreases in weight may compromise both the health and physical performance of the athlete.

Adolescent athletes often resort to faddish weight loss methods. These diets usually promote the elimination of important food groups (such as milk and starches) and a drastic reduction in calories. Following these regimens results in muscle deterioration and water loss, rather than the desired fat loss. Some adolescent athletes become so concerned with decreasing body fat that they resort to near starvation diets and excessive physical training. These practices impair athletic performance and adversely effect growth and development. There are cases of both male and female adolescent athletes that have developed such great aversions to food that they manifest the symptoms of anorexia nervosa.

High school wrestlers look for quick weight loss methods to qualify for weight classes. As a result they often resort to dehydration. This method of weight loss reduces strength and endurance and can impair performance by 20-30%. The side effects of repeated dehydration range from fatigue to circulatory collapse. This can also include poor growth as growth hormone production may be decreased.

Before an adolescent athlete embarks on a weight loss program, his or her percentage of body fat should be determined. The appropriate amount of weight to be lost can be calculated based on desired percentage of body fat. The athlete must understand that controlling the percentage of body fat is more important than weighing a specific number of pounds.

A loss of 1-2 pounds per week can safely be achieved by increasing exercise and making low calorie food choices. Generally, a male adolescent athlete should consume a minimum of 2000 Kcals per day. For a female, this should be 1500-1600 Kcals per day. The goal of weight loss is losing fat, not muscle.

Weight gain also takes time and planning. It is not easy for an athlete who is already consuming a high calorie diet to further increase calories to gain weight. A 1- 1½ pound weight gain per week requires eating 500-800 calories more per day. For the athlete already consuming close to 4,000 calories, this is easier to do by eating 6 meals a day. More basic food is necessary. There is no need for the athlete to consume an excessive amount of protein or special supplements.

The goal of gaining weight is to add muscle, not fat. To prevent an increase in percentage of body fat while gaining weight, the athlete must train vigorously.

Caffeine

Some studies show that moderate caffeine intake (130 mg or 1 c. coffee), improves performance and increases endurance. It is believed to work by increasing the mobilization of fat for fuel, thereby sparing glycogen.

More research is needed before the use of caffeine can be promoted. Side effects vary with the individual, but caffeine ingestion, especially greater than 300 mg, may cause insomnia, restlessness, and diuresis. Young athletes, who are not used to drinking caffeinated beverages, are particularly susceptible to these effects.

Alcohol

Use of alcohol by adolescents should be discouraged in general. Alcohol consumption is not recommended before, during, or immediately after competition. Muscles cannot use alcohol for energy and it may impair performance. In addition to decreasing reaction time, alcohol interferes with voluntary and involuntary reflexes, impairs responsiveness and coordination, and acts as a diuretic.

References

1. Baer JT, Taper LF. Amenorrheic and eumenorrheic adolescent runners: Dietary intake and exercise training status. J Am Dietetic Assoc. Vol. 92, No. 1, Jan 1992, pp 89-91.
2. Bergen-Cico OK, Short SH. Dietary intakes, energy expenditures, and anthropometric characteristics of adolescent female cross-country runners. J Am Dietetic Assoc. Vol. 92, No. 5, May 1992, pp 611-612.
3. Clark N. Nancy Clark's Sports Nutrition Guidebook. Leisure Press. Illinois 1990.
4. Food Power - A Coach's Guide to Improving Performance. National Dairy Council. Rosemount, IL 1994.
5. Loosli AR. Nutritional Intake in Adolescent Athletes. Pediatric Clinics of North America. Vol. 37, No. 5, Oct. 1990, pp 1143-1153.
6. Meredith CN, Frontera WR. Adolescent Fitness. Adolescent Medicine. Vol. 3, No. 3, Oct. 1992, pp 391-404.
7. Narins DM et al. "Nutrition and the Growing Athlete" Pediatric Nursing. May/June 1983, pp 163-168.
8. Nevin-Folino NL. Sports Nutrition for Children and Adolescents. as found in: Handbook of Pediatric Nutrition. edit. Queen PM, Lang CE. Aspen Publishers Inc., Maryland 1993, pp 187-204.
9. Recommended Daily Allowance. 10th ed. National Academy of Sciences. Washington DC 1989.
10. Risser WL et al. "Iron deficiency in female athletes: Its prevalence and impact on performance." Medicine and Science in Sports and Exercise, 1988, pp 116-121.

Nutrition Considerations for the Pregnant Adolescent

Teenage pregnancy and childbearing have been issues of growing concern in the United States. Teenage pregnancy, birth, and abortion rates are higher in this country than in any comparable developed country, and this is particularly true among younger adolescents. More than one million teenagers become pregnant each year and approximately half of them give birth.

Health Implications

Adolescent pregnancy has been associated with significant medical and health risks.

1. For adolescents age 15 and younger, there is an increased incidence of iron deficiency anemia, pregnancy-induced hypertension, cephalo-pelvic disproportion, and abruptio-placentae.
2. Most young teens get no prenatal care in the first trimester, 20 percent get none before the third trimester.
3. Adolescents who conceive less than three years after menarche are at greater risk for poor pregnancy outcome.
4. There is a higher likelihood of such problems as genitourinary tract infection, pre-eclampsia, anemia, and inadequate or excessive weight gain during pregnancy.
5. There are higher risks of complications during labor for younger mothers.
6. Adolescents are 30 to 50 percent more likely to have low birth weight babies than women in their twenties. Low birth weight is a major factor associated with infant mortality and is also related to physical and mental handicaps.
7. Babies of young teens are more likely to die in the first year than those born to mothers in their twenties.
8. Forty percent of those teens who give birth as teenagers have another child within two years. Since perinatal risks increase with each additional birth, older teens may be at greater risk in a repeat pregnancy than younger girls who are pregnant for the first time.

Nutritional Risks

Maternal and fetal nutritional status can be compromised by any number of factors that may characterize the pregnant woman. Nutritional assessment of the pregnant adolescent should include identification of these factors. According to the American College of Obstetricians and Gynecologists, the pregnant woman is likely to be at nutritional risk if at the onset of pregnancy:

1. She is an adolescent (particularly 15 years of age or less).
2. She has had three or more pregnancies within two years.
3. She has a history of poor obstetric or fetal performance.
4. She is economically deprived (an income less than the poverty line or a recipient of local, state, or federal assistance, such as Medicaid or the USDA food programs, such as WIC).
5. She is following a bizarre or nutritionally restrictive diet.
6. She is a heavy smoker, drug addict, or an alcoholic.
7. She has a therapeutic diet for chronic systemic disease.
8. She weighed, on her first prenatal visit to the doctor, less than 85 percent or more than 120 percent of standard weight for her age, height, and state of maturity.

A pregnant woman is very likely to be a nutritional risk if *during* pregnancy:

1. She has low or deficient hemoglobin (Hgb)/hematocrit (HCT)(low is Hgb less than 11.0 g, HCT less than 33; deficient is Hgb less than 10.0 g, HCT less than 30).
2. She has inadequate weight gain, or any weight loss during pregnancy, or a gain of less than two pounds (one kilogram) per month in the second and third trimesters.
3. She has excessive weight gain during pregnancy - more than two pounds (1 kilogram) per week.
4. She is planning to breast-feed her infant and, therefore, has increased nutritional demands.

Maternal Growth and Nutrition Issues

The critical biologic difference between the pregnant adolescent and the pregnant adult is the adolescent's normal potential for ongoing linear growth and acquisition of lean body mass. The greater the amount of uncompleted growth at conception, the greater are the nutritional needs of the adolescent and fetus.

Gynecologic age (GA), the difference between chronologic age and age at menarche (onset of menses), has been used as an indirect measure of physiologic immaturity and growth potential. A pregnant teenager with a GA of two years or less will still be in a period of appreciable growth. It is likely that these teenagers will be 15 years or younger. While maximal height and weight gain occurs prior to menarche (mean U.S. age is 12.8 years), growth does not cease until four to seven years later. In adult healthy women, heights and weights exceed those at menarche by 4.3 to 10.6 cm (2-4 in) and 5-10 kg (11-22 lbs). Almost all residual growth occurs in the first two years after menarche. Those who have achieved full growth, usually complete by four years after menarche, are considered to be comparable to adult women in their prenatal nutritional needs.

Nutritional Requirements

Nutrient requirements for pregnant adolescents are based on incremental additions of the nutrients recommended for pregnant adult women to the nutrient requirements for non-pregnant adolescents.

Recommended Nutrient Intake for Pregnant Adolescents

Nutrients	Age: 11 - 18 years
Energy (Kcal) (a)	2500 - 2700
Protein (g)	60
Calcium (mg)	1200
Phosphorus (mg)	1200
Iron (mg) (b)	30
Magnesium (mg)	320 - 340
Iodine (mcg)	175
Zinc (mg)	15
Copper (mg)	2
Vitamin A (mcg RE)	800
Vitamin D (mcg)	10
Vitamin E (mg a - TE)	10
Vitamin C (mg)	60 - 70
Niacin (mg NE)	17
Riboflavin (mg)	1.6
Thiamin (mg)	1.5
Folate (mcg)	370 - 400
Vitamin B 6 (mg)	2.0 - 2.2
Vitamin B 12 (mcg)	2.2

(a) Second and third trimester

(b) When diagnosed with anemia (a hemoglobin concentration below 11.0 g/dl first and third trimester or below 10.5 g/dl during the second trimester), the recommended iron dosage is increased to 60-120 mg elemental iron/day until normal hemoglobin levels are attained.

Recommended Total Weight Gain Ranges for Pregnant Adolescents {Using Prepregnancy Body Mass Index (BMI)}

Weight for Height Category	Recommended Total Gain *	
	Kg	lb
Underweight (BMI <19.8)	12.5 - 18	28 - 40
Normal Weight (BMI 19.8 - 26.0)	11.5 - 16	25 - 35
Overweight (BMI >26-29)	7.0 - 11.5	15 - 25
Very Overweight (BMI >30)	7.0 - 9.1	15 - 20

* Young adolescents should strive for gains at the upper end of the recommended range.

Nutritional Assessment

Adolescent females, in general, are at risk for nutritional problems, and pregnancy places an adolescent at even greater risk. Because of this, and the importance of nutrition in the course and outcome of pregnancy, all pregnant adolescents should have a formal assessment of their nutritional state at the beginning of their prenatal care, and have ongoing surveillance throughout the pregnancy. A complete nutritional assessment should include evaluation of dietary, anthropometric, biochemical, and clinical data as well as relevant medical, obstetric, and psycho-social history.

Once the nutritional assessment has been completed, nutrition risk factors and the identification of overt or potential nutrition problems should be evident. For review, warning signs of nutrition problems are listed below.

Warning Signs of Nutritional Problems in Pregnant Adolescents
MEDICAL/OBSTETRIC FACTORS
1. Adolescent with a gynecological age of less than three.
2. A previous pregnancy.
3. History of poor obstetric or fetal performance.
4. Chronic systemic disease.
5. Past or present eating disorder: anorexia or bulimia nervosa.
6. Heavy smoker.
7. Alcohol or drug use.
8. Underweight or overweight prior to pregnancy.
9. Persistent nausea or vomiting during pregnancy.
10. Inadequate weight gain during pregnancy.
11. Excessive weight gain during pregnancy.
12. Iron deficiency anemia or other nutritional deficiencies.

PSYCHO-SOCIAL FACTORS
13. Economically deprived.
14. Living alone or in an unstable family or other environment.
15. Little family or peer support.
16. Denial or unacceptance of the pregnancy.
17. Significant emotional stress or depression.
18. Fear of gaining weight.

NUTRITION/DIETARY FACTORS
19. Inadequate refrigeration or cooking facilities.
20. Cultural or religious dietary restrictions.
21. Frequent eating away from home.
22. Poor appetite.
23. Limited or monotonous diet.
24. Irregular meal patterns or skipping meals.
25. History of frequent dieting.
26. Exclusion of a major food group or groups.
27. Binge eating episodes.
28. Eating of non-food substances (pica).
29. Non-traditional dietary pattern, such as vegetarianism.
30. Overuse of nutritional supplements.

Approaches to Nutritional Counseling

- Set the stage for successful counseling by establishing rapport with the adolescent.
- Individualize the nutritional goals in counseling.
- Set specific and realistic nutritional goals.
- Explore with the adolescent her feelings about her pregnancy and her attitude about food. Help her to understand the reasons for her food choices and help her to evaluate these.
- Identify and work toward dispelling myths about food and pregnancy, particularly those that are harmful.
- Identify her motivation for maintaining positive food practices or for dietary change. These may include not only better health, but also appearance, feeling better, and a positive-self-concept. through nutrition, help promote a positive self-concept of the adolescent as an individual and as a mother.
- Translate food nutrition into the adolescent's lifestyle.
- Provide breakfast ideas that are quick and convenient. Encourage the adolescent to develop her own ideas. If she dislikes standard breakfast fare, offer unconventional alternatives.
- Identify nutritious snacks that she can eat as substitute for low nutrient density snack foods. For those who do not like to eat much at one meal, suggest frequent snacks during the day.
- For adolescents who enjoy fast foods, provide tips on how to "round out" a fast food meal, or how to "pick up" nutrients missing in the fast food meal in other foods eaten during the day.
- When counseling those who follow unusual or fad diets, reinforce the positive aspects of the diet while addressing those practices which may be harmful. Make recommendations for modifying a diet within the framework of what is acceptable to the adolescent, without causing undue stress. Use dietary supplements where appropriate.
- Inform the adolescent of the possible consequences of smoking, drug and alcohol use, and caffeine intake on her health and her baby's health.
- Involve the family in counseling sessions. encourage them to provide support and to improve access to nutritious food in the home.
- Identify foods that are fortified with nutrients that the adolescent omits or undereats, i.e., if she doesn't like milk, suggest using calcium fortified orange juice.

Recommended Daily Food Pattern for Pregnant Adolescents

Predominant Nutrient	Food	Servings
Calcium	Milk and milk products (cheese, ice cream, yogurt), soy products	4 or more
Protein, zinc, iron, pyridoxine	Meat, fish, poultry, eggs, dried beans, nuts	3 or more (7 oz.)
Vitamin C, folacin, pyridoxine	Citrus fruits and juices, green leafy vegetables, peppers	1 or more
Vitamin A, folacin, pyridoxine	Green leafy vegetables, yellow vegetables-carrots, sweet potatoes, squash	1 or more
Other vitamins and minerals	All fruits and vegetables	2 or more
Vitamin B complex, energy, zinc	Whole or enriched grains, breads, cereals	5 or more
Energy	Unsaturated fats and sugars	As needed

Size of servings:
Bread: 1 slice
Cereal or grain: 1/2 to 3/4 cup
Fruits and vegetables: 1/2 cup
Fruit juice: 4-6 ounces
Milk: 8 ounces
Milk products: 1 thin slice, or 1/2 cup
Meat, fish, or poultry: 2 to 3 ounces, or 2 to 3 thin slices
Eggs, legumes, or nuts*: 2 eggs*, 4 tablespoons peanut butter*, 1 to 1 1/2 cups cooked legumes
   *These foods have ½ the amount of protein per serving as meat, thus the normal serving size is
   doubled for teens.

From Frank, DA. J Calif Perinatal Assoc;3(1):21-26, 1985.

Breastfeeding During Adolescence

Biologically, the adolescent is capable of breastfeeding. No differences in quality or quantity of milk have been associated with material age. However, the nutritional needs of the adolescent during lactation will be greater than those of the adult woman for calories, protein, niacin, and thiamin.

The health and psychological benefits of breastfeeding for both mother and infant are widely recognized and have been extensively documented in the scientific literature and include nutritional, immunological, and psychological benefits for the infant. Disadvantages to the adolescent mother include: 1)total responsibility for feeding; 2) limited ability to leave the baby in the care of a surrogate mother; and 3) limited use of alcohol, cigarettes, and other drugs and medications such as oral contraceptives.

Adolescent mothers who are interested in breastfeeding should be encouraged and given support. However, many adolescent mothers may feel that they lack the psychological support or environment needed. The adolescent mother should be supported in whatever infant feeding choice they make.

References:

1. Frank, DA, Gibbons, M, Schlossman, N. Nutrition in adolescent pregnancy. J Calif Perinatal Assoc 1985:3(1):21.
2. Gutierrez, Y:. Nutrition during teenage pregnancy. Pediatr Annl 1993;22:2:99-108.
3. Institute of Medicine. Committee on Nutrition Status during Pregnancy and Lactation, Food and Nutrition Board, Nutrition during Pregnancy. National Academy Press, 1990 and 1992.
4. Rees, JM, Lederman, SA. Nutrition for the pregnancy adolescent. Adol Med 1992;3(3):439-457.
5. Skinner, JD. Food and nutrient intake of white, pregnant adolescents. J Am Diet Assoc 1992;92(9):1127-1129.
6. Story, M, Alton, I. Nutrition and the Pregnant Adolescent. Cont Nutr 1992;17(5).
7. Story, M, ed. Nutrition Management of the Pregnant Adolescent. US Dept HHS, Natl Clearinghouse, 1990.

Patient Resources

1. La Leche League International-Breastfeeding Support Group, 847-519-7730. To answer breastfeeding questions and give names of leaders in your city.
2. Hennepin County WIC, 612-348-6100. Can get number to WIC programs in other parts of the cities from this number.

Nutritional Intervention In Eating Disorders
Description

We live in a culture in which "thinness" is a measure of more than body conformation, and dieting has become a national obsession. More specifically, the cultural norms for body weight are up to 30 pounds less than the upper range of acceptable weights for height identified by the medical community.

One of the consequences of these cultural standards is the rise in the prevalence of eating disordered behavior. Three psychiatric disorders, anorexia nervosa, bulimia nervosa, and binge eating disorder will be discussed her in detail.

Anorexia Nervosa

Anorexia nervosa is a syndrome characterized by an intense fear of becoming obese that does not diminish with weight loss, disturbances in body image perceptions, and extreme weight loss. This incidence of anorexia nervosa has doubled in the past two decades. Current prevalence data varies from 0.64 to 1.12 per 100,000. However, the disease is 10 times more prevalent in females than in males.

Anorexia nervosa commonly starts in adolescence. A young person begins dieting as a result of real or perceived overweight and then becomes obsessed with becoming thin. Weight loss is achieved either by severe dietary restriction or by periods of severe restriction alternating with periods of binge eating, followed by self-induced vomiting. Excessive physical activity is also common as a means of increasing caloric expenditure.

Diagnostic criteria for anorexia nervosa:
1. Refusal to maintain body weight at or above minimally normal weight for age and height (<85% expected weight).
2. Intense fear of gaining weight or becoming fat, even though underweight.
3. Disturbance in the way in which one's body or shape is experienced, undue influence of body weight or shape on self evaluation, or denial of the seriousness of the current low body weight.
4. In postmenarcheal females, amenorrhea, i.e., the absence of at least three consecutive menstrual cycles. (A woman is considered to have amenorrhea if her periods occur only following hormone administration.)

Individuals with anorexia nervosa resist attempts aimed at weight gain. They demonstrate little insight regarding their eating behavior and deny hunger and the need for food. They exhibit rigid and perfectionistic behaviors with regard to eating as well as to most other areas of their lives. Although this population exhibits a high need for interpersonal approval, they typically have poor social skills and are socially isolated.

Goals for Nutritional Management of Person with Anorexia Nervosa:
1. To help patients attain and maintain normal nutritional status and normal growth.
2. To assist patients in establishing normal eating behaviors.
3. To promote a normal attitude about food.
4. To help patients develop appropriate responses to hunger and satiety cues.

<u>Interventions</u>

Resolution of the starvation state and associated symptoms is one of the first steps. Some of the symptoms associated with starvation include:

- Obsessive thoughts about food
- Depressed mood or mood swings
- Poor concentration or difficulty with decision-making
- Social isolation
- Decreased metabolic rate

As starvation is reversed, individuals with anorexia nervosa are more able to process information cognitively. At this point they are ready to begin the second phase of intervention, which involves addressing the psycho-social issues underlying their eating behavior.

The goals of nutritional intervention also shift from providing a sufficient quantity of calories to looking at the quality and adequacy of intake. It is also desirable to begin identifying and challenging faulty beliefs and attitudes about foods, eating, and body weight.

To achieve the goals of intervention, you need to:

1. Set weight and growth expectations. For a child or a younger adolescent, set a goal weight that will allow them to grow at a normal rate; use a pediatric growth table. Weekly weight gain expectations are usually between 0.5 kg to 1.5 kg/week. Note that if patients have been purging, taking laxatives, or restricting fluids, patients should be forewarned that they may experience a rapid weight gain because of their dehydrated state.
2. Set appropriate calorie goals based on normal intakes for age. Nutritionally, patients need to be provided with sufficient calories to promote weight gain. Quality of calories, however, is **not** a priority here. Recent evidence has shown that although caloric needs may be very low initially owing to decreased basal metabolic rate, caloric needs may increase dramatically within two to three weeks of refeeding and may exceed the needs of normal women during weight gain. A gradual increase in caloric intake is recommended to prevent excessive edema. For example, if patients are extremely emaciated or have been eating very little, start with about 1200 calories for the first few days. Thereafter, increase calories once weight gain slows down, but only when patient is managing to eat meals. Most women patients need an additional 3,000 calories to achieve weight gain/goal weight. Once weight is achieved, calorie level can be reduced to maintain weight.
3. Encourage a meal pattern with a wide variety of normal foods.
4. Monitor eating behaviors; it may be best to have them eat in a group if they are inpatient.
5. Correct nutrition misinformation via ongoing education.
6. Ongoing weight maintenance follow-up is essential.

Bulimia Nervosa

Bulimia nervosa is a disease characterized by recurrent episodes of binge eating behavior followed by self-induced vomiting, laxative abuse, fasting, and/or excessive exercising as a means of compensating for the excessive caloric intake. During the eating binges, there is a feeling of lack of control over eating behavior. Although bulimic symptoms may occur as part of anorexia nervosa, individuals with bulimia nervosa are typically of normal weight. They also experience body image distortion and are preoccupied with body shape and weight. Reports of the prevalence of this syndrome vary from 4.5 percent to 18 percent of high school and college students, to 2 percent of females attending a family planning clinic.

Bulimia typically begins in late adolescence after individuals have experimented with a variety of weight loss techniques. Binges, which generally consist of eating large amounts of high-carbohydrate "junk" foods, are followed by purging or restricting behaviors. Bulimics, however, may also purge after moderate-sized meals. The preoccupation with food in terms of planning and carrying out binge eating episodes often interferes with the person's ability to hold a job as well as with social activities.

Unlike individuals with anorexia nervosa, people with bulimia nervosa view their bulimic behaviors as "out of control" and often seek help to eliminate them, although they are determined to maintain their weight below a self-imposed level.

Diagnostic Criteria for Bulimia Nervosa:
1. Recurrent episodes of binge eating. An episode is characterized by both of the following: a. eating in a discrete period of time (any 2 hour period) an amount of food that is definitely larger than most people would eat during a similar period of time and under similar circumstances. b. a sense of lack of control over eating during the episode (e.g., a feeling that one cannot stop eating or control what or how much one is eating).
2. Recurrent inappropriate compensatory behavior in order to prevent weight gain, such as self-induced vomiting; misuse of laxatives, diuretics, enemas, or other medications; fasting; or excessive exercise.
3. The binge eating and inappropriate compensatory behaviors both occur, on average at least twice a week for three months.
4. Self-evaluation is unduly influenced by body shape and weight.
5. The disturbance does not occur exclusively during episodes of anorexia nervosa.

Goals for Nutritional Management of Bulimia Nervosa:
The treatment goals for eating disorders are threefold:
1. Elimination of the effects of food deprivation.
2. Identification and reconstruction of faulty beliefs about food and body weight regulation.
3. Normalization of eating behaviors.

Interventions:
Intervention involves resolution of the food deprivation that results from the purging or compensating behaviors following binge eating and addressing the underlying psycho-social issues that serve as cues for bulimic behaviors. Much of the goals for management and interventions are the same as for anorexia nervosa.

The initial thrusts of treatment involves providing these individuals with structured eating guidelines that specify when to eat, what to eat, and how much to eat. A modified exchange system is particularly suitable for these purposes. Antidepressants have also been found to be extremely helpful in some cases. Patients should be advised to eat three meals daily at fairly regular times ($\pm$ 1 hour). Patients should also be advised to eat at least every 6 hours during the day. These two changes will result in fewer cravings of foods and more control while eating. Some of the popular press advocate only eating when hungry. However, hunger sensations are not reliable at the beginning of treatment. Patients will begin to experience hunger in the mornings after eating breakfast daily for 2 to 3 weeks.

Early in treatment, it has also been found desirable to avoid "binge" foods or those foods that seem to trigger binge eating behavior. However, as eating behavior becomes more normal, individuals are encouraged to incorporate small amounts of these foods into their meal plans, particularly in "safe" and supportive environments. Doing so not only reduces psychological cravings and feelings of deprivation, but also functions to reprogram more positive responses and thereby to prevent relapse when such foods are encountered.

Another important issue in eliminating the effects of food deprivation is to provide adequate calories. Patients frequently will request weight reduction meal plans. however, it is important that treatment is focused on eliminating bulimic behaviors rather than weight loss. Meal patterns should be calculated to maintain current weight. In the case of an obese patient, the meal pattern can be calculated to maintain a healthy weight somewhat below actual weight. In both cases this can be calculated by using BEE (actual or healthy weight) x 1.2-1.3. Bulimics have been demonstrated to have lower calorie needs for maintenance than controls, hence, the low activity factor. Patients should be provided with an individualized meal pattern to achieve weight maintenance. However, discussion of calorie levels should be avoided until patients are free of bulimic behavior.

Faulty beliefs and attitudes about foods, eating, and body weight also need to be identified and challenged as early in treatment as possible. Although some individuals with bulimia nervosa may be overweight when entering treatment, it is undesirable to promote weight loss greater than one-half pound per week. Dieting and the resultant sense of food deprivation is a strong cue for bulimic behaviors.

The provision of adequate calories in three meals daily often results in a significant reduction of bulimic behaviors. Psychotherapy will assist in the further elimination of symptoms.

Patients will have numerous misconceptions about food as it relates to body weight. Common ones include: "All fat should be eliminated." "You shouldn't eat desserts or sweets." "Combination foods such as hot dishes have hidden calories." "Pizza is fattening." "Salads are good foods," etc... Patients should be helped to look at these beliefs, the evidence they have to support them, and the functionality of the beliefs. Although it is prudent to have patients avoid any binge foods early in treatment, ultimately these foods need to be reintroduced in a structured setting. Recovery involves patients being able to eat all kinds of foods whether they voluntarily choose to eat them or not.

The final focus of nutritional intervention is the normalization of eating behaviors. This is demonstrated by patients being able to choose foods that are not only nutritionally adequate, but in a socially acceptable form, i.e., pizza vs. boiled eggs, saltine crackers, and raw vegetables.

Generally speaking, nutritional counseling in bulimia is more effective in a group setting. Not only do patients learn from other group members but the group setting diffuses much of the shame associated with the behaviors.

In working with bulimic patients, especially on an outpatient basis, it is important to have the patient assume responsibility for following the recommendations provided. Dietitians should avoid writing meal plans for patients, or being critical or shaming of noncompliant behavior. Instead, patients should be reminded of their own treatment goals and assisted in looking at the advantages and disadvantages of following professional recommendations. Consistent noncompliance should be reported to the patients psychotherapist for assessment of patient's readiness to change.

Binge Eating Disorder

Binge Eating Disorder (BED) is a syndrome of persistent and frequent binge eating that is not accompanied by the regular compensatory behaviors required for a diagnosis of bulimia nervosa. This syndrome is relatively new and probably affects millions of Americans. People with BED frequently eat large amounts of food while feeling a loss of control over their eating. This disorder is different from binge-purge syndrome (bulimia nervosa) because people with binge eating disorder usually do not purge afterward by vomiting or using laxatives.

Diagnostic criteria for binge eating disorder:
1. Recurrent episodes of binge eating. An episode of binge eating is characterized by both of the following:
2. Eating, in a discrete period of time (e.g., within any 2-hour period), an amount of food that is definitely larger than most people would eat in a similar period of time under similar circumstances.
3. A sense of lack of control over eating during the episode (e.g., a feeling that one cannot stop eating or control what or how much one is eating).
4. The binge eating episodes are associated with three (or more) of the following:
    *   Eating much more rapidly than normal.
    *   Eating until feeling uncomfortably full.
    *   Eating large amounts of food when not feeling physically hungry.
    *   Eating alone because of being embarrassed by how much one is eating.
    *   Feeling disgusted with oneself, depressed, or very guilty after overeating.

Goals for Management of BED:
1. Decreasing dietary restraint.
2. Modifying maladaptive thoughts, beliefs, and values related to eating, shape, and weight.

Interventions:
Intervention for BED is similar to interventions for other eating disorders. Psychologically the focus is on using cognitive behavioral therapy to target their tendencies both to overresrict and then overeat; in other words, it focuses on overall moderation of food intake. Structuring eating and assuring that breakfast and lunch meals are adequate is helpful. Individuals will also need psychotherapy to identify issues that trigger binge eating as well as to evaluate the consequences of binge eating behavior.

Nutrition interventions may include:
1. Normalization of eating. This includes the adoption of a regular eating (i.e., a plan for when eating occurs) and the minimization or elimination of binge episodes.
2. Overall moderation of food intake without the adoption of a rigid or inflexible rules, and the identification and modification of maladaptive thoughts and beliefs that perpetuate the eating pattern.
3. Relapse prevention training.
4. Encouragement to exercise consistently.
5. Although calorie monitoring is typically discouraged, it may be a helpful tool for clients to demonstrate "normal" eating.
6. Nutrition education, emphasizing the basics of goon nutrition.

Other methods of treatment include (1) interpersonal psychotherapy to help people examine their relationships with friends and family and to make changes in problem areas; (2) treatment with medications such as antidepressants may be helpful for some individuals; (3) self-help groups also may be a source of support.

Other Examples Of Eating Disorders Not Otherwise Specified

Some individuals may present with some symptoms, but don't meet all criteria for anorexia nervosa, bulimia nervosa, or binge eating disorder, yet they clearly have disordered eating patterns. These individuals may meet the DSM IV criteria for eating disorders not otherwise specified, which include:

1. For females, all of the criteria for Anorexia Nervosa are met except that the individual has regular menses.
2. All of the criteria for Anorexia nervosa are met except that, despite significant weight loss, the individual's current weight is in the normal range.
3. All of the criteria for bulimia nervosa are met except that the binge eating or inappropriate compensatory mechanisms occur at a frequency of less than twice a week or for a duration of less than 3 months.
4. The regular use of inappropriate compensatory behavior by an individual of normal body weight after eating small amounts of food (e.g., self-induced vomiting after the consumption of two cookies).
5. Repeatedly chewing and spitting out, but not swallowing, large amounts of food.

Summary

Treatment of eating disorders such as bulimia nervosa and anorexia nervosa has a strong nutritional component. Treatment for both disorders appears to be most effective when it includes a multifaceted approach of psychotherapy, family therapy, psychotropicmedications, and cognitive behavioral techniques in addition to nutritional therapy and counseling.

References:

1. Casper R, et al. Total daily energy expenditure and activity level in anorexia nervosa. Am Clin Nutr 1991;53:1143-50.

2. Keys A, Brozek J, Henschel A, Michelsen D, Taylor HL. The biology of human starvation. Minneapolis: University of Minnesota Press, 1950.

3. Havala T, Shront SE. Managing the complications associated with refeeding. Nutrition in Clinical Practice. 1990;5:28-29.

4. American Psychiatric Association (APA). Diagnostic and Statistical Manual of Mental Disorders (4th ed.). Washington, DC: 1994.

5. Story M. Nutritional management and dietary treatment in bulimia. J Am Dietetic Assoc 1986;86(4):517-519.

6. Omizo SA, Aiko Oda E. Anorexia nervosa: psychological considerations for nutrition counseling. J Am Dietetic Assoc 1988; 88(1)49-51.

7. Position of the American Dietetic Association. Nutrition intervention in the treatment of anorexia nervosa and bulimia nervosa. J Am Dietetic Assoc 1988;88(1) 68-71.

8. Pomeroy C, Mitchell M. Medical complications and management of eating disorders. Psychiatric Annals. 1989;19(9):488-493.

9. Krey S, Palmer K, Porcelli K. Eating disorders: the clinical dietitians changing role. J Am Diet Assoc. 1989;89(1):41-42.

10. Gwirtsman H, Kaye W, Obarzanek E, George D, Jimerson D, Ebert M. Decreased caloric intake in normal weight patients with bulimia. Am J Clin Nutr. 49:86-92, 1989.

11. Hadigan C, Kissileff H, Walsh T. Patterns of food selection during meals in women with bulimia. Am J Clin Nutr, 50:759-66, 1989.

12. Fairburn, Christopher and Terence Wilson. Binge Eating: Nature, Assessment and Treatment. Guilford Press. 1996.

13. Thompson, Kevin J. Body Image, Eating Disorders, and Obesity: An Integrative Guide for Assessment and Treatment. Published by American Psychological Association. 1996.

14. McFarland, B. Brief Therapy and Eating Disorders: A Practical Guide to Solution-Focused Work with Clients. Joint Publication in the Jossey-Bass Social and Behavior. Jossey Bass Publications. 1995.

15. Brownell, Kelly D, and Christopher G. Fairburn. Eating Disorders and Obesity: A Comprehensive Handbook. Guilford Press. 1996.

16. Garner, David and Paule E. Garfinkel. Handbook of Treatment for Eating Disorders. Guilford Press. 1997.

Consumer References

1. Berg, Frances J, et al. Afraid to Eat: Children and Teens in Weight Crisis. Published by Healthy Weight Journal. 1997.

2. Roth, Geneen. Breaking Free from Compulsive Eating. Plume. 1993.

3. Hollis, Judy. Fat is a Family Affair. Hazelden. 1996

4. Roth, Geneen. Feeding the Hungry Heart: The Experience of Compulsive Eating. Plume. 1993.

5. Bode, Janet. Food Fight: A Guide to Eating Disorders for Pre-teens and their Parents. Simon & Schuster. 1997.

6. Waterhouse, Debra. Like Mother, Like Daughter: How Women are Influenced by Their Mother's Relationship with Food and How to Break the Pattern. Hyperion. 1997.

7. Ruggles Radcliffe, Rebecca. Enlightened Eating: Understanding and Changing Your Relationship with Food. 1996.

8. Foreyt, John P. and G. Ken Goodrick. Living without Dieting: A Revolutionary Guide for Everyone Who Wants to Lose Weight.

9. Tribole, Evelyn and Elyse Resch. Intuitive Eating: A Revolutionary Program That Works.

10. Fairburn GC. Overcoming Binge Eating. Guildford Press. 1995.

Organizations Interested in Eating Disorders

AED: Academy for Eating Disorders
Montefiore Medical School - Adolescent Medicine
111 East 210th Street
Bronx, NY 10467
(718) 920-6782

AABA: American Anorexia/Bulimia Association
293 Central Park West, Suite 1R
New York, NY 10024
(212) 501-8351

ANAD: National Association of Anorexia Nervosa & Associated Disorders
P.O. Box 7
Highland Park, IL 60035
(847) 831-3438

ANRED: Anorexia Nervosa and Related Eating Disorders, Inc.
P.O. Box 5102
Eugene, OR 97405
(541) 344-1144

EDAP: Eating Disorders Awareness & Prevention
603 Stewart Street, Suite 803
Seattle, WA 98101
(206) 382-3587

IAEDP: International Association of Eating Disorders Professionals
123 NW 13th Street, #206
Boca Raton, FL 33432-1618
(800) 800-8126

MEDA: Massachusetts Eating Disorders Association, Inc.
1162 Beacon St.
Brookline, MA 02146
(617) 738-6332

NEDO: National Eating Disorders Organization (Affiliated w/Laureate Eating Disorders Program)
6655 S. Yale Avenue
Tulsa, OK 74136
(918) 481-4044

OA: Overeaters Anonymous Headquarters
P.O. Box 44020
Rio Rancho, NM 87174-4020
(505) 891-2664

Organizations Interested in Size Esteem

AHELP: Association for the Health Enrichment for Large People
P.O. Drawer C
Radford, VA 24143
(703) 731-1778

Council on Size & Weight Discrimination, Inc.
P.O. Box 305
Mt. Marion, NY 12456
(914) 679-1209, Fax: (914) 679-1206

Largely Positive
P.O. Box 17223
Glendale, WI 53217

Largesse: The Network for Size Esteem
P.O. Box 9404
New Haven, CT 06534
(203) 787-1624

NAAFA: National Association to Advance Fat Acceptance, Inc.
P.O. Box 188620
Sacramento, CA 95818
(800) 442-1214

P.L.E.A.S.E: Promoting Legislation & Education About Self-Esteem, Inc.
91 S. Main St.
West Hartford, CT 06107
(860) 521-2515

Websites Related to Eating Disorders

National Institute of Mental Health at http://www.nimh.gov/

American Academy for Child and Adolescent Psychiatry at http://www.aacap.org/web/aacap

European Council on Eating Disorders http://psyctc.sghms.ac.uk/eat-d/eced2.htm

Anorexia Nervosa and Related Eating Disorders, Inc. at http://www.lifetimetv.com/Health Nutrition/Women'sWellness/eating_disorders/eresoun.htm

The American Anorexia/Bulimia Association at
http://www.social.com/health/nhic/data/hr0100/hr0123.html

New York Online Access to Health at http://noah.cuny.edu/wellconn/eatdisorders.html

NUTRITION FOR CHILDREN WITH SPECIAL HEALTH CARE NEEDS

Children with Special Health Care Needs

The phrase "children with special health care needs" describes those who were previously identified as handicapped, retarded, crippled, or having developmental disabilities. Children at high risk with chronic illness such as acquired immunodeficiency syndrome (AIDS), cocaine babies, prenatal exposure to chemicals, and ventilator dependent children are also included in this term. This broad range of chronic illness and conditions of physical impairment is estimated to have a prevalence of 10 to 20 percent, and shows evidence of increasing.

The identifiable etiologies include chromosomal abnormalities, congenital abnormalities, inherited metabolic disorder, specific syndromes, and neuromuscular dysfunction. Some individuals may present with more than one condition, ie., cerebral palsy and seizures, Down Syndrome and congenital heart disease.

Most children with special health care needs require the same nutrients as any individual, yet the needs can be influenced by the condition and/or its treatment. The beneficial effects of nutritional intervention include (a) prevention of retardation or further disability by dietary treatment, i.e., in phenylketonuria and other metabolic disorders, (b) health promotion, thus increasing the quality of life, decreasing the frequency of illness and the cost of medical services, (c) nutrition adequacy, thus allowing the individuals to attain good health, grow appropriately and perform to their optimal capacity in an educational or work setting.

Factors that affect the nutritional condition of children with special health care needs include:
- Altered growth rate
- Altered energy needs
- Feeding problems (physical and/or behavioral)
- Metabolic disorders
- Medication-nutrient interaction
- Constipation/diarrhea
- Lack of nutrition or feeding related knowledge of caregivers
- Unusual feeding behaviors
- Abnormal motor patterns
- Limited attention span
- Limitations in eating independence
- Oral-facial anomalies.

As the population of children with special health care needs has changed, so has the provision of care. The emphasis is on family-centered and community-based care. In a 1989 position paper on nutrition services for children with special health care needs, the American Dietetic Association recommended nutrition services that are coordinated, interdisciplinary, family-centered, culturally sensitive, and community based. This implies the provision of nutrition services in difference settings than the traditional medical model. The care will be provided in family homes, schools, child care settings, and other community agencies. Because the children are at increased risk they require early screening and periodic monitoring.

Caring for these children most often requires an interdisciplinary approach, with the child and family as essential members of this collaborative effort. Only when the knowledge and skills of all professionals and the family are coordinated can the child reach optimal potential.

Additionally, early intervention is key. Public Law 99-457, the Education of the Handicapped Act Amendments of 1986, expands education for children with special needs. Agencies have developed comprehensive, coordinated, multidisciplinary, interagency systems to provide early intervention services for infants and toddlers. Nutrition services are an area of need for many of these children and providing them at an early age can promote better health and prevent some problems in the future.

Comprehensive nutrition assessment may require specialized knowledge, skills and tools. The dietary analysis, biochemical and clinical components are fairly straightforward pediatric assessments. In addition, it is important to be aware of the socio-economic status and feeding behaviors of the patient or client. Medication/food interaction should be assessed. Anthropometric determinants are standard for the pediatric population, but the technique, equipment and growth grids may differ for these special populations. In addition, a feeding evaluation may be necessary.

Anthropometric measurements may be difficult to obtain. Whenever possible, standard equipment and techniques should be used to obtain and record serial length/height, weight and head circumference. For children with severe physical conditions, it may be impossible to get a standing measurement. In this case, other estimations may be used, such as arm span, sitting height, crown-rum, knee height, or arm length. Specialized growth grids are available for Down Syndrome and Turner Syndrome.

The process of feeding/eating may need to be assessed by an interdisciplinary team, and may include:

- A speech-language pathologist to assess the oral structure and sensitivity as well as oral-motor ability.
- An occupational therapist to assess the hand and mouth functioning and the needs for special feeding devices.
- A physical therapist to assess positioning needs.
- A registered dietitian to assess the nutritional adequacy of the diet and the appropriateness of food textures and fluid intake.
- A social worker to complete a psycho-social assessment of the patient/client and their family group.
- A psychologist to assess the behavioral aspects of the feeding problem.
- A radiologist to complete videofluoroscopy study and assess the swallowing mechanism.

Successful feeding may involve the use of special eating utensils or seating equipment, modifications of food texture and consistency, or use of commercial products such as thickening agents.

Planning for feeding children with special health care needs must be individualized to include realistic recommendations for kilocalorie and nutrient intakes, and food textures, as well as for developing feeding skills. The goal for all children is to provide as normal a diet as possible with as much self-sufficiency with regard to eating as the condition will allow.

Professional References

1. American Dietetic Association. Position of the American Dietetic Association: Nutrition Services for Children with Special Health Care Needs. J Am Dietetic Assoc 1989; 89:1133.
2. Ekvall SW, Pediatric Nutrition in Chronic Diseases and Developmental Disorders: Prevention, Assessment, and Treatment. Oxford University Press 1993.

Cerebral Palsy

Description

Cerebral Palsy is a generic descriptive term to describe a child with a congenital non-progressive neuromotor disorder. It is not a medical diagnosis with a single etiology or common natural history.

Classifications:

Spastic: Increased stretch reflexes, increased muscle tone, and weakness of the involved musculature. Seventy percent of cerebral palsy individuals are spastic.
  - A. **Hemiparesis:** Both extremities on the same side are spastic.
  - B. **Tetraparesis:** Spasticity on all four extremities.
  - C. **Spastic Diplegia:** Greater involvement in the lower limbs than the upper extremities, most common in low birth-weight and premature infants.
    1. **Hypertonic**
    2. **"Atonic"**
  - D. **Paraparesis:** Both legs are involved, yet the upper extremities are not affected.
  - E. **Monoparesis** and **triparesis**.

Dyskinetic: Impairment of volitional activity by uncontrolled and purposeless movements tending to disappear during sleep.
  - A. **Athetosis:** Characterized by slow, wormlike, writhing movement usually involving all four extremities, this is seen in 15 percent of cerebral palsy children.
  - B. **Other dyskinesis.**

Ataxia: Characterized by incoordination and balance problems, affected individuals have a wide-based gait.

Mixed type: The condition when both athetosis and spasticity exist in one person, which frequently occurs.

Nutrition Related Problems

1. Slow neuromotor development, slow growth in height, delayed bone development.
2. Feeding difficulties:
   - Long feeding time
   - Tonic bite reflex
   - Choking due to poor integration of the suckle swallow reflex and increased gag reflex
   - Tongue thrust
   - Poor lip and tongue control
   - High arched palate
   - Chewing difficulties
   - Abnormal intraoral sensation
   - Delayed self-feeding
3. Poor dentition, including sever malocclusion, bruxism, and caries.
4. Varied energy requirement due to excessive or inadequate physical activity.
5. Constipation, resulting from decreased peristaltic movement, abnormal muscle tone, lack of ambulatory activity, or medication.
6. Medication/nutrient interaction. Long-term users of certain anticonvulsants may develop folic acid, calcium and vitamin D deficiency with a small incidence of vitamin B12 deficiency.

Nutrition Management

1. Determination of ideal body weight

   For infants and children, NCHS weight for height growth chart is used to determine ideal body weight range. For young adults with spastic quadriplegia or low muscle mass, the ideal body weight is determined by subtracting 15 percent from the ideal body weight for normal people. For diplegic or hemiplegic individuals, subtract 5 to 10 percent.

2. Energy requirements

   Caloric requirements vary according to the type of cerebral palsy and the severity of the neuromuscular involvement. The goal is to ensure adequate growth and prevent extremes of underweight or overweight.

   Requirements for a child with spastic cerebral palsy are small due to their limited physical activity. However, involuntary muscle movement and other complications such as seizures of illness will increase caloric requirements. A current recommendation is to determine caloric needs on the basis of body height. For children 5 to 11 years of age with milk to moderate involvement, 13.9 kcal/cm is recommended, and 11.1 kcal/cm is recommended for children with severe involvement.

   Children with athetosis have involuntary motor activities resulting in extra energy expenditure and possible inadequate actual food intake. These individuals tend to be underweight and may develop vitamin/mineral deficiencies secondary to limited amount of food intake. Calories should be increased with nutrient dense foods.

3. Maintaining ideal body weight with adequate nutrient intake

   In order to prevent an over- or under-weight condition, the individual's anthropometric measurements should be monitored regularly, with caloric changes as indicated. When a limited caloric intake is needed to achieve or maintain the ideal body weight, it is essential to supply a diet with adequate levels of vitamins, minerals, and protein. Use of vitamin/mineral supplements may be required in some cases.

4. Dental problems

   All dietary measures to prevent dental caries should be considered. In severe cases of malocclusion, soft foods should be recommended. Bruxism (grinding teeth) may be managed by a reward system in some cases.

   Baby bottle tooth decay (BBTD) can be prevented by not placing the child in bed with a bottle or allowing the bottle after one year of age. If the child's developmental stage indicated the need for a bottle past one year, the teeth should be cleaned with a gauze pad after feeding.

5. Management of feeding problems

   A team approach is necessary to manage feeding problems. Nutritional intervention strategies include the following:
   a. An alternate route of enteral feeding (primarily gastrostomy) is recommended when:
      - Aspiration is diagnosed through a videofluoroscopy study. (To ensure safe feeding.)
      - The individual has difficulty drinking or only aspirates when drinking. (To ensure adequate fluid intake.)
      - The individual has difficulty ingesting solid foods, or only aspirates when eating solid foods. (To ensure adequate caloric intake.)

- When oral feeding is such a physically and emotionally draining activity to both the individual and the caregiver, gastrostomy feeding is recommended for supplemental nutrition to ensure adequate nutritional intake and quality feeding interaction. If the child's oral feeding skills improve, gastrostomy feeding can be discontinued.

b. Change of food texture/temperature.
- Thickened fluids can be used to facilitate drinking. The fluids can be thickened with baby cereal, unflavored gelatin, applesauce, dehydrated baby foods, or commercial thickening agents.
- When the child is ready for a higher level feeding skill, the food texture needs to be upgraded in time to promote such feeding skill. It is important to recognize the readiness cues to proceed and not keep the child on low texture foods any longer than necessary.
- Food with two textures is usually more difficult to handle orally than food with one texture, ie, apple versus peeled apple
- Some cerebral palsy children may be temperature sensitive. They may prefer cold or warm foods.

c. Change of feeding time.
- For children who tire easily, small but frequent feedings may be more appropriate.

6. Management of constipation

High fiber intake or the use of unprocessed wheat bran with increased fluid intake is recommended. For children with ambulatory ability, increased physical activity should also be suggested. In acute cases of constipation, a medical intervention such as laxatives, stool softeners, enemas, and mineral oil may be required. Medical interventions should be used only to solve the acute problem because when used continuously, it may lead to more loss of intestinal motility with eventual dependency on those methods. When mineral oil is used, it should not be taken with or near meal time, and should be on a short-term basis to prevent possible loss of fat soluble vitamins.

7. Long-term users of anticonvulsants may have altered metabolism and absorption of Vitamins D, K, Folate, B12 B6 calcium, alkaline phosphatase and phosphorus.

Vitamin and mineral supplements may be needed both for prevention and treatment if vitamin/mineral deficiencies are identified.

Client Resources

1. For information on local affiliates contact the United Cerebral Palsy Association, 1660 L Street, NW, Suite 700, Washington, DC, 20036-5602; 1-800-USA-5UCP.

Cleft Lip and/or Palate
Description

A cleft is an opening in the lip, the hard palate or the soft palate. These openings are normally present early in fetal development but close before birth. Cleft lip is a unilateral or bilateral separation of the upper lip and frequently the dental ridge as well, occurring during the fifth week of fetal development. Clefts of the palate may occur in the bony hard palate or soft palate or in both at approximately the seventh or eighth week of development. There can also be a combination of cleft lip and cleft palate.

A related condition is the submucous cleft, a cleft involving the muscles of the soft palate and part of the hard palate. The palate may look whole, but if there is an absence of bone in the hard palate or muscle tissue in the midline of the soft palate, it is termed a submucous cleft. Bifid or notched uvula usually accompanies this condition, along with hypernasal voice quality. Feeding is not a major problem, but milk may come through the nose, which should be seen as an indication to examine for a submucous cleft. Since diagnosis is frequently overlooked until the preschool years when hypernasal speech is apparent, referral of children with nasal milk loss can accelerate early diagnosis.

Incidence

Approximately 5,000 children are born with cleft lip or palate in the United States each year. Differences do exist in the incidence of cleft lip, cleft palate, and cleft lip and palate among races and sexes. It is frequently reported that some type of cleft occurs in approximately one in every 700 births in the white population, more often among Orientals and certain groups of American Indians, and less frequently among blacks. More males than females have cleft lip with or without cleft palate, with a left-sided cleft being more frequent than a right-sided cleft. Clefts of the hard and soft palate or of the soft palate only are less frequent than is cleft lip with or without cleft palate and occurs in about one out of every 2,200 live births, affecting more females than males.

Treatment and Management

Closure of clefts is accomplished through a sequence of staged surgical procedures. While surgical repair and reconstruction timetables vary significantly throughout the country, the goal is to facilitate eating and speaking while improving appearance with a minimum of scarring and promoting normal facial growth.

The first treatment is surgical repair of the lip usually within the first month. Palate repair is done at approximately one year of age, before there has been much speech development. As the child matures, there may be many surgical revisions, dental procedures, speech therapy, otologic care and possibly psychological therapy. Intervention, treatment and family support are complicated, so it is highly recommended that the children be followed routinely by a multidisciplinary team. Over 200 cleft palate treatment teams practice in the United States.

Nutritional Considerations

The challenge immediately after birth is to reassure the parents that the child can be fed an adequate diet with no compromise in growth or health. Depending on the location (lip, hard palate, soft palate or combination) and the extent of the opening (bilateral or unilateral), feeding may or may not be a problem. When feeding is difficult, it is a mechanical problem in that the child is unable to suck adequately because negative pressure cannot be achieved. Nutrient needs of children with cleft lip/palate are the same as those of other children and they will experience the same appetite fluctuations, taste preferences and food quirks.

The importance of good nutrition for these children is:
- to build up resistance to infection
- to acquire the necessary weight needed for surgery
- to build up strength the child needs to meet the stress of surgery
- to promote healing after surgery
- to promote healthy oral structures.

For these reasons, it is recommended that a nutrition assessment including anthropometric measurements and dietary analysis be a routine part of the team evaluation.

Factors to Be Considered in Nutritional Evaluation

Sucking

The first problem to present itself may be insufficient suction. However, a baby with a cleft lip and palate will start to suck when a nipple is placed in his or her mouth, just as any newborn baby does. This occurs because the sucking and swallowing reflexes are present even though the muscles are not able to operate as efficiently because of the cleft. Poor sucking causes fatigue and subsequent insufficient formula or breast milk to satisfy the baby's appetite and nutrient needs.

Swallowing

Swallowing problems may occur in infants with the Pierre Robin sequence, pharyngeal or esophageal abnormalities, or central nervous system problems. Infants with cleft lip/palate as their sole health condition swallow normally, but, because they may swallow excess air, need to be burped more frequently to decrease nasal regurgitation and possible aspiration.

Positioning

The most successful position for feeding is in a semi-sitting position (60-90 degree angle) to allow gravity to assist with swallowing. An infant should never be put to bed with a bottle, since this habit can lead to ear infections and if continued past one year of age can also contribute to tooth decay. In addition to the position of the child's body, the position of the nipple is important. Some children are more successful at sucking when the liquid is directed toward the cheek, rather than the back of the throat.

Growth

Slow weight gain has occasionally been reported during the first few months of life. When it occurs, this lag may be due to early feeding difficulties, frequent upper respiratory infections, middle ear disease, repeated surgical procedures, psychosocial dynamics, or some combination.

There are reports in the literature of a higher incidence of growth hormone deficiency in children with cleft lip/palate. Although some children have been successfully treated with growth hormone, this concept does not have total agreement. Even though research cannot currently resolve the debate, it is highly recommended that growth be routinely measured and plotted on a growth chart as a method of screening for growth disorder and referral, if indicated.

Growth may also be affected by surgical procedures. A slowdown of growth may occur if normal eating is impossible due to extensive surgery or prolonged healing. In addition, surgeries that may affect nasal air flow can affect food intake. It has been observed that children who are mouth breathers sometimes have diminished interest in food, which may be due to inability to smell the food as well as the great difficulty in coordinating chewing, swallowing, and breathing.

Dentition

Many children with cleft conditions have an oral structure that can compromise adequate nutrition. Malocclusion, crowding and bite problems can make eating difficult and may limit types and textures of food.

Dietary Management in Infancy

Feeding is an immediate and traumatic concern for the family. The methods of feeding vary, depending on the type and extent of cleft as well as the philosophy of the hospital staff. In addition, early discharge of newborns may hinder the family from learning the types of equipment and/or techniques for feeding the baby. Hospital discharge should be delayed until the child can feed successfully in approximately thirty minutes and the parent is confident about the feeding. If the child has difficulty sucking or swallowing, it may be a cause of great anxiety and frustration for the adults doing the feeding.

There are many approaches to feeding babies with cleft lip/palate, and parents need to be assured there is no right or wrong method. The goal is to find a method that allows the child to consume the liquid in a reasonable amount of time with few, if any, physical problems. In time, most infants learn methods of compensating for the physical defect. Some children squeeze or chew the nipple; others learn to direct it to the area where the most suction can be obtained.

There may be a good deal of trial and error before achieving the perfect feeding situation. Even then, it usually changes as the child grows. A feeding method that works at birth may not be appropriate as the child matures and develops greater strength. Each child is different and the parents should be guided toward allowing enough time to feed, to the development of a relaxed feeding atmosphere, and to a willingness to adapt and change with their infant.

Most babies can be breastfed or bottlefed, but occasionally babies who have an exceptionally wide cleft or accompanying other conditions or syndromes may need to be fed by tube feeding or gavage. Ascepto syringe is often the methods chosen by the surgeon after surgery.

Some babies may need to have a prosthetic feeding appliance inserted. An obturator (dental plate usually made of dental acrylic) can be constructed to fit an individual baby's mouth. It artificially restores the hard palate until surgery can be performed and often improves the feeding situation.

Breast feeding children with cleft lip or palate has traditionally been discouraged because of anticipated failure to obtain good suction and fear that it would have deleterious effects after surgery. However, many women have successfully nursed their children. A baby with a cleft lip may be able to obtain adequate suction because the soft breast tissue may mold to the open area between the mouth and nose better than a firmer bottle nipple. A baby with a bilateral cleft of the palate may have more difficulty breast feeding and it may not be successful.

Because of the benefits of breastfeeding, mothers should be made aware of all the options so they can make an informed decision. In addition to breastfeeding or formula, the choices for the mother are to express her milk with a breast pump and give it in a bottle, or use a lactation aid device.

Some Recommendations for Bottle Feeding

1. Commercial bottles and nipples designed for children with cleft lip and/or palate. Available from the major formula manufacturers.
2. Standard commercial products include:
   a. Cross-cut preemie nipple. The nipple walls are softer and compress more easily, but may also collapse.
   b. Soft regular nipples with cross-cut or enlarged holes.
3. Modifications of existing infant feeding equipment include:
   a. Playtex® bottle with opening on side enlarged to allow for squeezing of bag containing formula.
   b. Regular nipple with additional holes added.
   c. Nipple softened by boiling
   d. Plastic bottle that has had the bottom removed and a plastic liner inserted. The bag compresses as the child sucks and thus avoids excess air intake,
   e. Plastic bottle that has been softened by boiling or previous use. This is usually too large for a newborn but works well when the baby is older.
   f. Inverted Playtex® nipple that creates a longer nipple.

Dietary Management During Preschool Years

Types of milk and addition of solid foods should progress at the same rate as for any child. Spoon feeding and cup drinking should be started at the same age as other children. Solids should always be fed by spoon and never from a bottle or commercial syringe-type infant feeder unless it is prescribed for a unique situation. Spoon feeding and finger foods are all activities that contribute to a healthy diet, as well as strengthening the oral-facial muscles.

Hard and sticky foods or small particles that may become lodged in the palate opening should be avoided. Occasionally acid or spicy foods may cause irritation. Since all toddlers can so easily experience food asphyxiation, foods that are small, round, slippery or tough should be avoided or only given in a supervised setting. See the section on choking prevention.

Dietary Management During Childhood and Adolescence

Depending on the degree of oral involvement, severe malocclusion can occur. There may be a cross-bite, missing and/or supernumerary teeth, and dental crowding and rotations. The diets of come children may be compromised by their inability to masticate a wide variety of foods. The child should be asked how well s/he can chew and which foods cause problems. The foods may need to be modified, cut smaller or moistened, or, until better dental closure is obtained, a substitute may be used.

Some older children may breathe through their mouth due to reduced nasal airway, ie, too wide a pharyngeal flap or deviated septum. This causes a very dry mouth and difficulty in coordinating chewing, swallowing, and breathing. Often, these children complain of excessive effort in eating or reduced taste due to a poor sense of smell.

Dietary Management During Hospitalization

The post surgical diets and feeding methods are usually dictated by the surgical team and/or hospital protocol and thus vary throughout the country. The purpose should be to maintain adequate nutritional status during the recovery period without a compromise in health or growth. The post-surgical diet advances from liquid to solids, and the routine or oral surgical progression can usually be followed. It may be advisable to increase the caloric density of the food as well as to institute small frequent feedings. If an older child must remain on semi-solids for an extended period, such as following bone graft surgery, a nutritional supplement may be indicated. Nutrition and feeding education for family is imperative if the child is going home on any special dietary regimen or with new feeding equipment.

Professional References

1. American Cleft Palate Educational Foundation, 1218 Grandview Avenue, University of Pittsburgh, PA 15261.
2. Balluff, MA, Udin, RD. Using a feeding appliance to aid the infant with a cleft palate. Ear, Nose, Throar J, 1986, 65:316.
3. Paradise, JL, McWilliams, BJ, Elster, B. Feeding of infants with cleft palate. Pediatrics, 1984, 74:316.

Client Resources

1. American Cleft Palate Association. Hotline 1-800-24-CLEFT.
2. Minnesota Department of Health. Feeding Young Children with Cleft Lip and Palate. Minneapolis, 1990.

Down Syndrome
Description

Down Syndrome, trisomy 21, is a chromosomal disorder affecting 1 in 660 live births. There is a high incidence of cardiac anomalies accompanying Down Syndrome and mild to moderate mental retardation.

Nutritional Related Problems

Varied growth patterns. Individuals with Down Syndrome are growth retarded compared with the normal population. The deficient growth rate is most marked in infancy and again in adolescence. There is also a tendency toward overweight beginning in late infancy and throughout the growing years. The rate of weight gain proceeds more rapidly than gains in height. Down Syndrome specific growth charts are available to monitor these individuals.

The degree of mental retardation may result in delayed progress in advancement of feeding skills. Hypotonicity (decreased muscle tone), which may result in difficulties in sucking, chewing, and swallowing. The hypotonicity may also affect the peristaltic movement, the muscle control of the bowel, and may lead to constipation.

Oral problems may include:
- A narrow and/or short palate
- Tongue protrusion, drooling, and poor lip closure
- Delayed tooth eruption, malocclusion and bruxism
- Mouth breathing because of a narrow nasal passage

Nutritional Management

Most children can be helped by early intervention in group or individual settings. An interdisciplinary team focusing on developmental readiness, adequate nutrition, parental interaction and physical growth should provide the stimulus necessary to progress as effectively as possible.

The focus should be adequate nutrient intake. Because the behaviors and/or developmental readiness may limit varied nutrient intake, care should be taken to assure adequacy of all nutrients. This is especially true if calories are being limited.

The child should advance in feeding skills and food textures as close to normal as possible. If constipation becomes a problem, a diet high in giver and fluids with an increase in physical activity is recommended.

Feeding problems have been identified in some children. They may be slow to advance to more textures or eat a limited amount of food. This can compromise the nutritional adequacy. Behavioral situations and parental expectations can also affect the developmental progress.

Serial monitoring of growth will alert the care providers to possible early interventions necessary to prevent obesity. Caloric intake needs to be adjusted if the child is gaining weight too rapidly. Suggested energy needs of children with Down Syndrome:

16.1 kcal/cm: male 1-3 years
14.3 kcal/cm: female 1-3 years

Percentile Charts for Down Syndrome Children

These charts provide standards for infants and children with Down Syndrome. They are based on longitudinal data and include children with congenital heart disease.

The percentile curves correct both for the average smaller size of Down Syndrome children at the various ages and for their slowed growth velocity, which renders the curves "flatter" than expected to conform better to percentile channels on these charts than those given on normal charts. However, because deficiencies in growth velocity occur at varying times and are of widely different magnitudes, a child may not remain in a single growth channel on the Down Syndrome chart.

Downward percentile shifts are most apt to occur between 6 and 24 months. While such shifts may still occur after 36 months, they are far less common. A small number of Down Syndrome children (approximately 10 percent) grown in a normal fashion, ie, their growth conforms better to percentile channels represented on normal growth charts.

Children with mild or severe heart disease show greater growth deficiencies than those without or with only mild heart disease. Velocity of growth for cardiac children is comparable to those without after about 36 months of age, through the size difference established by that time is never made up. As with normal children with heart disease, noticeable catch-up growth follows surgical repair of the lesion.

Weight gain for children with Down Syndrome is more rapid than height growth. This often results in overweight by 36 months of age. The etiology of this problem is not well understood, but may relate to decreased physical activity. Because the percentile plots reflect this trend, these charts should always be used in conjunction with charts for normal growth.

Professional References

1. Cronk, C, Crocker, AC, *et al.* Growth Charts for Children with Down Syndrome: 1 Month to 18 Years of Age. *PEDS,* 1988, 81:102.
2. Cloud, HH: Developmental Disabilities in Handbook of Pediatric Nutrition, Queen, PM; Lang, CE (eds). Aspen Publishers, Inc., Gaithersburg, MD, 1993, pp 400-421.

Client Resources

1. National Down Syndrome Congress, 1605 Chantilly Drive, Suite 250, Atlanta, GA, 1-800-232-6372.

Prader-Willi Syndrome

Prader-Willi Syndrome was originally described in 1956 by A. Prader, a. Labhart and H. Willi. It is a rare birth defect that results in initial hypotonia, hypogenitalism and later obesity through compulsive eating. Chromosome 15 is missing in about one-half of the individuals with Prader-Willi Syndrome. It is estimated that there are 10,000-23,000 people with Prader-Willi Syndrome worldwide and it is seen in 1 in 15,000 live births in the United States.

Prominent physical symptoms of Prader-Willi Syndrome include: Failure-to-thrive as an infant, hypotonia, hypogenitalism, mental retardation, small hands and feet, short stature, poor coordination, near-sightedness, almond-shaped eyes, straight hair and obesity. The obesity, if left uncontrolled, can lead to scoliosis, diabetes, and respiratory and cardiovascular problems. As the child grow, their behavior is more temperamental and scratching and picking at sores on hands is common.

A team of parents, pediatrician/family-practitioner, registered dietitian, endocrinologists, psychologist/psychiatrist, physiatrist, social worker, special education teachers and nurses is a positive way of working with children and adults with Prader-Willi Syndrome. In the United States, seven clinics specialize in care for these patients.

The following is a list of ways to control food storage to maximize weight control:
- Lock cabinets with food in them.
- Lock refrigerator and freezer.
- Lock medicine cabinet.
- Lock liquor cabinet.
- Lock cleaning supplies.
- Check kitchen frequently.
- Check plants with berries on them.
- Once meal preparation begins, someone must remain in the kitchen at all times.
- No food in rooms other than the kitchen.
- All eating is done at the table.
- No sugar, jelly or jam on the table.,
- Clear food and wash dishes promptly.
- No gum, mints or cough drops in pockets or purse.
- No unsupervised eating.
- Discuss issue with relatives and neighbors.
- Monitor portion size.

It is estimated that a person with Prader-Willi Syndrome requires 8-9 calories per centimeter of height for gradual weight loss and 10-11 calories per centimeter of height for weight maintenance. A registered dietitian should establish a meal pattern following the exchange system, *see the section on weight management*, and educate all parties involved with the client's meal preparation. Weekly weights and a routine exercise program should be followed.

Professional References
1. Ekvall SW, Pediatric Nutrition in Chronic Diseases and Developmental Disorders: Prevention, Assessment, and Treatment. Oxford University Press 1993: 157-159.
2. Hoffman CJ, Aultman D, Pipes P. A Nutrition Survey of and Recommendations for Individuals with Prader-Willi Syndrome Who Live in Group Hones. J Am Dietetic Assoc 1992; 92:823-830, 833.

Client Resources

National Office, Prader-Willi Syndrome Association
6490 Excelsior Blvd., E-102
St. Louis Park, MN 55426
612/926-1947
FAX 612/928-9133

Spina Bifida
Description

Spina bifida is a collective term used to describe a defect in the spinal column caused by abnormal fetal development in early pregnancy. Myelomeningocele is a type of spina bifida in which an opening in the neural tube and a sac containing nervous tissue protrudes from the back. Other general terms for spinal column defects are neural tube defects, and myelodysplasia. Myelomeningocele usually is associated with varying degrees of muscle weaknesses and paralysis in the lower body, depending on where the lesion occurs. Lesions occurring higher on the spinal column result in greater paralysis than those occurring at a lower lever. Individuals with higher spinal cord defects often lack ambulatory activity.

Other conditions associated with spina bifida include:
- Bladder and bowel incontinence
- Loss of sensation in the lower body
- Hydrocephalus, which is treated by surgical placement of a shunt to drain excess fluids from the head. If not treated, the head becomes enlarged due to fluid accumulation.
- Mental retardation
- Spontaneous fractures
- Trophic ulcers
- Deformities of the lower extremities
- Obesity
- Epilepsy, which occurs in 10 to 30 percent of patients

Growth

Growth may be affected as a result of atrophy of the lower extremities, abnormal vertebral growth, musculoskeletal deformities, renal disease, malnutrition, frequent hospital admission, and hydrocephalus. Obesity is a significant variable and prevention is important. Since leg contractures and scoliosis are common, measuring in the conventional manner may not yield accurate results.

Measurement of Height

Arm span has been found to correlate directly with standing height in normal children and can be used for height on NCHS growth charts. Arm span is measured from the tip of the middle finger on one hand to the tip of the middle finger on the other hand, with arms outstretched as far as possible. For children with decreased leg muscle mass due to myelomeningocele, the arm span to height ration is adjusted as follows:

- Height = 0.9 x armspan (for persons with high lumbar and thoracic level defects and without any leg muscle mass)
- Height - 0.95 x armspan (for persons with mid and low lumbar level defects and without any leg muscle mass)
- Height = 1.0 x armspan (for persons with sacral level defects who have minimal or no leg muscle mass loss)

Measurement of Weight

A child can be weighed by him or herself with an appropriate scale, including a baby scale, a wheelchair scale, a chair scale, or a bed scale. If no scale is available for weighing the child alone, a small child can be weighed while being held by an adult and then subtracting the adult's weight. This method should be used on a limited basis as its accuracy is highly questionable. For larger children and adolescents, there may not be a satisfactory method to monitor weight. In these cases, serial measurements of skinfold thickness can offer a way to monitor changes in fat stores.

Visual assessment is an essential part of the clinical assessment of obesity. In persons with paralysis of leg muscles, body fat may be accumulated in the upper body while the legs look very thin.

Nutritional Management

Energy Requirement

Short stature, lack of activity, and decreased basal metabolic rate all contribute to the decreased caloric requirement and thus increased risk for obesity. The energy requirement is frequently considered to be 50 percent of the caloric level of a normal child. Seven (7) kcal/cm is used for weight loss.

Obesity

Obesity has been viewed as an additional handicap to children with spina bifida. The handicap is manifested in the following ways:

Increased difficulty in ambulatory ability even with bracing and in independently transferring in and out of a wheelchair.

Increased risk of skin breakdown and pressure sores.

Increased difficulty for care providers.

The prevention of obesity through nutrition counseling when the child is young is vital. For very young children, the goal should be a decrease in the rate of weight gain. Intervention for obesity requires the same approach as that for any other individual. Individualized diet, activity, and eating behavior must all be addressed.

Constipation

Neurogenic bowel (abnormal central nervous system control of the bowels) is the primary cause of constipation in individuals with myelomeningocele. Other factors include inactivity, lack of fiber and fluid intake, and certain drugs that decrease intestinal motility, ie, anticholinergic medicines used to treat neurogenic bladder. A bowel management program should include regular toileting, increased fiber and fluid intake, and medical treatment when necessary.

Urinary Tract Infections (UTI)

Neurogenic bladder may result in chronic incomplete emptying of the bladder, which may lead to frequent urinary tract infections and ultimately result in kidney damage. A bladder management program which includes regular emptying of the bladder, adequate water intake, and medical treatment of any UTI, is vital to the prevention and treatment of urinary tract infections. A vitamin C supplement to acidify the urine and thus decrease bacterial growth is an effective way to prevent UTIs. The amount prescribed should be determined individually by increasing the dose gradually until the urine pH drops to below 6. Using an acid-ash diet to acidify the urine is not currently advocated. Such a diet is high in meats, eggs, fats, and cereal products and low in fruits and vegetables. This diet is contradictory to a diet required for the prevention and treatment of constipation and obesity. In addition, such a diet may be nutritionally inadequate for this population.

Professional References

1. Ekvall SW, pediatric Nutrition in Chronic Disease and Developmental Disorders: Prevention, Assessment, and Treatment. Oxford University Press 1993.

Client Resources

1. Spina Bifida Association of America, 1700 Rockville Pike, Suite 540, Rockville, MD 20852, 1800-621-3141.

Nutritional Problems of Children with Special Health Care Needs

PROBLEM	MAY RESULT FROM	MAY RESULT IN	INTERVENTION STRATEGIES
Feeding problems	Anatomic condition Delayed problems Behavior problems Parent-child interaction Seizures Poor suck/swallow/chew Malocclusion/caries/oral sensitivity Abnormal reflexes Down Syndrome Cerebral Palsy Cleft lip/palate	Malnutrition Overnutrition	Proper positioning Proper utensils Proper feeding techniques Modified food texture Appropriate food temperatures
Overweight	Growth retardation Hypotonia Decreased BMR Some medications High caloric intake Decreased activity Inappropriate feeding/eating practices Prader-Willi Syndrome Spina Bifida Down Syndrome	Obesity Poor motor development Poor self-image	Decrease caloric intake Increase activity Routine growth checks Behavior modification
Underweight	High energy needs Hypotonia Low caloric intake Frequent illness Environmental issues Impaired oral/motor function Cerebral Palsy	Severe malnutrition	Increase caloric intake Supplementation Increase frequency of eating
Refusal to eat or loss of appetite	Food of incorrect texture Severe illness Behavioral problems Poor positioning Tiredness Sensitive mouth area Some medications	Marked weight loss Malnutrition	Overcoming causes of poor eating Behavior modification

PROBLEM	MAY RESULT FROM	MAY RESULT IN	INTERVENTION STRATEGIES
Constipation	Spina Bifida Down Syndrome Spastic Cerebral Palsy Decreased activity Low fiber intake Some medications Inadequate fluid intake Abnormal muscle tone Abnormal Anatomy	Severe pain and bleeding Lack of appetite	Increase Fluid Increase fiber and texture Increase physical activity Stool softener Toileting schedule
Vomiting	Overfeeding Illness Stress Digestion problems Gastroesophageal reflux Medications Rumination	Dehydration Hospitalization Weight loss	Change diet if needed Encourage fluids Position child correctly Alter food volume Behavior modification
Excessive fluid loss or poor intake of fluid	Heavy drooling Some medications Problems in drinking and swallowing fluids	Dehydration Constipation	Position child correctly Encourage fluids Enteral feeding of fluids Thickening agent Correct glass/cup
Vitamin and Mineral Deficiency	Limited dietary intake Drug-nutrient interactions		Supplement as indicated
Drug-nutrient interaction	Anti-convulsants Tranquilizers Stimulants Spasmolytics Diuretics	Appetite fluctuation GI disturbances Dental/gum problems Altered absorption, metabolism, and/or excretion	Appropriate supplement Awareness of timing drugs and food Adjust caloric intake Increase fiber and fluid
Pica (eating non-food items such as dirt, clay, old paint chips)	Increased need to suck Emotional factors Mental retardation	Lead poisoning Anemia (low iron in blood) These can lead to learning and physical problems	Good nutrition with a diet rich in protein, iron and calcium Supervision of child Medication
Aspiration while swallowing	Cerebral Palsy Epilepsy Poor neuromuscular coordination while swallowing	Frequent pneumonia Malnutrition	Gastrostomy feeding Avoiding small round foods

Nutritional Problems of Children with Special Health Care Needs, continued

PROBLEM	MAY RESULT FROM	MAY RESULT IN	INTERVENTION STRATEGIES
Pronounced dental problems	Delayed tooth eruption Medications Poor oral hygiene Frequent sugary snacks Poor tooth enamel Malocclusion Bruxism Excessive continuation of bottle Down Syndrome Oral facial anomalies	Poor and painful chewing Decreased food intake	Good dental hygiene Decrease sweet snacks Avoid bottle in bed Orthodontics, peri-odontics Adjust texture of diet Fluoride supplement

(Modified with permission from "Nutrition for Children with Special Needs." 1985, United Cerebral Palsy of Minnesota, Inc.)

* Intervention strategies indicate minor changes that may alleviate the problem. Long-term or serious problems require in-depth assessment, counseling and follow-up by appropriate health professionals (frequently an interdisciplinary team).

ENTERAL AND PARENTERAL NUTRITION SUPPORT

Enteral Nutrition
Infant Formula Selection

Types of Infant Formulations

Clinical Condition	Formula Description
Premature Infant (LBW, VLBW, ELBW)	Premature formula with cow's milk protein, whey; MCT, soy, coconut oils; syrup solids, cornstarch, lactose; additional vitamins (D), minerals (Ca, P, Mg), trace elements
Discharged Premature Infant	Infant formula with additional calories, protein, minerals (Ca, P, Zn), vitamins (D)
Term Infant	Infant formula with cow's milk protein; soy, coconut, palm olein, sunflower oils; lactose; vitamins, minerals and trace elements
Cow's Milk Protein Sensitivity, Diarrhea, Lactose intolerance, Galactosemia	Lactose-free soy protein isolate formula with corn syrup solids, sucrose; soy, coconut, palm olein, sunflower, safflower oils; vitamins, minerals, trace elements; with or without fiber
Primary or Secondary Lactose Intolerance	Lactose-free soy protein isolate formula or Lactose-free cow's milk protein formula with corn syrup solids; palm olein, soy, coconut, sunflower oils; vitamins, minerals (trace)
Renal Disease	Cow's milk protein formula with low renal solute load, low electrolytes content, and reduced minerals (Ca, P, Mg, Fe, Mn)
Steatorrhea associated with bile acid deficiency, Liver disease, Ileal resection or Lymphatic anomalies, Cystic Fibrosis	Infant formula with major fat source from MCT oil either with cow's milk protein or protein hydrolysate
Cow's milk and Soy protein sensitivity, severe protein allergies; abnormal nutrient digestion, absorption and/or transport; intractable diarrhea and/or severe protein-calorie malnutrition	Protein hydrolysate or free amino acid formula which is both lactose-free and sucrose-free with some MCT oil
Inborn Errors of Metabolism	Metabolic infant formula with modified specific nutrient(s)

Practical Clinical Questions Raised
- A. Should we be trying to mimic human milk? And is it possible?
- B. How much of an added nutrient is sufficient but not excessive? And what form should be used?
- C. Since infant formula is the major beverage consumed during the first year of life, what are the potential impacts later in life?
- D. For infants on tube feeding, how will infant formula nutrients be utilized differently from healthy term infants?

Flowchart to select infant formulas based on bowel function

Premature Infant→   Yes→   Premature Formula
↓

No
↓

Normal Term Infant→   Yes→   60/40 Whey/Casein or Casein Formula
↓

No
↓

Primary or Secondary Lactose Intolerance or Casein Sensitive→   Yes→   Lactose-Free Soy Protein Isolate Formula (Sucrose and Com-free also available)
↓

No
↓

Organ Dysfunction→
(eg. Renal, Cardiac)   Yes→   Low Electrolyte/ Renal Solute Load Formula
↓

No
↓

Severe Steatorrhea Associated with Bile Acid Deficiency.   →
Ileal Resection or Lymphatic Anomalies   Yes→   Infant Formula with MCT oil
↓

No
↓

Sensitive to Casein and Soy Protein Abnormal Nutrient Absorption, Digestion and Transport,   →
Severe Intractable Diarrhea or Protein Calorie Malnutrition   Yes→   Hypoallergenic, Hydrolyzed Casein with MCT oil (Also Lactose- and Sucrose-free)

Flowchart to select adult formulas for children over 1 year of age, based on bowel function

Capable and Willing to Consume Oral Supplement→	Yes→	Flavored, Milk-based or Soy-Isolate Formula
↓		
No		
↓		
Gastrostomy Feeding, Intact GI Tract with → Normal Digestion and Absorption	Yes→	Blenderized Formula
↓		
No		
↓		
Nasogastric or Transpyloric Feeding, → Normal Digestion and Absorption with or without Steatorrhea	Yes→	Polymeric Formula
↓		
No		
↓		
Moderately Impaired Pancreatic and Small → Bowel Function	Yes→	Chemically Defined Formula
↓		
No		
↓		
Severe Malabsorption Nutrient Imbalance → Inborn Errors of Metabolism	Yes→	Modular Formula
↓		
No		
↓		
Trauma or Organ → Failure	Yes→	Modified Polymeric Formula or Specialized Protein Formula

Accessing the Gastrointestinal Tract for Enteral Feeding

The appeal of enteral feedings continues to grow as feeding techniques and safe, practical gastrointestinal access improves. Following is a review of the most common enteral feeding routes.

Nasogastric (NG) and Oral Gastric (OG)

This is still the most frequently employed feeding method. Disadvantages include delayed development of oral motor functions, mechanical problems such as tube dislodging, or malpositioning and occlusion of the tube; physical problems such as diarrhea, aspiration, esophageal, and mucosal erosion; metabolic problems such as hypoglycemia and hypophosphatemia (in malnourished persons).

Common indications for us of an NG or OG feeding tube include prematurity, cardiorespiratory distress, neurologic dysfunction, congenital abnormalities of head, neck, or GI tract, malabsorption, short-term coma, conditions of hypermetabolism, and refusal to take formula and/or food. Monitoring for aspiration, dislodgment of tube and occlusion of the airway in small infants is essential.

Nasoduodenal/ Nasojejunal

This feeding access method is advocated for patients who would be placed at risk if fed intragastrically. Patients considered to have significant potential for feeding aspiration include patients with any of the following:

- Mechanical ventilators
- Neurological deficits
- Impaired gag reflex
- Gastroesophageal reflux
- Respiratory problems
- Debilitation
- Severe malnourishment

The patient may still be at risk for aspiration of gastric contents; however, when positioned properly, the transpyloric feeding site offers a safer alternative to intragastric feeding. The nasoduodenal or nasojejunal tubes must be monitored to ensure correct placement. X-ray tube is indicated. Feeding residuals may still be checked. If the feeding tube is in the correct position, residuals should be of very low amounts. If larger residuals develop, the tube has most likely slipped back into the stomach. Assessing residuals may not be possible due to collapse of the small bore, pliable feeding tubes. Monitoring abdominal girths is generally recommended with transplyoric enteral feeding.

Needle Catheter Jejunostomy (NCJ)

Needle Catheter Jejunostomy (NCJ) is a temporary feeding jejunostomy. It can be used for feeding in the immediate post-operative period, since the small bowel maintains its absorptive capabilities. It does not go through a period of "post-surgical ileus" as does the stomach and large bowel. Nasogastric decompression is often required post-surgically, and with the NCJ, early enteric feeding is still possible during this period. The NCJ can easily be removed once the patient is tolerating oral nutrition.

Standard polymeric, preferably isotonic, feeding formulas are well tolerated. The NCJ usually has a small lumen. Conscientious flushing of the NCJ with water 4 to 6 times per day is essential to maintain patency of the tube.

Contraindications for NCJ include Crohn's disease of the small intestine, extensive adhesions, radiation enteritis, ascites, profound immunosuppresion, coagulopathy, and anastomosis distal to the NCJ.

Jejunostomy

There is renewed interest in feeding jejunostomies, particularly in the patient who is undergoing an upper gastrointestinal surgery. The catheter may be simply sutured into place, as in NCJ, for temporary nutrition; or if more permanency is indicated, a silicone catheter with two sets of "wings" for anchoring and dacron cuff may be used.

Polymeric isotonic formulas are generally satisfactory for use in proximal jejunal feedings. Exceptions might be pancreatic disease, when more distal jejunal feedings are required, or reduced gastrointestinal absorption capabilities, in which case a hydrolyzed or an elemental, low-fat formula may be beneficial. Particular care needs to be taken to ensure control of formula contamination. Since the stomach is bypassed, the patient does not benefit from the bactericidal effects of gastric hydrochloric acid.

A feeding pump is routinely used to control continuous formula delivery and to optimize jejunal tolerance. Bolus feedings are not recommended for this feeding route. Over a period of time, adaptation to cyclic feedings is possible. Contraindications of jejunostomies include those listed under NCJ.

Gastrostomy

There are two general types of gastrostomies: temporary and permanent. A temporary gastrostomy uses serosa-lined channel, while a permanent gastrostomy uses gastric mucosa. Using the serosal lining allows for more rapid closure after removing the tube, while using gastric mucosa allows the tube to be removed without spontaneous closure. The percutaneous endoscopic gastrostomy (PEG) is a nonoperative technique for placing a gastrostomy. A standard Nasogastric feeding tube can also be slipped through some PEGs to allow for intraduodenal or intrajejunal feeding, combined with gastric decompression.

Technical complications of gastrostomies are usually related to intraperitoneal leakage or bleeding around the enterostomy. Other complications may include gastroesophageal reflux of the formula, and aspiration pneumonia. The most common complication with the gastrostomy is cellulitis at the ostomy site. Contraindications to gastrostomy feedings include severe gastroesophageal reflux and poor gastric emptying. A Nissen fundoplication may be performed at the time of gastrostomy placement to control reflux and allow for gastric feeding.

Gastrostomies do take advantage of the stomach's ability to adjust to varying volumes and osmolalities. The stomach's own infectious protection, hydrochloric acid, is also utilized. In addition delivering feeding formula intragastrically also provides the stomach with a good protective buffer.

Professional references

1. Caldwell CK, Caldwell MD, Zitarelli ME, Pediatric Enteral Nutrition IN Enteral and Tube Feeding 2nd Ed. Rombeau & Caldwell (eds), W.B. Saunders Co., Philadelphia, PA, 1990. pp. 325-360.
2. Guenter P, Jones S, Jacobs DO, et al. Administration and Delivery of Enteral Nutrition In Enteral and Tube Feeding 2nd Ed. Rombeau & Caldwell (eds), W.B. Saunders Co., Philadelphia, PA, 1990. pp. 192-203.
3. Guidelines for the Use of Parenteral and Enteral Nutrition in Adult and Pediatric Patients. JPEN 17(4):27SA-49SA, 1993.
4. Hohenbrink K. Pediatrics IN Nutrition Support Dietetics Core Curriculum, 2nd Ed, American Society for Parenteral and Enteral Nutrition, 1993. pp. 163-192.
5. Ideno KT. Enteral Nutrition IN Nutrition Support Dietetics Core Curriculum, 2nd Ed, American Society for Parenteral and Enteral Nutrition, 1993. pp. 71-104.
6. Lingard CD. Enteral Nutrition IN Handbook of Pediatric Nutrition, Queen & Lang (eds), Aspen Publishers, Inc., Gaithersburg, MD, 1993. pp. 249-278.
7. Moore MC, Greene HL. Tube Feeding of Infants and Children. Peds Clin. N. Am. 1985; 32(2): 401-417.
8. Sinden AA, Dillard VL, Sutphen JL. Enteral Nutrition IN Pediatric Gastrointestinal Disease, Walker, et al. (eds), B.C. Decker, Inc., Philadelphia, PA, 1991. pp. 1623-1638.
9. Warman KY. Enteral Nutrition Support of the Pediatric Patient IN Pediatric Nutrition 2nd Ed., Hendricks & Walker (eds.), B.C. Decker, Inc., Philadelphia, PA, 1990. pp. 72-109.

Enteral Nutrition Monitoring (In the Hospital Setting)

Enteral nutritional support may be associated with mechanical, gastrointestinal, or metabolic complications. In order to avoid these complications, a patient's metabolic status, feeding tolerance, and fluid and electrolyte balance, must be carefully monitored. A protocol providing guidelines for uniform care should be established in order to ensure that these parameters are properly monitored. Following is a list of suggested guidelines to be included in a protocol.

1. Tube placement should be verified with a chest X-ray or a flat plate of the abdomen prior to starting the tube feeding and whenever tube placement is in question.
2. Clean technique during preparation, storage, and administration of the feeding is crucial.
3. The head of the bed should be elevated 30 to 40 degrees when feeding into the stomach. Keep the patient elevated throughout the feeding and for approximately one hour after stopping the feeding. This will help prevent gastric reflux and aspiration.
4. Gastric residuals should be monitored each feeding or every two (2) hours initially and every six (6) to eight (8) hours later. Residuals are checked with every feeding in low birth weight infants. Residuals should be reinstilled to prevent fluid and electrolyte imbalance.
   - As a general rule, the feeding should be withheld and the physician contacted if the residual is greater than the amount delivered in the past two (2) hours or > 150% of the volume per hour with continuous feedings.
   - The residual should be rechecked in one to two hours. If it remains elevated, contact the physician.
   - For bolus or intermittent feeding schedules, gastric residuals should be checked before each feeding. Hold feedings for residuals >50% of the previous bolus feeding.

5. Urine glucose and ketone, or preferably blood glucose, should be checked
   - Every four to eight hours for 48 hours in the nondiabetic patient. This may be discontinued after 48 hours if it is consistently negative.
   - Every four to eight hours throughout the duration of the therapy in diabetic patient if needed.
6. Formula hang time should not exceed hospital policy; however, as a rule, it should not be longer than 12 hours. Hanging a four- to eight-hour supply of feeding at one time is optimal.
7. The feeding tube should be flushed with water before and following each intermittent feeding or delivery of medications and at least four to six times a day for continuous feedings. This will clear the tube, reducing the incidence of tube occlusion. Additional water can be used for the flush if needed by the patient for fluid support.
8. The feeding bag and tubing should be changed daily to reduce the risk of excessive bacterial growth.
9. Monitor the patient's status daily in regard to the tube feeding. Watch for adverse reactions such as nausea, vomiting, cramping, distention, constipation, and diarrhea.
10. Monitor the frequency of stools and the gastric residual volumes daily.
11. Have the patient weighed each day initially; then two to three times per week after the patient is stable. This allows more accurate assessment of adequate calorie and fluid support.
12. Input and output should be recorded daily to assist in fluid balance monitoring.
13. The frequency of monitoring a patient's biochemical profile will be influenced by the disease state as well as by the severity of the disease state. Generally, baseline lab values should be drawn within the first 24 to 48 hours of the tube feeding, then every three to four days.

Abnormal values should be monitored more frequently until they are within normal limits. Lab data to be monitored may include the following:

- Serum electrolytes
- Blood glucose
- BUN
- Creatinine
- Albumin
- Transferrin (if available)
- Phosphorus
- Magnesium
- CBC with differential lymphocyte count
- Calcium
- Other lab values (such as liver function tests) may also be indicated.
- Nitrogen balance studies may be performed as needed to determine the adequacy of protein.

14. Monitor medications for drug/nutrient interactions and/or possible drug-related feeding intolerance. Follow where drugs are being delivered -- IV, p.o., feeding tube, etc. Refer to updated sources for drug compatibilities with enteral formulas, medication osmolalities, and possible drug induced metabolic complications. (See reference 9).

15. Initiate a calorie count when a patient begins oral support. The patient should be consuming approximately one-half to two-thirds of their nutritional support needs orally prior to totally discontinuing the tube feeding. Cyclic or nocturnal tube feeding may be desired to supplement p.o. capabilities.

Professional references

1. Caldwell CK, Caldwell MD, Zitarelli ME. Pediatric Enteral Nutrition IN Enteral and Tube Feeding 2nd Ed. Rombeau & Caldwell (eds), W.B. Saunders Co., Philadelphia, PA, 1990. pp. 325-360.
2. Guenter P, Jones S, Jacobs DO, et al. Administration and Delivery of Enteral Nutrition In Enteral and Tube Feeding 2nd Ed. Rombeau & Caldwell (eds), W.B. Saunders Co., Philadelphia, PA, 1990. pp. 192-203.
3. Guidelines for the Use of Parenteral and Enteral Nutrition in Adult and Pediatric Patients. JPEN 17(4):27SA-49SA, 1993.
4. Hohenbrink K. Pediatrics IN Nutrition Support Dietetics Core Curriculum, 2nd Ed, American Society for Parenteral and Enteral Nutrition, 1993. pp. 163-192.
5. Ideno KT. Enteral Nutrition IN Nutrition Support Dietetics Core Curriculum, 2nd Ed, American Society for Parenteral and Enteral Nutrition, 1993. pp. 71-104.
6. Lingard CD. Enteral Nutrition IN Handbook of Pediatric Nutrition, Queen & Lang (eds), Aspen Publishers, Inc., Gaithersburg, MD, 1993. pp. 249-278.
7. Moore MC, Greene HL. Tube Feeding of Infants and Children. Peds Clin. N. Am. 1985; 32(2): 401-417.
8. Sinden AA, Dillard VL, Sutphen JL. Enteral Nutrition IN Pediatric Gastrointestinal Disease, Walker, et al. (eds), B.C. Decker, Inc., Philadelphia, PA, 1991. pp. 1623-1638.
9. Thomson CA, LaFrance RJ. Pharmacotherapeautics IN Nutrition Support Dietetics Core Curriculum, 2nd Ed, American Society for Parenteral and Enteral Nutrition, 1993. pp. 433-457.
10. Warman KY. Enteral Nutrition Support of the Pediatric Patient IN Pediatric Nutrition 2nd Ed., Hendricks & Walker (eds.), B.C. Decker, Inc., Philadelphia, PA, 1990. pp. 72-109.

Feeding Tube Type and Selection

1. Soft, pliable, biocompatible material (such as polyurethane or silicone). These will not react with the patient's gastrointestinal secretions as the polyvinylchloride (PVC) tubes do. The PVC tubes will stiffen with age and may contribute to patient discomfort, rhinitis, pharyngitis, esophagitis, or ulceration.
2. Radiopaque to allow for radiographic confirmation of correct placement.
3. Stylet or guidewire that is easily withdrawn after placing the feeding tube. The likelihood of the stylet to accidentally come through the feeding port should be minimal.
4. The tube should be self-lubricating when wet for ease of tube insertion and removal of stylet.
5. It should be compatible with the feeding bag and extension tubing.

6. Weighed tubes have not been shown to be consistently effective in spontaneous passage distal to the pylorus. Therefore, selection of the tube and bolus size should be based on patient comfort and ease of insertion.
7. Longer feeding tube lengths (43-inch and longer) are required for nasoduodenal feedings in adults. Thirty-six- length is usually seen in intragastric feedings.
8. An 8- to 10-French tube size is the largest size tube ever needed for delivering any feeding formulas.

Not advised

Large-bore nasogastric tubes used for decompressing the gastrointestinal tract are not advised and should not be used for long-term nutriture. If a large nasogastric tube is in position, it may be prudent to convert this from suction or drainage to low volume feedings. This will allow you to evaluate patient tolerance of enteral feedings for a couple of days before changing to a regular feeding tube. The large, stiff nature of these tubes also allows for more accurate gastric residual checks in the initial stages of enteral feeding.

Using large trans-nasal tubes for any length of time is not advised because they may cause these complications: rhinitis, pharyngitis, otitis media, poor cough, atelectasis, increased upper respiratory secretions, increased gastroesophageal reflux, and increased risk of feeding aspiration.

Feeding Tube Placement

Nasoduodenal intubation may be accomplished under fluoroscopy. With the guidewire or stylet still in the lumen of the feeding tube, the radiologist is able to manipulate the end of the feeding tube through the pylorus into the duodenum. Another means of intubation involves a gastroenterologist using an endoscope to carry the feeding tube into the duodenum. Relying on gastrointestinal motility to pass the weighted tip of the feeding tube into the duodenum is unpredictable and not routinely successful.

A secondary advantage to intragastric feeding is that it is able to control gastric pH and provide a degree of protection from stress ulcers. Nasoduodenal feedings have not been found to adequately protect against ulcers. A nasogastric tube for delivering antacid therapy and monitoring pH may still be indicated. The histamine H_2 receptor inhibitors (Tagamet, Zantac, etc.) may also provide adequate protection from ulcers. NCJ can be done at the time of laparotomy or upper abdominal surgery. It is positioned distal to the ligament of Treitz (the gastrointestinal landmark that separates the duodenum from the jejunum).

There is renewed interest in feeding jejunostomies, particularly in the patient who is undergoing an upper gastrointestinal surgery. The Stamm and the Witzel are examples of temporary gastrostomies. A tube such as a mushroom, Malecot, or Foley catheter is used. The Janeway is a permanent gastrostomy. A stoma is created. The percutaneous endoscopic gastrostomy (PEG) is a nonoperative technique for placing a gastrostomy. It is done with the aid of a gastroscope and local anesthesia around the area of incision. This procedure may carry less risk to the patient than traditional surgical gastrostomies and is gaining popularity. A standard nasogastric feeding tube can also be slipped through some PEGs to allow for intraduodenal or intrajejunal feeding, combined with gastric decompression.

Possible Complications Associated with Enteral Nutrition

COMPLICATION	POSSIBLE CAUSES	POSSIBLE TREATMENT/ PREVENTION
DIARRHEA	Rapid formula administration Hyperosmolar formula	Initiate feedings at low rate. Use continuous infusion rather than bolus feeding, or extend infusion time for the bolus feeding. Do not increase rate and strength simultaneously. Temporarily reduce rate and/or strength. Switch to isotonic formula if using a hyperosmolar feeding.
	Severe Malnutrition	Use TPN to improve nutrition before enteral feeding. Use elemental formula requiring less digestion if the patient has first failed to tolerate an isotonic feeding.
	Malabsorption	Change formula to: Lactose free (if lactose intolerant) Low fat content (for fat malabsorption) Fiber containing formula to slow transit time Part of fat as MCT (for fat malabsorption) Avoid MCT in large amounts (can contribute to osmotic diarrhea). Elemental diet (For gastrointestinal pathology). Additional pancreatic enzyme therapy (for compromised pancreatic function).
	Bacterial overgrowth of small bowel	Consider keeping gastric pH less than 4 to help reduce risk of bacterial overgrowth (may not always be appropriate). May require appropriate antibiotic treatment before feedings can be resumed.
	Contaminated formula or equipment	Replace formula. Use clean technique during formula preparation and handling. Store open formula in the refrigerator (covered). Dispose of formula open longer than 24 hours. Do not hang more than 4 to 8 hours feeding at one time, and rinse bag and tubing with water before refilling. Clean equipment daily. (or replace equipment) Perform routine cultures/ monitoring of formulas and preparation areas.
	Bolus of cold formula	Bring formula to room temperature before administering.
	Toxins in gastrointestinal tract	Check for toxins, and begin appropriate drug therapy.
	Antibiotic therapy	Check for stools for C. Difficile. If diarrhea is due to toxin such as Clostridium difficile, anti-diarrheal agents should not be used. In very severe cases, drug therapy may be indicated to treat the C. deficit. IV nutrition may be needed during this time.

COMPLICATION	POSSIBLE CAUSES	POSSIBLE TREATMENT/ PREVENTION
DIARRHEA, Continued	Administration of hypertonic electrolyte solution. Magnesium containing compounds and antacids, Sorbitol containing medications such as elixirs, Phosphorus supplements, and Hyperosmolar medications.	Check the form of medication and route of delivery: 1. Suggest that medications not be mixed with the tube feeding formula. Medication should be given as a bolus; however, dilute the medication with water (if the medication is hyperosmolar) to improve patient tolerance. 2. Where in the gastrointestinal tract is the medication being delivered -- stomach, jejunum, duodenum? Is this appropriate for the best drug action and patient tolerance? 3. Would smaller, more frequent doses improve tolerance? 4. Would changing the form of medication help? Can a syrup form be changed to a form less hypertonic? Does the medication contain sorbitol? 5. Consult with pharmacist to problem solve.
	Fecal impaction- stooling around the impaction	Remove the impaction. The patient may need stool softeners if it is a high impaction.
	Sepsis	Evaluate for underlying sepsis and treat.
	Idiopathic	If pathalogical (organic, bacterial, etc.) and the reason for the diarrhea is not evident, judicious use of anti-diarrheal agents may be indicated. Avoid overuse of these. Controlling stooling to 2 or 3 stools per day is a reasonable goal.
	Low-residue formula	Consider a fiber-supplement formula.
CONSTIPATION	Medications, immobility, low-residue Dehydration	Adequate fluids, change to formula containing fiber, bowel program, or further evaluation of gastrointestinal function.
CRAMPING, DISTENTION, BLOATING, NAUSEA, DIARRHEA	Concurrent administration of medications, or electrolyte imbalance	Check the form of medication and route of delivery (see the same under "Diarrhea").
	Inappropriate rate or strength	Begin and progress formula gradually. Do not increase rate and strength simultaneously. Use continuous infusion rather than bolus feeding, or extend bolus infusion time.
	Bolus of cold formula	Bring formula to room temperature before administering it.
	Malabsorption	Reduce the percentage of calories from carbohydrate or change to low fat or elemental type of formula.
	High-MCT feeding	Administer MCT gradually over entire feeding period.
	Rapid refeeding	Initiate feedings at low rate

COMPLICATION	POSSIBLE CAUSES	POSSIBLE TREATMENT/ PREVENTION
GLUCOSE INTOLERANCE HYPERGLYCEMIA, GLYCOSURIA	Metabolic stress with insulin resistance, diabetes mellitus	Administer insulin; possibly decrease the rate until blood glucose is under better control. Resume adequate support as soon as possible.
GASTRIC RETENTION OR INADEQUATE GASTRIC EMPTYING	High-fat formula	Change formula to one with a lower fat content, having <30-40% total calories from fat.
	Gastroparesis	Feed beyond pylorus, nasoduodenal tube, or jejunostomy. Reduce infusion rate.
	Inappropriate patient position/ immobility	Increase mobility and/or elevate the head of the bed to 30-45 degrees. If this is not possible, position patient on right side for enhanced gastric emptying. Hold the feeding 2 to 8 hours, and resume it at a lower rate.
	Medications (opiates, anticholinergics)	Consider adding medication which stimulates gastric emptying.
	Non-functioning gastrointestinal tract	Use parenteral route.
HYPERGLYCEMIC, HYPEROSMOLAR, HYPERTONIC DEHYDRATION	Inadequate insulin	Monitor blood and urine glucose levels on a regular basis. Provide insulin as needed.
	Use of high-protein and/or high-electrolyte formula, resulting in a high renal solute load	Increase free water. Assess for excess fluid losses. Dilute the formula, and increase the feeding volume, or bolus water down the feeding tube.
	Inadequate fluid intake or excessive losses	Decrease renal solute load (protein and electrolytes). Monitor fluid intake and output.
RESPIRATORY INSUFFICIENCY EXACERBATED BY CO_2 RETENTION	Excess CO_2 production from a high-carbohydrate formula	Increase the percentage of calories from fat, and control the carbohydrate load.
	Overfeeding	Reassess caloric goal. Reduce total calories in regimen.
GASTRIC REFLUX, PULMONARY ASPIRATION	Improper placement of feeding tube	Identify the tube placement before initiating feedings using X-ray. Monitor the tube position every 4 to 8 hours. Consider coloring formula blue for ongoing monitoring (it will show up in pulmonary secretions if patient is aspirating some formula).

COMPLICATION	POSSIBLE CAUSES	POSSIBLE TREATMENT/ PREVENTION
GASTRIC REFLUX, PULMONARY ASPIRATION Continued	Large-bore tube	Change to a smaller bore tube (<10F for children, or less in infants).
	Patient is lying flat	Elevate the head of the bed 30 degrees or more at all times. If the patient needs to be supine for any reason, hold the feeding 30 to 60 minutes before the procedure.
	Impaired gag reflex, altered gastric motility	Feed beyond pylorus. Nasoduodenal or nasojejunal feeding tube or jejunostomy.
	Bolus feeding	Change to a continuous-drip feeding.
	Reflux owing to respiratory treatments (percussion, postural drainage)	Hold tube feeding 30-60 minutes prior to therapy.
ELECTROLYTE DISORDERS	Insufficiency of heart, liver, kidney; dilutional states, diuretic therapy, refeeding syndrome, malabsorption, excess fluid & electrolyte losses, drug/nutrient interaction	Monitor electrolytes and fluid status. Monitor daily weights. Adjust electrolytes and/or fluids as necessary. Evaluate for alternative formulas or medications to avoid drug nutrient interactions.
TUBE DISPLACEMENT	Coughing, vomiting	Replace tube and confirm placement with X-ray.
NASOPHARYNGEAL DISCOMFORT, IRRITATION, SINUSITIS, OTITIS MEDIA	Large or rigid feeding tube	Use small bore, soft, pliable (silicone or polyurethane) tube. Consider gastrostomy or jejunostomy sites for long term feeding (>30 days).
MUCOSAL EROSION	Large bore, rigid tube	Remove tube or replace it with a smaller, softer one.
OBSTRUCTED TUBE	Inadequately crushed medication	Give medications as liquids or make sure they are finely ground and completely dissolved in water. Do not add medications to the feeding container. Administer all medications as a bolus. Flush the feeding tube with 20 to 30 ml of water before and after administering medications.

COMPLICATION	POSSIBLE CAUSES	POSSIBLE TREATMENT/ PREVENTION
OBSTRUCTED TUBE, Continued	Residual feeding accumulation, protein coagulation	Use infusion pump.

Mix the formula appropriately.

Flush the tube with 20 to 30 ml of water every 6 to 12 hours or after each feeding.

For Declogging Tube:

1. Pancreatic enzymes: mix 1 Viokase tablet with one 325 mg tablet of sodium bicarbonate (to adjust pH), and add 5 ml water. Instill solution into tube, and allow to sit up to 30 minutes. Irrigate tube with water to remove tube.

2. Food-grade enzymes: meat tenderizer or papain dissolved in water might help dissolve the obstruction.

Never attempt to put the guide wire or stylet back down the tube if the tube is still in the patient.

References:

1. Ideno KT. Enteral Nutrition IN Nutrition Support Dietetics Core Curriculum, 2nd Ed., American Society for Parenteral and Enteral Nutrition, 1993. pp. 71-104.
2. Kohn CL, Keitney JK. Techniques for evaluating and managing diarrhea in the tube-fed patient: a review of the literature. Nutrition in Clinical Practice 1987; (dec.):250-7.
3. Warman KY. Enteral Nutrition Support of the Pediatric Patient IN Pediatric Nutrition 2nd Ed., Hendricks & Walker (eds.), B.C. Decker, Inc., Philadelphia, PA, 1990. pp. 72-109.

Selected Enteral/Infant Formulas

The tables on the following pages represent the composition of selected enteral formulas. Product information has been verified with the manufacturers' representatives from the companies listed below and is the most accurate data available as of April 1994.

1. Medical Nutritionals (MA528 10/96) Mead Johnson & Company, Evansville, IN 47721. Used with permission.
2. Pediatric Product Handbook (L-B6-12/95) Mead Johnson & Company, Evansville, IN 47721. Used with permission.
3. Product Handbook, May 1996 (D365) Ross Products, Division of Abbot Laboratories, Columbus, OH 43215-1724. Used with permission.
4. Enteral Products & Services Guide (164-197) 1997 Sandoz Nutrition Corporation, Minneapolis, MN 55416. Used with permission.
5. Enteral Product Reference Guides (N20110-02/97) Nestle Clinical Nutrition, Deerfiled, IL 60015-1760. Used with permission.
6. Nutrient Comparison Chart (5/95NP-003R3) Carnation Good Start and Follow Up Formulas, Carnational Nutritional Products, U.S.A.
7. Enteral Nutrition Products Ready Reference (9/95) McGaw, Inc., Irvine, CA 92714-5895. (Values for Hepatic-Aid and Immun-Aid). Used with permission.
8. Modulars Nutritional Information (1/93) Corpak, Inc., Wheeling, IL 60090.
9. Product Guides (Nov. 1995) Scientific Hospital Supplies (SHS), Gaithersburg, MD 20884. Used with permission.
10. Composition of Medical Foods for Infants, Children, and Adults with Metabolic Disorders (G680, February 1996) Ross Products Division, Columbus, OH 43215-1724.
11. Product Guide (6/96) Nutrition Medical, Minneapolis, MN 55442.

Note: Because formula compositions may change, dietitians should rely on new product information for complete and accurate content of formulas. The tables on the following pages are not intended to be a complete list, but representative of tube feedings used in the community. Brand names used do not constitute an endorsement of any particular product.

KEY FOR ALL ENTERAL FORMULA CHARTS

AA	Amino Acids	MAL	Maltodextrin
ALB	Albumin	MCT	Medium Chain Triglycerides
ARG	Arginine	Men.O.	Menhaden Oil
BCAA	Branch Chain Amino Acids	Mod.S.	Modified Starch
Can.O.	Canola Oil	MS	Monosaccharides
CAS	Caseinate (sodium and/or calcium)	NFDM	Nonfat Dry Milk
Coc.O.	Coconut Oil	NP Cal	Nonprotein Calories
C.O.	Corn Oil	Oleo	Oleo
CS	Corn Starch (modified) or Corn Syrup Solids	O.B.O.	Oenothera Biennis Oil
Egg Alb	Egg Albumin	Pal.O.	Palm Oil
EWS	Egg White Solids	PN.O.	Peanut Oil
Fruc	Fructose	RAF	Refined Animal Fat
GAL	Galactose	Saf.O.	Safflower Oil
GLN	Glutamine	Sar.O.	Sardine Oil
GOS	Glucose Oligosaccharides	SOY	Soy Protein Isolate
GP	Glucose Polymers	Soy H.	Soy Protein Hydrolysate
GUA	Enzymatically Modified Guar	Soy O.	Soy Oil
HC	Hydrolyzed Casein	SPS	Soy Polysaccharide
HCS	Hydrolyzed Corn Starch	Star	Starch
HL	Hydrolyzed Lactalbumin	Struc	Structured Lipid
HOSO	High Oleic Safflower/Sunflower Oil	SUC	Sucrose
HW	Hydrolyzed Whey (no casein)	Sug	Sugar
HWC	Hydrolyzed Whey & Casein	Sun.O.	Sunflower Oil
LAC	Lactose	T.S.	Tapioca Starch
Lactalb	Lactalbumin	WP	Whey Protein

STANDARD AND TUBERIZED FORMULAS
Nutrient Analysis per 1000 ml

Product (Manufacturer)	PRO	SOURCES FAT (MCT:LCT)	CHO	Kcal /ml /oz	mOsm/ kg H2O	Non-PRO Cal:N	PRO g/l %	FAT g/l %	CHO g/l %	Na mEq/l mg/l	K mEq/l mg/l	Cl mEq/l mg/l	Ca mg/l	Phos mg/l	Mg mg/l	Fe mg/l
Compleat® Regular Formula (Sandoz/Novartis)	Beef NFDM	C.O. Beef	MAL, Frt, Veg, LAC 4.2g Dietary Fiber/1000ml	1.07 32	450	131:1	43.0 16.0	43.0 36.0	130.0 48.0	56.5 1300	35.9 1400	31.4 1100	670	1200	270	12
Compleat® Pediatric (Sandoz/Novartis)	Beef, CAS	HOSO Soy O. Sun.O MCT - Beef	HCS Frt/Veg	1.0 30	380	142.1	38.0 15.0	39.0 35.0	126.0 50.0	30.0 680	39.0 1520	20.0 720	1000	1000	188	13.2
Compleat® Modified Formula (Sandoz/Novartis)	Beef, CAS	Can.O. Beef	MAL, Veg, Frt 4.2g Dietary Fiber/1000ml	1.07 32	300	131:1	43.0 16.0	37.0 31.0	140.0 53.0	43.4 1000	35.9 1400	31.4 1100	670	870	270	12
Ensure w/ Fiber® (Ross)	CAS, SOY	C.O.	HCS, SUC, SPS* *14.4g dietary fiber per 1000 ml	1.10 33	480	148:1	39.7 14.5	37.2 30.5	162.0 55.0	36.8 845	43.4 1693	38.6 1350	719	719	288	13.0
Ensure® (Ross)	CAS, SOY	C.O.	CS, SUC	1.06 31	555	153:1	37.2 14.1	25.8 22.0	169.0 63.9	36.8 845	40.0 1564	37.3 1310	1268	1268	423	19.0
Fiberlan (Nutrition Medical)	CAS	C.O. MCT 50:50	MAL SPS* *14g dietary fiber per 1000 ml	1.2 35.5	310	125:1	50.0 17.0	40.0 53.0	160.0 53.0	44.0 1012	44.0 1716	NA	NA	NA	NA	NA
Fibersource® (Sandoz/Novartis)	CAS	MCT Can.O. 50:50	HCS SPS* *10g dietary fiber per 1000ml	1.2 35.5	390	151:1	43.0 14.0	41.0 30.0	170.0 56.0	47.8 1100	46.2 1800	31.4 1100	670	670	270	12
Isocal® (Mead J.)	CAS, SOY	Soy O. MCT 20:80	MAL	1.06 32	270	167:1	34.2 13.0	44.4 37.0	135.0 50.0	23.0 530	34.0 1320	30.0 1060	634	528	211	9.5

NOTE: Formulas may change composition. These values are current as of 6/1/97. Check with manufacturers for updated information. All values used with permission.

STANDARD FORMULAS AND BLENDERIZED
(continued)
Nutrient Analysis per 1,000 ml

Product (Manufacturer)	PRO	SOURCES FAT (MCT:LCT)	CHO	Kcal /ml /oz	mOsm/ kg H₂O	Non-PRO Cal:N	PRO g/l %	FAT g/l %	CHO g/l %	Na mEq/l mg/l	K mEq/l mg/l	Cl mEq/l mg/l	Ca mg/l	Phos mg/l	Mg mg/l	Fe mg/l
Isolan® (Nutrition Medical)	CAS	C.O. MCT (50:50)	MAL	1.06 / 31	300	141:1	40.0 / 15.0	36.0 / 31.0	144.0 / 54.0	39.0 / 897	34.0 / 1326	NA	NA	NA	NA	NA
IsoSource® (Sandoz/Novartis)	CAS SOY	Can.O. MCT (50:50)	HCS	1.2 / 35.5	360	148:1	43.0 / 14.0	41.0 / 30.0	170.0 / 56.0	52.2 / 1200	43.6 / 1700	31.4 / 1100	670	670	270	12.0
Jevity® (Ross)	CAS	HOSO Can.O. MCT (20:80)	HCS SPS* *14.4 g dietary fiber per 1000 ml	1.06 / 31	371	125:1	44.3 / 17.0	34.7 / 29.0	154.4 / 54.3	40.4 / 930	40.0 / 1570	37.4 / 1310	909	758	303	13.7
Nutren 1.0® (Nestle)	CAS	Can.O. MCT, C.O. (24:76)	MAL CS	1.0 / 30	300-390	131:1	40.0 / 16.0	38.0 / 33.0	127.0 / 51.0	38.0 / 876	32.1 / 1252	30.8 / 1200	668	668	268	12.0
Nutren 1.0® w/Fiber (Nestle)	CAS	Can.O. MCT,C.O. (24:76)	MAL CS,SPS* *14 g dietary fiber per 1000 ml	1.0 / 30	303-412	131:1	40.0 / 16.0	38.0 / 33.0	127.0 / 51.0	38.0 / 876	32.1 / 1252	30.8 / 1200	668	668	268	2.0
Nutrilan® (Nutrition Medical)	CAS	C.O. MCT (20:80)	MAL SUC,GP	1.06 / 31	520	149:1	38.0 / 14.0	37.0 / 31.0	143.0 / 54.0	30.0 / 690	34.0 / 1326	NA	NA	NA	NA	NA
Osmolite® (Ross)	CAS, SOY	HOSO, Can.O. MCT (20:80)	MAL	1.06 / 31	300	153:1	37.2 / 14.0	34.9 / 29.0	151.1 / 57.0	27.8 / 640	26.1 / 1020	24.2 / 850	530	530	212	9.5

NOTE: Formulas may change composition. These values are current as of 6/1/97. Check with manufacturers for updated information. All values used with permission.

STANDARD FORMULAS AND BLENDERIZED
(continued)
Nutrient Analysis per 1,000 ml

Product (Manufacturer)	PRO	SOURCES FAT (MCT:LCT)	CHO	Kcal /ml /oz	mOsm/ kg H₂O	Non-PRO Cal:N	PRO g/l %	FAT g/l %	CHO g/l %	Na mEq/l mg/l	K mEq/l mg/l	Cl mEq/l mg/l	Ca mg/l	Phos mg/l	Mg mg/l	Fe mg/l
PediaSure® (Ross)	CAS WP	HOSO Soy O. MCT (20:80)	HCS SUC	1.0 30	345	185:1	30.0 12.0	49.7 44.0	110.0 44.0	16.5 380	33.5 1310	28.9 1010	970	800	200	14.0
PediaSure w/Fiber® (Ross)	CAS WP	HOSO Soy O. MCT (20:80)	HCS SUC SPS* *5.0g dietary fiber per 1000ml	1.0 30	345	185:1	30.0 12.0	49.7 44.0	113.5 44.0	16.5 380	33.5 1310	28.6 1010	970	800	200	14.0
ProBalance® (Nestle)	CAS	C.O. MCT	MAL SPS* *10 g dietary fiber per 1000 ml	1.2 35.5	350–450		54.0 18.0	40.6 30.0	156.0 52.0	33.2 763	40.0 1560	37.0 1296	1250	1000	400	18.0
Resource® Standard (Sandoz/Novartis)	CAS, SOY	C. O.	HCS SUC	1.10 31	430	154:1	37.0 14.0	37.0 32.0	140.0 54.0	38.7 890	41.0 1600	40.5 1000	530	530	210	9.5
Resource® Fruit Box (Sansoz/Novartis)	WP	NA	HCS Sug	0.76 23	700	131:1	37.0 20.0	NA	150.0 80.0	13.0 295	2.4 93	28.0 930	570	680	210	9.5
Sustacal Basic® (Mead J)	CAS SOY	Soy O.	CS SUC	1.06 31	500	153:1	37.0 14.0	35.0 30.0	148.0 56.0	37.0 850	40.0 1560	37.4 1310	530	530	210	9.7
Sustacal® w/Fiber (Mead J)	CAS, SOY	C.O.	MAL Sug, SPS* *10.6 g Dietary fiber per 1000 ml	1.06 31	480	120:1	46.0 17.0	35.2 30.0	139.0 53.0	31.0 720	36.0 1390	39.7 1390	845	704	282	12.7
Ultracal® (Mead J)	CAS	Can.O. MCT (40:60)	MAL	1.06 31	310	128:1	44.0 17.0	45.0 37.0	123.0 46.0	40.0 930	41.0 1610	41.0 1440	850	850	340	15.2

NOTE: Formulas may change composition. These values are current as of 6/1/97. Check with manufacturers for updated information. All values used with permission.

SELECTED ENTERAL FORMULAS
CALORIE- AND/OR PROTEIN-DENSE
Nutrient Analysis per 1,000 ml

Product (Manufacturer)	SOURCES PRO	SOURCES FAT (MCT:LCT)	SOURCES CHO	Kcal /ml //oz	mOsm/kg H₂O	Non-PRO Cal:N	PRO g/l / %	FAT g/l / %	CHO g/l / mg/l	Na mEq/l / mg/l	K mEq/l / mg/l	Cl mEq/l / mg/l	Ca mg/l	Phos mg/l	Mg mg/l	Fe mg/l
Comply® (Mead J)	CAS	C.O.	HCS MAL, SUC	1.5 / 45	460	131:1	60.0 / 16.0	60.0 / 36.0	180.0 / 48.0	52.1 / 1200	47.0 / 1850	48.0 / 1700	1200	1200	480	22.0
Deliver 2.0® (Mead J)	CAS	Soy.O. MCT (30:70)	CS	2.0 / 60	640	145:1	75.0 / 15.0	102.0 / 45.0	200.0 / 40.0	35.0 / 800	43.0 / 1700	34.0 / 1200	1000	1000	400	18.2
Ensure®High Protein (Ross)	CAS, SOY	Saf.O	MALT SUC	1.06 / 31	610	92:1	50.4 / 21.3	25.0 / 24.0	129.4 / 54.7	52.6 / 1209	53.5 / 2085	45.2 / 1585	1042	1042	417	18.8
Ensure® Plus (Ross)	CAS, SOY	C.O.	MALT, CS, SUC	1.5 / 45	690	146:1	54.9 / 14.7	53.3 / 32.0	200.0 / 53.3	45.6 / 1050	49.8 / 1941	54.3 / 1899	705	705	283	12.7
Ensure® PlusHN (Ross)	CAS, SOY	C.O.	MALT SUC	1.5 / 45	650	125:1	62.6 / 16.7	50.0 / 30.0	200.0 / 53.3	49.6 / 1184	54.0 / 1818	45.3 / 1606	1055	1055	423	19.0
Entrition®0.5 (Nestle)	CAS SOY	C.O.	MALT	0.5	120	NA	NA	17.5 / 14.0	68.0 / 54.5	15.2 / 350	15.4 / 600	12.8 / 500	250	250	100	4.5
Entrition® HN (Nestle)	CAS SOY	C.O.	MAL	1.0 / 30	300	117:1	44.0 / 17.6	41.0 / 36.8	114.0 / 45.6	36.7 / 845	40.5 / 1579	44.0 / 1540	770	770	308	13.9
Fibersource HN® (Sandoz/Novartis)	CAS	MCT Can.O. (50:50)	HCS *SPS *6.8g dietary fiber per 1000 ml	1.2 / 35.5	390	118:1	53.0 / 18.0	41.0 / 30.0	160.0 / 52.0	47.8 / 1100	46.2 / 1800	31.4 / 1100	670	670	270	12
Isocal® HN® (Mead J)	CAS SOY	Soy.O. MCT (40:60)	MAL	1.06 / 31	270	125:1	44.0 / 17.0	45.0 / 37.0	123.0 / 46.0	40.4 / 930	41.0 / 1610	41.0 / 1440	850	850	340	15.2
IsoSource® HN (Sandoz/Novartis)	CASCan.O. SOY	HCS MCT (50:50)	1.2	330 / 35.5	116:1	53.0	41.0 / 18.0	160.0 / 30.0	47.8 / 52.0	43.6 / 1100	31.4 / 1700	670 / 1100	670	270	12.0

NOTE: Formulas may change composition. These values are current as of 6/1/97. Check with manufacturers for updated information. All values used with permission.

CALORIE- AND/OR PROTEIN-DENSE
(continued)

Nutrient Analysis per 1,000 ml

Product (Manufacturer)	PRO	SOURCES FAT (MCT:LCT)	CHO	Kcal /ml /oz	mOsm/ kg H₂O	Non-PRO Cal:N	PRO g/l %	FAT g/l %	CHO g/l %	Na mEq/l mg/l	K mEq/l mg/l	Cl mEq/l mg/l	Ca mg/l	Phos mg/l	Mg mg/l	Fe mg/l
IsoSource®1.5 (Sandoz/Novartis)	CAS	MCT, Can O. Soy O.	HCS, Sug, SPS, GUA	1.5 / 45	650	116:1	68.0 / 18.0	65.0 / 38.0	170.0 / 44.0	57.0 / 1300	54.0 / 2100	45.0 / 1600	1100	1100	430	19.0
IsoSource VHN® (Sandoz/Novartis)	CAS SOY	Can. O. MCT (19:81)	HCS GUA SPS	1.0 / 30	300	77:1	62.0 / 25.0	29.0 / 25.0	130.0 / 50.0	60.1 / 1300	41.0 / 1600	40.0 / 1400	800	800	320	14.0
Magnacal® Renal (Mead J)	CAS	Soy O. MCT	MAL, SUC	2.0 / 60	570	154:1	75.0 / 15.0	101.0 / 45.0	200.0 / 40.0	34.8 / 800	32.6 / 1270	33.7 / 1180	1010	800	200	18.0
Nitrolan® (Nutrition Medical)	CAS	C.O. MCT (50:50)	MAL	1.24 / 37	310	104:1	60.0 / 19.0	40.0 / 29.0	160.0 / 52.0	38.0 / 874	38.0 / 1482	NA	NA	NA	NA	NA
Nutren 1.5® (Nestle)	CAS	MCT Can.O. C.O. (48:52)	MAL	1.5 / 45	430	131:1	60.0 / 16.0	67.6 / 39.0	169.2 / 45.0	50.9 / 1170	48.0 / 1872	49.7 / 1740	1000	1000	400	18.0
Nutren 2.0® (Nestle)	CAS	MCT Can.O. C.O. (73:27)	CS MAL SUC	2.0 / 60	710	131:1	80.0 / 16.0	106.0 / 45.0	196.0 / 39.0	56.5 / 1300	49.2 / 1920	53.6 / 1876	1340	1340	536	24.0
Osmolite HN® (Ross)	CAS, SOY	HOSO Can.O. MCT (20:80)	MALT	1.06 / 31	300	125:1	44.3 / 16.7	34.7 / 29.0	143.9 / 54.3	40.4 / 930	40.2 / 1570	41.1 / 1440	758	758	304	13.7
Promote® (Ross)	CAS SOY	HOSO Can.O. MCT (20:80)	HCS SUC *Promote w/Fiber contains 14.4 g/liter blend of oat & soy fibers	1.0 / 30	340	75:1	62.5 / 25.0	26.0 / 23.0	130.0 / 52.0	43.4 / 1000	50.8 / 1980	36.2 / 1260	1200	1200	400	18.0
Protain XL® (Mead J)	CAS	MCT C.O.	MAL *SPS	1.0 / 30	340	NA	57.0 / 22.0	30.0 / 27.0	129.0 / 50.0	40.0 / 920	45.1 / 1760	38.1 / 1350	800	800	320	18.0

NOTE: Formulas may change composition. These values are current as of 6/1/97. Check with manufacturers for updated information. All values used with permission.

477

CALORIE- AND/OR PROTEIN-DENSE
(continued)
Nutrient Analysis per 1,000 ml

Product (Manufacturer)	PRO	SOURCES FAT (MCT:LCT)	CHO	Kcal /ml /oz	mOsm/ kg H_2O	Non-PRO Cal:N	PRO g/l %	FAT g/l %	CHO g/l %	Na mEq/l mg/l	K mEq/l mg/l	Cl mEq/l mg/l	Ca mg/l	Phos mg/l	Mg mg/l	Fe mg/l
Replete® (Nestle)	CAS	C.O.	MAL CS	1.0 30	350	75:1	62.5 25.0	34.0 30.0	113.2 45.0	38.0 876	38.5 1500	37.1 1300	1000	1000	400	18.0
Replete w/Fiber® (Nestle)	CAS	Can.O. MCT (25:75)	MAL CS, SPS* *14g dietary fiber per 1000 ml	1.0 30	310	75:1	62.5 25.0	34.0 30.0	113.0 45.0	38.0 876	38.5 1500	37.1 1300	1000	1000	400	18.0
Resource Plus® Liquid (Sandoz/Novartis)	CAS, SOY	C. O.	HCS SUC	1.5 45	600	146:1	55.0 15.0	53.0 32.0	200.0 53.0	56.5 1300	53.8 2100	45.7 1600	710	710	320	14.0
Sustacal® Plus (Mead J.)	CAS	C.O.	CS, Sug	1.5 45	630	134:1	60.9 16.0	57.5 34.0	190.0 50.0	37.0 850	38.0 1480	35.8 1268	850	850	338	15.2
TraumaCal® (Mead J)	CAS	Soy.O. MCT (30:70)	CS SUG	1.5 45	490	91:1	82.4 22.0	68.5 40.0	142.0 38.0	52.0 1200	36.0 1400	45.3 1606	750	750	200	9.0
TwoCal HN® (Ross)	CAS	C.O. MCT (20:80)	MALT SUC	2.0 60	690	125:1	83.7 16.7	90.9 40.1	217.3 43.2	63.3 1456	62.8 2456	46.5 1649	1052	1052	421	19.0
Ultralan® (Nutrition Medical)	CAS SOY	MCT C.O. (50:50)	MAL	1.5 45	540	131:1	60.0 16.0	50.0 30.0	202.0 54.0	51.0 1173	49.0 1911	NA	NA	NA	NA	NA

NOTE: Formulas may change composition. These values are current as of 6/1/97. Check with manufacturers for updated information. All values used with permission.

ELEMENTAL, SEMI-ELEMENTAL, OR PEPTIDE
Nutrient Analysis per 1,000 ml

Product (Manufacturer)	PRO	SOURCES FAT (MCT:LCT)	CHO	Kcal /ml /oz	mOsm/ kg H₂O	Non-PRO Cal:N	PRO g/l %	FAT g/l %	CHO g/l %	Na mEq/l mg/l	K mEq/l mg/l	Cl mEq/l mg/l	Ca mg/l	Phos mg/l	Mg mg/l	Fe mg/l
Alitraq (Ross)	SOY.H. GLN* WP,HL ARG	MCT Saf.O. (53:47) *14g GLN per 1000ml	MALT Fruc	1.0 / 30	575	94:1	52.5 / 21.0	15.5 / 13.0	165.0 / 66.0	43.5 / 1000	30.8 / 1200	37.1 / 1300	733	733	267	15.0
Criticare HN® (Mead J.)	HC AA	Saf. O.	MAL, CS	1.06 / 31	650	149:1	38.0 / 14.0	5.3 / 4.5	220.0 / 81.5	27.0 / 630	34.0 / 1320	30.0 / 1060	530	530	210	9.5
Crucial (Nestle)	HC ARG	MCT Fish Oil (50:50)	MAL CS	1.5 / 45	490	NA	93.8 / 25.0	67.6 / 40.0	135.0 / 36.0	50.8 / 1168	48.0 / 1872	49.7 / 1740	1000	1000	400	18.0
L-Elemental (Nutrition Medical)	AA	Saf.O	MAL	1.0 / 30	630	149:1	38.2 / 15.3	2.8 / 2.5	205.6 / 82.2	460	780	NA	NA	NA	NA	NA
L-Elemental Plus (Nutrition Medical)	AA	Soy O.	MAL	1.0 / 30	650	115:1	45.0 / 18	6.7 / 6	190.0 / 76	610	1056	NA	NA	NA	NA	NA
Neocate One+ (SHS)	AA	Saf.O. MCT (35:65)	CS SUC MAL	1.0 / 45	725	NA	25.0 / 10.0	35.0 / 32.0	146.0 / 58.0	8.7 / 200	23.8 / 930	10.0 / 350	620	620	90	7.7
Peptamen (Nestle)	HW	MCT Sun.O. (70:30)	MAL Star	1.0 / 30	270	131:1	40.0 / 16.0	39.0 / 33.0	127.0 / 51.0	21.7 / 500	32.1 / 1252	28.5 / 1000	800	700	400	12.0
Peptamen VHP (Clintec)	HW	MCT Soy.O. (70:30)	MAL SUC,CS	1.0 / 30	300	NA	62.5 / 25.0	39.2 / 33.0	104.4 / 42.0	24.3 / 560	38.5 / 1500	28.6 / 1000	800	700	300	18.0
Perative (Ross)	HC HL,ARG	Can.O. MCT,C.O. (40:60)	HCS	1.3 / 38.5	385	97:1	66.7 / 20.5	37.1 / 25.0	177.2 / 54.5	45.9 / 1055	44.4 / 1730	47.0 / 1646	869	869	347	15.6
Pro-Peptide (Nutrition Medical)	HW	MCT Sun.O.	MAL Star	1.0 / 30	270	131:1	40:0 / 16.0	39.2 / 33.0	127.2 / 51.0	21.7 / 500	32.0 / 1252	NA	NA	NA	NA	NA

NOTE: Formulas may change composition. These values are current as of 6/1/97. Check with manufacturers for updated information. All values used with permission.

479

SELECTED ENTERAL FORMULAS
ELEMENTAL, SEMI-ELEMENTAL, OR PEPTIDE
Nutrient Analysis per 1,000 ml

Product (Manufacturer)	PRO	SOURCES FAT (MCT:LCT)	CHO	Kcal /ml /oz	mOsm/ kg H₂O	Non-PRO Cal:N	PRO g/l %	FAT g/l %	CHO g/l %	Na mEq/l mg/l	K mEq/l mg/l	Cl mEq/l mg/l	Ca mg/l	Phos mg/l	Mg mg/l	Fe mg/l
Pro-Peptide Vanilla (Nutrition Medical)	HN	MCT Sun.O	MAL Star	1.0 30	380	131:1	40.0 16.0	39.2 33.0	127.2 51.0	21.7 500	32.0 1252	NA	NA	NA	NA	NA
Pro-Peptide VHN (Nutrition Medical)	HW	MCT Soy.O.	MAL Star	1.0 30	300 360	75:1	62.4 25.0	39.2 33.0	104.4 42.0	24.3 360	38.5 1500	NA	NA	NA	NA	NA
Reabilan® (Nutrition Medical)	HWC	MCT, OB.O. Soy.O. (40:60)	MAL, T.S.	1.0 30	350	175:1	31.5 12.5	39.0 35.0	131.5 52.5	30.4 702	32.0 1252	56.3 2002	499	499	251	10
Reabilan® HN (Elan)	HWC	MCT, OB.O. Soy O. (40:60)	MAL, T.S.	1.33 39	490	117:1	58.2 17.5	54.0 35.0	158.0 47.5	43.5 1000	42.4 1661	70.4 2499	451	499	331	13.3
SandoSource® Peptide (Sandoz/Novartis)	CAS AA	MCT Soy O.	HCS	1.0 30	490	100:1	50.0 20.0	17.0 15.0	160.0 65.0	52.0 1200	41.0 1600	27.0 470	570	570	230	10.0
Tolerex® (Sandoz/Novartis)	AA	Saf.O.	MAL	1.0 30	550	282:1	21.0 8.0	1.5 1.0	230.0 91.0	20.4 470	31.0 1200	27.1 950	560	560	220	10.0
Travasorb® HN (Nestle)	HL	MCT Sun.O	GOS	1.0 30	560	126:1	45.0 18.0	13.4 12.0	175.0 70.0	40.0 921	30.0 1170	39.0 1365	500	500	200	9.0
Travasorb MCT (Nestle)	HL CAS	MCT Sun.O.	CS	1.0 30	250	NA	45.0 18.0	33.0 30.0	123.0 50.0	15.2 350	25.6 1000	34.7 1215	500	500	200	9.0

NOTE: Formulas may change composition. These values are current as of 6/1/97. Check with manufacturers for updated information. All values used with permission.

Nutrient Analysis per 1,000 ml

Product (Manufacturer)	PRO	SOURCES FAT (MCT:LCT)	CHO	Kcal /ml /oz	mOsm/ kg H₂O	Non-PRO Cal:N	PRO g/l %	FAT g/l %	CHO g/l %	Na mEq/l mg/l	K mEq/l mg/l	Cl mEq/l mg/l	Ca mg/l	Phos mg/l	Mg mg/l	Fe mg/l
Travasorb® STD (Nestle)	HL	MCT Sun.O. (60:40)	GOS	1.0 / 30	560	202:1	30.0 / 12.0	13.4 / 12.0	190.0 / 76.0	40.0 / 921	30.0 / 1170	42.9 / 1500	500	500	200	9.0
Vital® HN (Ross)	HW, Meat, SOY AA	Saf.O. MCT (45:55)	HCS, SUC	1.0 / 30	500	125:1	41.7 / 16.7	10.8 / 9.4	185.0 / 73.9	24.6 / 566	35.9 / 1400	29.5 / 1032	667	667	267	12.0
Vivonex® Pediatric (Sandoz/Novartis)	AA	MCT Soy.O.	MAL Mod S	0.8 / 24	360	200:1	24.0 / 12.0	24.0 / 35.0	130.0 / 63.0	17.0 / 400	31.0 / 1200	28.0 / 1000	970	800	200	10.0
Vivonex Plus® (Sandoz/Novartis)	AA (30% BCAA)	Soy O.	MAL ModS	1.0 / 30	650	115:1	45.0 / 18.0	6.7 / 6.0	190.0 / 76.0	26.6 / 610	28.2 / 1100	27.0 / 940	560	560	220	10.0
Vivonex® T.E.N. (Sandoz/Novartis)	AA (33% BCAA)	Saf. O.	MAL Mod S	1.0 / 30	630	149:1	38.0 / 15.0	2.8 / 3.0	210.0 / 82.0	20.0 / 460	20.0 / 780	23.1 / 820	500	500	200	9.0
E028 Extra® (SHS) *Values per 100 grams of powder	AA	Veg. Fats Coc.O.	SUC CS	0.85 / 24	636	NA	12.5 / 12.0	17.5 / 36.0	55.0 / 52.0	13.3 / 305	11.9 / 466	9.4 / 333	188	200	82	4.2
Advera® (Ross)	Soy H. CAS	Can.O. MCT Saf.O. (20:80)	MALT SPS* *8.9g dietary fiber per 1000 ml	1.28 / 38	505	108:1	60.0 / 18.7	22.8 / 15.8	215.6 / 65.5	44.0 / 1013	65.0 / 2532	42.2 / 1477	1083	1083	338	19.1
Amin-Aid® (R & D Laboratories)	AA	Soy O.	MAL SUC	2.0 / 60	700	800:1	19.4 / 4.0	46.2 / 21.2	365.6 / 74.8	<15	<6					

NOTE: Formulas may change composition. These values are current as of 6/1/97. Check with manufacturers for updated information. All values used with permission.

SELECTED ENTERAL FORMULAS
SPECIALTY

Product (Manufacturer)	PRO	SOURCES FAT (MCT:LCT)	CHO	Kcal /ml /oz	mOsm/ kg H₂0	Non-PRO Cal:N	PRO g/l %	FAT g/l %	CHO g/l %	Na mEq/l mg/l	K mEq/l mg/l	Cl mEq/l mg/l	Ca mg/l	Phos mg/l	Mg mg/l	Fe mg/l
Citrotein® (Sandoz/Novartis)	EWS	Soy O.	SUC HCS	0.67 20	480 - 490	76:1	41.0 25.0	1.6 2.0	120.0 73.0	29.1 670	14.1 550	22.6 790	1100	1100	420	38.0
DiabetiSource (Sandoz/Novartis)	CAS Beet	HOSO Can.O.	MAL Fruc	1.0 30	360	100:1	50.0 20.0	49.0 44.0	90.0 36.0	43.0 1000	28.0 870	31.0 1100	670	87	270	12.0
Glucerna® (Ross)	CAS	HOSO Can.O.	HCS Fruc *SPS	1.0 30	375	150:1	41.8 16.7	54.4 49.0	95.8 34.3	40.4 930	40.2 1570	41.1 1440	704	704	282	12.7
Glytrol (Nestle)		Can.O HOSO MCT	MALT CS Fruc	1.0 30	380	NA	45.0 18.0	47.5 42.0	100.0 40.0	740	1400	1200	720	720	286	12.8
Hepatic-Aid® II (McGaw)	AA (46% BCAA)	Soy O.	MAL SUC	1.2 35.5	560	148:1	44.1 15.0	36.2 27.7	168.5 57.3	<15	<6					
Immun-Aid® (McGraw)	Lactalb ARG<GLN (35% BCAA)	Can.O. MCT (50:50)	MAL 30	1.0	460	52:1 32.0	80.0 20.0	22.0 48.0	120.0 575	25.0 1055	27.0 888	25.1	500	500	200	9.0
Impact® (Sandoz/Novartis)	CAS ARG	Struc Pal.O. Sun.O. Men.O.	HCS	1.0 30	375	71:1	56.0 22.0	28.0 25.0	130.0 53.0	47.8 1100	36.0 1400	37..1 1300	800	800	270	12.0
Impact® 1.5 (Sandoz/Novartis)	Cas ARG	Struc Men.O.	HCS	1.5 45	550	71;1	80.0 22.0	69.0 40.0	140.0 38.0	56.0 1280	43.0 1680	45.0 1600	960	960	320	12.0

*14.4 g dietary fiber per 1000 ml

NOTE: Formulas may change composition. These values are current as of 6/1/97. Check with manufacturers for updated information. All values used with permission.

Product (Manufacturer)	PRO	SOURCES FAT (MCT:LCT)	CHO	Kcal /ml /oz	mOsm/ kg H_2O	Non-PRO Cal:N	PRO g/l %	FAT g/l %	CHO g/l %	Na mEq/l mg/l	K mEq/l mg/l	Cl mEq/l mg/l	Ca mg/l	Phos mg/l	Mg mg/l	Fe mg/l
Impact w/Fiber® (Sandoz)	CAS ARG	Struc Pal.O. Sun.O. Men.O.	HCS *SPS Guar *10g dietary fiber per 1000ml	1.0 30	375	71:1	56.0 22.0	28.0 25.0	140.0 53.0	47.8 1100	36.0 1400	37.1 1300	800	800	270	12.0
L-Elemental Hepatic (Nutrition Medical)	AA (46% BCAA)	S.O.	MAL SUC	1.2 35.2	560	148:1	44.1 15.0	36.2 27.7	168.5 57.3	< 345 < 15	<195 < 15					
Lipisorb® (Mead J)	CAS	MCT Soy O. (85:15)	MAL SUC	1.35 40	630	125:1	57.0 17.0	57.0 35.0	161.0 48.0	59.0 1350	43.0 1690	62.0 2200	850	850	340	15.2
Nepro® (Ross)	CAS	MCT CO Can.O.	C.S. SUC	2.0 60 HOSO	635	155:1	69.9 14.0	95.8 43.0	215.6 43.0	36.2 834	26.7 1042	24.6 1001	1355	688	208	19.0
Nutrihep® (Nestle)	AA WP (50% BCAA)	MCT Can.O. C.O. (66:34)	MAL Mod.S.	1.5 45	690	194:1	40.0 11.0	21.2 12.0	289.5 77.0	13.9 320	33.8 1320	42.8 1500	1000	1000	400	18.0
Nutrivent® (Clintec)	CAS	Can.O. MCT,C.O. (40:60)	MAL SUC	1.5 45	450	116:1	68.0 18.0	94.8 55.0	100.8 27.0	50.9 1170	48.0 1872	49.7 1740	1200	1200	480	18.0
Pulmocare® (Ross)	CAS	Can.O. MCT C.O.,HOSO (20:80)	MAL SUC	1.5 45	475	125:1	62.6 16.7	93.2 55.0	105.5 28.0	57.0 1310	44.4 1730	48.2 1688	1055	1055	423	19.1
Renal Diet (Nestle)	CAS	Can.O. MCT	MAL Mod.S.	2.0 60	600	NA	34.4 6.9	82.4 35.0	290.4 58.1							

NOTE: Formulas may change composition. These values are current as of 6/1/97. Check with manufacturers for updated information. All values used with permission.

SELECTED ENTERAL FORMULAS
SPECIALTY

Product (Manufacturer)	PRO	SOURCES FAT (MCT:LCT)	CHO	Kcal /ml /oz	mOsm/ kg H2O	Non-PRO Cal:N	PRO g/l %	FAT g/l %	CHO g/l %	Na mEq/l mg/l	K mEq/l mg/l	Cl mEq/l mg/l	Ca mg/l	Phos mg/l	Mg mg/l	Fe mg/l
Resource® Diabetic (Sandoz/Novartis)	CAS SOY	HO Soy.O.	HCS Fruc	1.06 31	450	104:1	63.0 24.0	47.0 40.0	99.0 36.0	42.0 970	29.0 1100	26.0 910	930	930	210	9.5
Respalor® (Mead J)	CAS	Can.O. MCT (30:70)	CS SUC	1.5 45	580	102:1	76.0 20.0	71.0 41.0	148.0 39.0	55.2 1270	37.9 1480	48.2 1690	710	710	280	12.7
Suplena® (Ross)	CAS	HOSO Soy O.	MALT SUC	2.0 60	600	393:1	30.0 6.0	95.6 51.0	255.2 43.0	34.0 783	28.6 1116	26.5 926	1385	728	211	18.9
Travasorb MCT® (Clintec)	Lactalb CAS	MCT Sun.O. (80:20)	CS	1.0 30	250	101:1	49.6 20.0	33.0 30.0	122.8 50.0	15.2 350	25.6 1000	34.7 1215	500	500	200	9.0

NOTE: Formulas may change composition. These values are current as of 6/1/97. Check with manufacturers for updated information. All values used with permission.

SELECTED ENTERAL FORMULAS
MODULAR

CARBOHYDRATE

Product (Manuf.)	CHO SOURCE	Kcal
Modual® (Mead J.) (powder)	MAL	3.8/g
L.C. (liquid) (Corpak)	CS	2.75/ml
Polycose® Liquid (Ross)	GP	2/ml
Polycose Powder (Ross)	GP	4.0/g

PROTEIN

Product (Manuf.)	PRO SOURCE	Kcal	% of wt. that is PRO
*Casec® (Mead J.) (powder)	CAS	3.7/g	90
*Pro-Mix RDP® (powder) (Corpak) Trace of lactose	Whey	3.6/g	75
PROMOD® (Ross) (powder)	Whey	4.2/g	75
Elementra® (Clintec) (powder)	HW	3.8/g	79
Aminess® (Clintec) (Tablets)	Essential AA + HIS	3.0/tab 0.69 g pro/tab	85

FAT

Product (Manuf.)	FAT SOURCE	Kcal	Fat g/ml
MCT Oil® (Mead J.)	Coc. O.	7.7/ml	0.94
Microlipid® (Mead J)	Saf. O.	4.5/ml	0.5
Duocal® Fat & Carbohydrate (SHS) (powder)	HC, C.O. Coc.O. MCT	4.9/g	0.22 g fat/ 0.73g CHO/g

NOTE: Formulas may change composition. These values are current as of 6/1/97. Check with manufacturers for updated information. All values used with permission.
* Products contain some sodium, potassium, phosphorus, calcium, and other minerals.

SELECTED INFANT FORMULAS
STANDARD MILK-BASED FORMULAS
Nutrient Analysis per 1000 ml

Product (Manufacturer)	PRO	SOURCES FAT	CHO	Kcal /ml /oz	mOsm/ kg H2O	RSL mOsm/l	PRO g/l %	FAT g/l %	CHO g/l %	Na mEq/l mg/l	K mEq/l mg/l	Cl mEq/l mg/l	Ca mg/l	Phos mg/l	Mg mg/l	Fe mg/l
Human	Whey Casein	Milk Fat	Lactose	0.68 20.0	290	75	11.0 6.0	39.0 52.0	72.0 42.0	7.8 180	13.5 525	12.0 420	280	140	35	0.3
Whole Cow Milk	Casein Whey	Butter Fat	Lactose	0.65 19.0	285	226	34.5 21.0	34.5 49.0	48.4 30.0	21.7 500	40.0 1560	29.0 1030	1225	956	134	0.5
Goat Milk	Casein	Butter Fat	Lactose	0.70 21.0	300	N/A	36.7 21.0	42.6 54.0	46.0 25.0	22.4 515	54.0 2105	N/A	1375	1140	145	0.5
Enfamil® (Mead J)	WP NFDM	Pal.O. Soy.O. Coc.O. HOSO	Lactose	0.67 20.0	300	134	15.0 9.0	35.8 48.0	73.7 44.0	7.9 182	18.7 730	12.0 426	527	358	54	4.7 or 12
Follow Up® (Carnation)	NFDM	Pal.O. Soy.O. Coc.O. HOSO	CS Lactose	0.67 20.0	326	121	17.6 10.8	26.0 35.1	88.0 52.8	11.3 260	23.0 900	17.0 600	900	600	56	12.7
Similac® (Ross)	NFDM	Soy.O Coc.O	Lactose	0.67 20.0	300	96	14.5 9.0	36.5 49.0	72.3 42.0	8.0 183	18.2 710	12.2 433	495	379	41	1.5 or 12
Similac Neocar® Power Standard Dilution 22	WP NFOM	Soy.O HOSO Coc.O	CS Lactose	0.74 22.0	290	131	19.3 10.0	40.9 49.0	76.6 41.0	10.7 246	27.1 1056	15.8 558	781	461	67	13.4
Similac® and Similar w/Iron 24	NFOM	Soy.O Coc.O	Lactose	0.81 24.0	380	146	22.0 11.0	42.8 47.0	85.3 42.0	12.0 276	27.5 1071	18.6 658	725	568	57	1.8 or 14
Similar 27	NFOM	Soy.O Coc.O	Lactose	0.91 27.0	410	164	24.7 11.0	48.1 47.0	95.9 42.0	13.5 310	30.9 1205	20.9 740	822	639	64	2.0

NOTE: Formulas may change composition. These values are current as of 6/1/97. Check with manufacturers for updated information. All values used with permission.

STANDARD SOY-BASED FORMULAS

Nutrient Analysis per 1000 ml

Product (Manufacturer)	SOURCES PRO	FAT	CHO	Kcal /ml /oz	mOsm/ kg H₂O	RSL mOsm/l	PRO g/l %	FAT g/l %	CHO g/l %	Na mEq/l mg/l	K mEq/l mg/l	Cl mEq/l mg/l	Ca mg/l	Phos mg/l	Mg mg/l	Fe mg/l
Alsoy (Carnation)	SOY CAS WP	Soy.O	SUCR MAL Potato	0.67 20.0	270	130	21.0 12.3	37.2 49.1	67.6 40.0	12.2 281	20.1 784	14.9 523	683	422	74	12.7
Isomil® (Ross)	SOY	Soy.O. Coc.O	C.S. SUC	0.67 20.0	230	110	16.6 10.0	36.9 49.0	69.6 41.0	12.9 297	18.7 730	11.8 419	710	507	51	12.2
Isomil DF (Ross)	SOY	Soy.O. Coc.O.	C.S. SUC *SPS	0.67 20.0	240	115	18.0 11.0	36.9 49.0	68.3 40.0	12.9 297	18.7 730	12.0 419	710	507	51	12.2
Isomil SF® 20 (Ross)	SOY	Soy.O. Coc.O	HCS.	0.67 20.0	180	115	18.0 11.0	36.9 49.0	68.3 40.0	12.9 297	18.7 730	12.0 419	710	507	51	12.2
Prosobee® (Mead J.)	SOY	Pal.O., Soy.O. Coc.O. HOSO	C.S.	0.67 20.0	200	129	20.0 12.0	35.0 48.0	67.0 40.0	10.4 240	20.8 812	15.3 541	710	561	74	12.2

*SPS   6 g Dietary Fiber per 1000ml

NOTE: Formulas may change composition. These values are current as of 6/1/97. Check with manufacturers for updated information. All values used with permission.

487

SELECTED INFANT FORMULAS
SPECIALTY FORMULAS
Nutrient Analysis per 1000 ml

Product (Manufacturer)	SOURCES PRO	FAT (MCT:LCT)	CHO	Kcal /ml /oz	mOsm/ kg H2O	RSL mOsm/l	PRO g/l %	FAT g/l %	CHO g/l %	Na mEq/l mg/l	K mEq/l mg/l	Cl mEq/l mg/l	Ca mg/l	Phos mg/l	Mg mg/l	Fe mg/l
Alimentum® (Ross)	H.C.	MCT, Saf.O. Soy.O. (50:50)	SUC T.S.	0.67 / 20.0	370	123	18.6 / 11.0	37.5 / 48.0	68.9 / 41.0	12.9 / 297	20.5 / 798	15.3 / 541	710	507	51	12.2
Good Start® (Carnation)	HW	Pal.O. Coc.O. Soy.O. HOSO	LAC MAL	0.67 / 20.0	265	101	16.0 / 9.8	34.0 / 46.0	73.0 / 44.2	7.0 / 160	16.9 / 660	11.0 / 390	430	240	45	10.0
Lactofree (Mead J)	Milk Pro Isolate	Pal.O. Soy.O. Coc.O. HOSO	C.S.	0.67 / 20.0	200	100	15.0 / 9.0	35.8 / 48.0	70.3 / 42.0	8.7 / 200	19.1 / 744	12.8 / 453	554	372	54	12.2
L-Elemental Pediatric (Nutrition Medical)	AA	MCT Soy.O	MAL ModS	0.8	360		24.0 / 12.0	24.0 / 25.0	130.0 / 63.0	17.0 / 400	31.0 / 1200.0					
Nutramigen® (Mead J)	H.C.	C.O. Soy.O. HOSO	C.S. ModS	0.67 / 20.0	320	125	18.8 / 11.0	34.0 / 45.0	74.0 / 44.0	13.6 / 312	19.1 / 744	16.4 / 573	635	426	73	12.2
Peptamen Junior (Nestle)	HW	MCT C.O. Can.O	C.S.	1.0 / 30	260	NA	30.0 / 12.0	38.5 / 33.0	137.5 / 55.0	20.0 / 460	33.8 / 1320	30.9 / 1080	1000	800	200	14.0
Portagen® (Mead J)	CAS	MCT C.O. (86:14)	C.S. SUC	0.67 / 20.0	230	200	23.0 / 14.0	32.0 / 40.0	77.0 / 46.0	15.9 / 365	21.3 / 833	16.3 / 573	625	469	135	12.5
Pregestimil® (Mead J)	H.C.	MCT, C.O. Soy.O. HOSO (55:45)	C.S. ModS	0.67 / 20.0	320	123	18.8 / 11.0	37.5 / 48.0	69.6 / 41.0	11.5 / 264	18.9 / 737	16.4 / 581	635	426	74	12.7
Similac PM 60/40® (Ross)	WP CAS	Soy.O. Coc.O.	Lactose	0.67 / 20.0	280	93	15.0 / 9.0	37.8 / 50.0	68.9 / 40.7	7.0 / 160	14.9 / 580	11.3 / 399	379	189	41	1.5
Similac RCF® (Ross)	SOY	Soy.O Coc.O.		0.67 / 20.0	NA	131	19.7 / 12.0	35.5 / 47.0	68.3 / 41.0	12.8 / 293	18.5 / 720	12.0 / 413	700	500	50	1.5

(Values based on 20 cal/oz with added CHO)

NOTE: Formulas may change composition. These values are current as of 6/1/97. Check with manufacturers for updated information. All values used with permission.

PREMATURE FORMULAS
Nutrient Analysis per 1000 ml

Product (Manufacturer)	PRO	SOURCES FAT (MCT:LCT)	CHO	Kcal /ml /oz	mOsm/ kg H₂O	RSL mOsm/l	PRO g/l %	FAT g/l %	CHO g/l %	Na mEq/l mg/l	K mEq/l mg/l	Cl mEq/l mg/l	Ca mg/l	Phos mg/l	Mg mg/l	Fe mg/l
Enfamil Premature® 20 (Mead J)	WP / NFDM	MCT / Soy. O. Coc. O. (40:60)	C.S. / LAC	0.67 / 20.0	260	176	20.0 / 12.0	34.4 / 44.0	74.0 / 44.0	11.5 / 264	17.8 / 696	16.2 / 575	1105	552	46	1.7 o / 12.0
Enfamil Premature® 24 (Mead J)	WP / NFDM	MCT / Soy.O. Coc.O. (40:60)	C.S. / LAC	0.81 / 24.0	310	152	24.3 / 12.0	41.3 / 44.0	88.9 / 44.0	13.7 / 316	21.4 / 834	19.5 / 689	1337	672	55	2.0 o / 14.6
Similac Special Care® 20 (w/iron) (Ross)	NFDM / WP	MCT / Soy.O. Coc.0 (50:50)	HCS / Lactose	0.67 / 20.0	239	124	18.3 / 10.6	36.7 / 47.8	71.6 / 41.6	12.7 / 291	22.3 / 872	15.5 / 548	1217	676	81	2.5 or / 12.2
Similac Special Care® 24 (Ross)	NFDM / WP	MCT / Soy. O. Coc.O. (50:50)	HCS / Lactose	0.81 / 24.0	280	149	22.0 / 11.0	44.1 / 47.0	86.1 / 42.0	15.2 / 349	26.8 / 1047	18.8 / 658	1462	812	97	3.0 or / 14.6
Similac Natuaral Care ® Human Milk Fortifier	NFDM / WP	MCT / Soy.O. Coc.O.	HCS / Lactose	0.81 / 24.0	280	149	22.0 / 11.0	44.1 / 47.0	86.1 / 42.0	15.2 / 349	26.8 / 1047	18.8 / 658	1705	853	98	3.0

NOTE: Formulas may change composition. These values are current as of 6/1/97. Check with manufacturers for updated information. All values used with permission.

SELECTED INFANT FORMULAS
ELECTROLYTE SOLUTIONS
Nutrient Analysis per 1000 ml

Product (Manufacturer)	SOURCES PRO	SOURCES FAT	CHO	Kcal /ml /oz	mOsm/ kg H2O	RSL mOsm/l	PRO g/l %	FAT g/l %	CHO g/l %	Na mEq/l mg/l	K mEq/l mg/l	Cl mEq/l mg/l	Ca mg/l	Phos mg/l	Mg mg/l	Fe mg/l
Infalyte (Mead J)			RiceSyrup Solids	0.13 3.8	200				30.0 100.0	50.0 1150	25.0 975	45.0 1575				
Pedialyte® (Ross)			Dextrose	0.1 3.0	250				25.0 100.0	45.0 1035	20.0 780	35.0 1243				
Rehydralyte® (Ross)			Dextrose	0.1 3.0	305				25.0 100.0	75.0 1725	20.0 780	65.0 2308				

NOTE: Formulas may change composition. These values are current as of 6/1/97. Check with manufacturers for updated information. All values used with permission.

SELECTED ENTERAL FORMULAS
METABOLIC FORMULAS FOR INFANTS AND CHILDREN
Nutrient Analysis per 100 grams Powdered Formula

Product (Manufacturer)	PRO	SOURCES FAT	CHO	Kcal	mOsm/ kg H2O	RSL mOsm/l	PRO g/l / %	FAT g/l / %	CHO g/l / %	Na mEq/l / mg/l	K mEq/l / mg/l	Cl mEq/l / mg/l	Ca mg/l	Phos mg/l	Mg mg/l	Fe mg/l
Calcilo® XD (Ross)	WP CAS	C.O. Coc.O.	LAC	513/ 100g	193/	69/	11.4 / 8.9	28.7 / 50.3	52.3 / 40.8	4.7 / 108	10.8 / 420	8.3 / 292	<50	128	31	9.2
Cyclinex-1® (Ross)	AA	Pal.O. Coc.O. Soy O.	HC	515/ 100g	220/	70/	7.5 / 6.0	27.0 / 47.0	52.0 / 47.0	9.4 / 215	19.4 / 760	11.7 / 415	650	455	50	10.0
Cyclinex-2® (Ross)	AA	Pal.O. Coc.O. Soy O.	HC	480/	276/	197/	15.0 / 12.5	20.7 / 38.5	40.0 / 49.0	51.1 / 1175	46.8 / 1830	37.4 / 1325	1150	1150	300	17.0
Flavonex® (Ross)			SUC	392/100g					98.0 / 100							
Glutarex-1® (Ross)	AA	Pal.O. Coc.O. Soy O.	HC	480/ 100g	273/ 100g	95/ 100g	15.0 / 12.5	23.9 / 45.0	46.3 / 42.5	8.3 / 190	17.3 / 675	9.2 / 325	575	400	45	9.0
Glutarex-2® (Ross)	AA	Pal.O. Coc.O. Soy O.	HC	475/ 100g	534/ 100g	219/ 100g	30.0 / 29.0	15.5 / 34.0	30.0 / 37.0	38.3 / 880	35.0 / 1370	26.5 / 940	880	880	225	13.0
HIST-1® (Mead J)	AA		SUC				51.0		17.0	46.5 / 1070	59.0 / 2300	47.1 / 1650	2400	1860	520	34.0
HIST-2® (Mead J)	AA		SUC				67.0		7.0	27.8 / 640	34.1 / 1330	28.3 / 990	1310	1010	156	15.0

NOTE: Formulas may change composition. These values are current as of 6/1/97. Check with manufacturers for updated information. All values used with permission.

METABOLIC FORMULAS FOR INFANTS AND CHILDREN
(continued)
Nutrient Analysis per 100 grams Powdered Formula

Product (Manufacturer)	PRO	SOURCES FAT	CHO	Kcal /ml /oz	mOsm/ kg H₂O	RSL mOsm/l	PRO g/l %	FAT g/l %	CHO g/l %	Na mEq/l mg/l	K mEq/l mg/l	Cl mEq/l mg/l	Ca mg/l	Phos mg/l	Mg mg/l	Fe mg/l
HOM-1® (Mead J)	AA		SUC				52.0		18.0	46.5 1070	59.0 2300	47.1 1650	2400	1860	520	34.0
HOM-2® (Mead J)	AA		SUC				69.0		5.0	27.8 640	34.1 1330	28.3 990	1310	1010	156	15.0
Hominex-1® (Ross)	AA	Pal.O. Coc.O. Soy O.	HC	480/ 100g	273/ 100g	98/ 100g	15.0 12.5	23.9 45.0	46.3 42.5	8.3 190	17.3 675	12.3 435	575	400	45	9.0
Hominex-2® (Ross)	AA	Pal.O. Coc.O. Soy O	HC	410/ 100g	545/ 100g	226/ 100g	30.0 29.0	15.5 34.0	30.0 37.0	38.3 880	35.0 1370	32.7 1160	880	880	225	13.0
I-Valex-1® (Ross)	AA	Pal.O. Coc.O. Soy O.	HC	480/	273/	95/	15.0 12.5	23.9 45.0	46.3 42.5	8.3 190	17.3 675	9.2 325	575	400	45	9.0
I-Valex-2® (Ross)	AA	Pal.O. Coc.O. Soy O	HC	410/	581/	220/	30.0 29.0	15.5 34.0	30.0 37.0	38.3 880	35.0 1370	26.5 940	880	880	225	13.0
Ketonex-1® (Ross)	AA	Pal.O. Coc.O. Soy O.	HC	480/	273/	95/	15.0 12.5	23.9 45.0	46.3 42.5	8.3 190	17.3 675	9.2 325	575	400	45	9.0
Ketonex-2® (Ross)	AA	Pal.O. Coc.O. Soy O.	HC	410/	545/	220/	30.0 29.0	15.5 34.0	30.0 37.0	38.3 880	35.0 1370	26.5 940	880	880	225	13.0
Lofenalac® (Mead J)	H.C.	C.O.	C.S. T.S.				15.0 13.0	18.0 35.0	60.0 52.0	9.6 220	12.1 470	9.1 320	430	320	50	8.6

NOTE: Formulas may change composition. These values are current as of 6/1/97. Check with manufacturers for updated information. All values used with permission.

METABOLIC FORMULAS FOR INFANTS AND CHILDREN
(continued)
Nutrient Analysis per 100 grams Powdered Formula

Product (Manufacturer)	SOURCES PRO	SOURCES FAT	SOURCES CHO	Kcal /ml /oz	mOsm/ kg H₂0	RSL mOsm/l	PRO g/l %	FAT g/l %	CHO g/l %	Na mEq/l mg/l	K mEq/l mg/l	Cl mEq/l mg/l	Ca mg/l	Phos mg/l	Mg mg/l	Fe mg/l
Low Methionine Diet® Powder (Mead J)	SOY	Pal.O. Soy O. Coc. O. HOSO	C.S.				15.5 12.0	28.0 49.0	51.0 39.0	8.0 185	16.2 630	12.2 430	480	380	56	9.7
Low Phe/Tyr Diet® Powder (Mead J)	H.C.	C.O.	C.S. T.S.				15.0 13.0	18.0 35.0	60.0 52.0	9.6 220	12.1 470	9.1 320	430	320	50	8.6
LYS-1® (Mead J)	AA		SUC				48.0		23.0	46.5 1070	59.0 2300	47.1 1650	2400	1860	520	34.0
LYS-2® (Mead J)	AA		SUC				64.0		12.0	27.8 640	34.1 1330	28.3 990	1310	1010	156	15.0
Mono-/Disaccharide Free Diet® Powder (Mead J)	H.C.	MCT C.O.	T.S.				22.0	33.0	33.0	14.8 340	22.1 860	19.4 680	740	490	86	14.8
MSUD-1® (Mead J)	AA		SUC				41.0		29.0	46.5 1070	59.0 2300	47.1 1650	2400	1860	520	34.0
MSUD-2® (Mead J)	AA		SUC				54.0		22.0	27.8 640	34.1 1330	28.3 990	1310	1010	156	15.0
MSUD Analog® (SHS)	AA	PN.O. RAF Coc.O.	C.S.				13.0 11.0	20.9 39.0	59.0 50.0	5.2 120	10.8 420	8.2 290	600	500	40	10.0
MSUD Diet Powder (Mead J)	AA	C.O.	C.S. T.S.				9.9 8.0	20.0 38.0	63.0 54.0	8.0 185	12.6 490	10.6 370	490	270	52	8.9
MSUD Maxamaid® (SHS)	AA	trace	SUC HCS				25.0 29.0	tr <0.5	62.0 71.0	25.0 580	22.0 840	13.0 450	810	810	200	12.0

NOTE: Formulas may change composition. These values are current as of 6/1/97. Check with manufacturers for updated information. All values used with permission.

493

METABOLIC FORMULAS FOR INFANTS AND CHILDREN
(continued)
Nutrient Analysis per 100 grams Powdered Formula

Product (Manufacturer)	PRO	SOURCES FAT	CHO	Kcal /ml /oz	mOsm/ kg H_2O	RSL mOsm/l	PRO g/l %	FAT g/l %	CHO g/l %	Na mEq/l mg/l	K mEq/l mg/l	Cl mEq/l mg/l	Ca mg/l	Phos mg/l	Mg mg/l	Fe mg/l
MSUD Maxamum (SHS)	AA	trace	SUC HCS				39.0 47.0	tr <1	45.0 53.0	24.0 560	18.0 700	16.0 560	670	670	285	23.5
OS-1® (Mead J)	AA		SUC				42.0		29.0	46.5 1070	59.0 2300	47.1 1650	2400	1860	520	34.0
OS-2® (Mead J)	AA		SUC				56.0		20.0	27.8 640	34.1 1330	28.3 990	1310	1010	156	15.0
Periflex® (SHS) (Per 100g powder)	AA		NA	17	NA	NA	20.0	17 37	40.5 300	13.0 1120	28.7 500	14.3	850	850	110	12.0
Phenyl-Free® (Mead J)	AA	C.O. Coc.O.	SUC C.s. T.s.				20.0 20.0	6.8 15.0	66.0 65.0	17.8 410	35.0 1370	26.6 930	510	510	152	12.2
Phenex-1® (Ross)	AA	Pal.O. Coc.O. Soy O.	HC	480/ 100g	270/	95/	15.0 12.5	23.9 45.0	46.3 42.5	8.3 190	17.3 675	9.2 325	575	400	45	9.0
Phenex-2® (Ross)	AA	Pal.O. Coc.O. Soy O.	HC	410/	521/	220/	30.0 29.0	15.5 34.0	30.0 37.0	38.3 880	35.0 1370	26.5 940	880	880	225	13.0
PKU-1® (Mead J)	AA		SUC				50.0		19.0	46.5 1070	59.0 2300	47.1 1650	2400	1860	520	34.0
PKU-2® (Mead J)	AA		SUC				67.0		7.0	27.8 640	34.1 1330	28.3 990	1310	1010	156	15.0
PKU-3® (Mead J)	AA		SUC				68.0		3.0	27.8 640	34.1 1330	28.6 1000	1310	1010	540	21.0
Pro-Phree® (Ross)		Pal.O. Coc.O. Soy O.	HC	520/	150/	43/	tr	31.0 54.0	60.0 46.0	10.9 250	22.4 875	9.9 350	750	525	63	11.9

NOTE: Formulas may change composition. These values are current as of 6/1/97. Check with manufacturers for updated information. All values used with permission.

METABOLIC FORMULAS FOR INFANTS AND CHILDREN
(continued)
Nutrient Analysis per 100 grams Powdered Formula

Product (Manufacturer)	SOURCES PRO	SOURCES FAT	SOURCES CHO	Kcal /ml /oz	mOsm/ kg H2O	RSL mOsm/l	PRO g/l %	FAT g/l %	CHO g/l %	Na mEq/l mg/l	K mEq/l mg/l	Cl mEq/l mg/l	Ca mg/l	Phos mg/l	Mg mg/l	Fe mg/l
Propimex-1® (Ross)	AA	Pal.O. Coc.O. Soy O.	HC	480/ 100g	276/	98/	15.0 12.5	23.9 45.0	46.3 42.5	8.3 190	17.3 675	12.3 435	575	400	45	9.0
Propimex-2® (Ross)	AA	Pal.O. Coc.O. Soy O.	HC	410/	545/	226/	30.0 29.0	15.5 34.0	30.0 37.0	38.3 880	35.0 1370	32.7 1160	880	880	225	13.0
Protein Free Diet® Powder (Mead J)		C.O.	C.s. T.s.					23.0 41.0	72.0 59.0	3.5 80	8.7 340	3.9 135	540	300	63	10.8
ProViMin® (Ross)	Casein	Coc.O.		313/	200/	493/	73.0	1.4	2.0	52.0 1200	84.0 3300	65.0 2300	2400	1700	200	40.0
RCF® (Ross)	SOY	Soy.O. Coc.O.	Added	0.67 20.0 Per 1000 ml			20.0 12.0	36.0 48.0	68.3 40.0	12.9 297	18.7 730	12.0 419	710	507	51	1.5
**diluted formula w/CHO added																
TYR-1® (Mead J)	AA		SUC				47.0		21.0	46.5 1070	59.0 2300	47.1 1650	2400	1860	520	34.0
TYR-2® (Mead J)	AA		SUC				63.0		12.0	27.8 640	34.1 1330	28.3 990	310	1010	156	15.0
Tyromex-1® (Ross)	AA	Pal.O. Coc.O. Soy O.	HC	480/	273/	98/	15.0 12.5	23.9 45.0	46.3 42.5	8.3 190	17.3 675	12.3 435	575	400	45	9.0
Tyrex-2® (Ross)	AA	Pal.O. Coc.O. Soy O.	HC	410/	245/	91/	30.0 29.0	15.5 34.0	30.0 37.0	38.3 880	35.0 1370	26.5 940	880	880	225	13.0

NOTE: Formulas may change composition. These values are current as of 6/1/97. Check with manufacturers for updated information. All values used with permission.

METABOLIC FORMULAS FOR INFANTS AND CHILDREN
(continued)
Nutrient Analysis per 100 grams Powdered Formula

Product (Manufacturer)	SOURCES PRO	SOURCES FAT	CHO	Kcal /ml /oz	mOsm/ kg H₂O	RSL mOsm/l	PRO g/l %	FAT g/l %	CHO g/l %	Na mEq/l mg/l	K mEq/l mg/l	Cl mEq/l mg/l	Ca mg/l	Phos mg/l	Mg mg/l	Fe mg/l
UCD 1 (Mead J)	AA		SUC				56.0		8.0	54.8 / 1260	71.8 / 2800	55.4 / 1940	2800	2200	0	40.0
UCD 2 (Mead J)	AA		SUC				67.0		6.0	27.8 / 640	34.1 / 1330	28.3 / 990	1310	1010	0	15.0
XLEU Analog (SHS)	AA	PN.O. RAF Coc.O.	C.S.				13.0 / 11.0	20.9 / 39.0	59.0 / 50.0	5.2 / 120	10.8 / 420	8.2 / 290	600	500	40	10.0
XLEU Maxamaid (SHS)	AA	trace	SUC HCS				25.0 / 29.0	tr	62.0 / 71.0	25.0 / 580	22.0 / 840	13.0 / 450	810	810	200	12.0
XLYS TRY Analog (SHS)	AA	PN.O. RAF Coc.O.	C.S.				13.0 / 11.0	20.9 / 39.0	59.0 / 50.0	5.2 / 120	10.8 / 420	8.2 / 290	600	500	40	10.0
XLYS TRY Maxamaid (SHS)	AA	trace	SUC HCS				25.0 / 29.0	tr	62.0 / 71.0	25.0 / 580	22.0 / 840	13.0 / 450	810	810	200	12.0
XLYS TRY Maxamum (SHS)	AA	trace	SUC HCS				39.0 / 47.0	tr	45.0 / 53.0	24.0 / 560	18.0 / 700	16.0 / 560	670	670	285	23.5
XMET Analog (SHS)	AA	PN.O. RAF Coc.O.	C.S.				13.0 / 11.0	20.9 / 39.0	59.0 / 50.0	5.2 / 120	10.8 / 420	8.2 / 290	600	500	40	10.0
XMET Maxamaid (SHS)	AA	trace	SUC HCS				25.0 / 29.0	tr	62.0 / 71.0	25.0 / 580	22.0 / 840	13.0 / 450	810	810	200	12.0

NOTE: Formulas may change composition. These values are current as of 6/1/97. Check with manufacturers for updated information. All values used with permission.

METABOLIC FORMULAS FOR INFANTS AND CHILDREN
(continued)
Nutrient Analysis per 100 grams Powdered Formula

Product (Manufacturer)	PRO	SOURCES FAT	CHO	Kcal /ml /oz	mOsm/ kg H2O	RSL mOsm/l	PRO g/l %	FAT g/l %	CHO g/l %	Na mEq/l mg/l	K mEq/l mg/l	Cl mEq/l mg/l	Ca mg/l	Phos mg/l	Mg mg/l	Fe mg/l
XMET Maxamum (SHS)	AA	trace	SUC HCS				39.0 47.0	tr	45.0 53.0	24.0 560	18.0 700	16.0 560	670	670	285	23.5
XMTVI Analog® (SHS)	AA	PN.O. RAF Coc.O.	C.S.				13.0 11.0	20.9 39.0	59.0 50.0	5.2 120	10.8 420	8.2 290	600	500	40	10.0
XMTVI Maxamaid (SHS)	AA	trace	SUC HCS				25.0 29.0	tr	62.0 71.0	25.0 580	22.0 840	13.0 450	810	810	200	12.0
XP Analog® (SHS)	AA	PN.O. RAF Coc.O.	C.S.				13.0 11.0	20.9 39.0	59.0 50.0	5.2 120	10.8 420	8.2 290	600	500	40	10.0
XP Maxamaid (SHS)	AA	trace	SUC HCS				25.0 29.0	tr	62.0 71.0	25.0 580	22.0 840	13.0 450	810	810	200	12.0
XP Maxamum (SHS)	AA	trace	SUC HCS				39.0 47.0	tr	45.0 53.0	24.0 560	18.0 700	16.0 560	670	670	285	23.5
XPHEN TYR Analog (SHS)	AA	PN.O. RAF Coc.O.	C.S.				13.0 11.0	20.9 39.0	59.0 50.0	5.2 120	10.8 420	8.2 290	600	500	40	10.0
XPHEN TYR Maxamaid (SHS)	AA	trace	SUC HCS				25.0 29.0	tr	62.0 71.0	25.0 580	22.0 840	13.0 450	810	810	200	12.0
XPTM Analog® (SHS)	AA	PN.O. RAF Coc.O.	C.S.				13.0 11.0	20.9 39.0	59.0 50.0	5.2 120	10.8 420	8.2 290	600	500	40	10.0

NOTE: Formulas may change composition. These values are current as of 6/1/97. Check with manufacturers for updated information. All values used with permission.

497

Total Parenteral Nutrition
Indications for Use

Parenteral nutrition is needed to maintain or restore body weight and to promote growth and development in patients who cannot obtain sufficient nutrients by either the oral or enteral routes. The limited reserves of a premature infant require initiation of TPN if enteral nutrition cannot be begun by the third day of life. It is characterized by the provision of the intravenous dextrose, amino acids, electrolytes, vitamins, minerals, and trace elements either with or without lipids.

Peripheral vs. Central Parenteral Nutrition

Peripheral parenteral nutrition is appropriate for only a one to two-week period of nutrition support because the maximum calorie intakes achievable via the peripheral vein rarely exceed maintenance calorie requirements. Maintenance nutrition support may not be achievable if the patient is fluid restricted. In contrast, central parenteral nutrition allows one to meet calorie and nitrogen requirements for both growth and maintenance because higher concentrations of glucose and amino acids are quickly diluted with the rapid central venous blood flow. With peripheral venous access, it is recommended that the osmolarity of the TPN solution be ≤900 mOsm/L to avoid thrombophlebitis.

Maximum Suggested Dextrose Concentrations:

Neonates	12.5%
Infants and Young Children <25kg	10.0%
Older Children	5.0%

*Note: When determining maximum dextrose concentration, the amino acid and electrolyte concentrations of the final solution must also be considered. To estimate osmolarity of the TPN solution, the following equation may be used:

$$(100 \times \% \text{ amino acid}) + (50 \times \% \text{ dextrose}) + (2 \times \text{mEq/L Na+}) + (2 \times \text{mEq/L K+}) +$$
$$(1.4 \times \text{mEq/L Ca++}) + (1 \times \text{mEq/L Mg++}) = \text{mOsm/L}$$

Limit Ca++ to 5-10 mEq/L
Limit K+ to 40 mEq/L

Determining Nutritional Requirements

Calorie requirements represent the energy intake necessary for maintenance, growth and activity. For Neonates:

    a. Maintenance Needs: 50-60 kcal/kg per day
    b. Growth Needs: 70-120 kcal/kg per day

For the hospitalized child, maintenance calories may increase by 50 to 100% with severe stress (infection, trauma). The energy necessary for activity varies considerably between infants and disease states, and therefore must be individualized. The calorie cost for growth is at least five calories per gram of weight gain; however, the present clinical condition of each patient must be considered. Growth may not be a feasible goal during the acute stress situation, or early in an intensive care unit stay. Once the child is stabilized, calorie needs should be reassessed to provide for normal or catch-up weight gains.

Assessing the need to use catch-up growth formulas:

    a. Assess gestational age (<37 weeks = preterm)
    b. Assess growth of head circumference (up to age 24-36 months)
    c. If preterm, determine corrected age (until 2 years) by subtracting number of weeks premature from 40 weeks. For example: 24 weeks premature, subtract 16 weeks from actual age.
    d. Plot child on National Center for Health Statistics (NCHS) growth chart (growth charts for special conditions exist for Down's and Turner's Syndromes and Prematurity)

1. If <5th or >95th percentile weight, length or height for age, further evaluation is needed.
2. If <10th or >90th percentile weight for length, further evaluation is needed.
   Length should be checked weekly for infants and monthly for toddlers. Note length lags 4-6 weeks behind weight gain.
e. Determine ideal weight for length (height) by:
   1. Finding where patient's length is at 50th percentile length for age on NCHS chart.
   2. Draw vertical line from this point down to weight for age graph.
   3. Ideal weight for length is where the line intersects the 50th percentile on the weight for age graph.
f. Determine the severity of under/over weight (Waterlow Classification). Actual weight divided by ideal weight for length = weight/length ratio:

0.9-1.1	Normal
0.8-0.89	Mild Malnutrition
0.7-0.79	Moderate Malnutrition
< 0.7	Severe Malnutrition

The most important indications of nutritional status in pediatrics are the serial measures of weight and length. Follow the trend of weight for length ratio. Note any major changes in percentiles on the growth charts (≥ 2 growth channels). Compare the average weight gain to the expected weight gain for normal growth as listed below:

Age	Rate of Gain
0-3 months	25-39 grams/day
3-6 months	20 grams/day
6-9 months	15 grams/day
12-18 months	8 grams/day
18-24 months	6 grams/day
2-7 years	38 grams/month
7-9 years	56-62 grams/month
9-11 years	67-77 grams/month
11-13 years	85-110 grams/month

Calorie needs may be calculated by several methods. The RDA guidelines may also be used, but generally overestimate energy needs for parenteral support in many patients. The following are general guidelines for assessing calorie needs:

1. Recommended Dietary Allowances (1989)

Age	Kcal/kg	Protein gms/day
Preterm	120-150	6.0-4.0
0-6 months	108	2.2
6-12 months	98	1.6
1-3 years	102	1.2
4-6 years	90	1.2
7-10 years	70	1.0
11-14 years (Female	47	1.0
11.14 years (Male	55	1.0
15-18 years (Female)	40	0.8
15-18 years (Male)	45	0.9

2. If patient determined to need catch-up calories for growth, the following calculation can be used:
   a. Plot child's height and weight on the NCHS growth chart.
   b. Determine at what age the present weight would fall at the 50th percentile. This equals child's weight age.
   c. Determine recommended calories for weight age using the RDA's.
   d. Determine the ideal weight at the 50th percentile for the child's percent age. This equals child's ideal weight for chronological age.
   e. Multiply the recommended calories for weight age by the ideal weight.
   f. Divide this value by the child's actual weight

$$\frac{\text{Catch-up growth requirement}}{\text{Kcal/kg per day}} = \frac{\text{Calories required for weight age} \times \text{Ideal Weight for Age}}{\text{Actual Weight (kg)}}$$

3. As a function of weight
   100 kcal/kg for each kg up to 10 kg plus
   50 kcal/kg for each kg from 10-20 kg plus
   20 kcal/kg for each kg greater than 20 kg
   **For teens ≥ 16 years old needs may be near that of adult or approx 25-30 kcal/kg/day

4. Basal Energy Expenditure Multiplied by stress Factors
   a. Calculate the basal energy expenditure (BEE).
      1. The Harris-Benedict Equation may be used to calculate the BEE for children >20-25 kg (or >6 years old).
         Infants kcal/day = 22.1 + (31.05 x wt) + (1.16 x ht)

         3-10 year olds (FAO/WHO formula)
         Males   BEE = 22.7 x wt(kg) + 495
         Females   BEE = 22.5 x wt(kg) + 499

         10-18 year olds
         Males   BEE = 17.5 x wt(kg) + 631
         Females   BEE = 12.2 x wt(kg) + 746

      2. Basal Energy Expenditure may also be predicted using the following general guidelines (adapted from Reference 11):

Weight	Kcal/kg/day
Up to 12 kg	55
12-17 kg (12-36 months)	50
17-23 kg	45
23-30 kg	40
31-40 kg	35
41-60 kg	30
> 60kg	25

   b. Multiply BEE by a stress factor. General guidelines for stress factors are (11):
      Basic Maintenance   1.1-1.3
      Sepsis   1.4-1.5
      Mild to moderate trauma   1.2-1.3
      Severe trauma   1.5-1.7
      Cardiac failure   1.15-1.25
      Long term growth failure   1.5-2.0
      Burns (relates to extent) 1.3-2.0

5. Special Considerations
   a. Congenital heart disease: 125/kcal/kg/day or more
   b. BPD (Bronchopulmonary dysplasia):   120-150 kcal/kg/day
                                            70-80 kcal/kg/day if infant
                                            >9 mo old w/activity level decreased
   c. Developmental delays: For decreased activity: 10-12 kcal/cm ht or 1.2 x BEE
                              For increased activity: 15 kcal/cm ht
   d. Cystic Fibrosis: 40-50% >RDA
   e. Anoxic CNS: Begin with 60-70% RDA and adjust based on weight gain
   f. Refeeding Syndrome: Begin with 80-100% BEE and increase every 2-3 days. Close
                              electrolyte monitoring required.
   g. Quadriplegic/   As low as 50% RDA
        Spina Bifida

Monitoring patterns of weight gain or loss is necessary for determining appropriate calories to be administered via total parenteral nutrition. In the case of long term TPN support, ongoing reassessment of length (or height), and weight to length ratios should be utilized to evaluate the appropriateness of weight gain.

Considerations for Carbohydrate Composition of TPN

Dextrose content of the parenteral solution should be advanced over two to three days to reduce intolerance. The usual method is to increase dextrose concentration while keeping the volume of the parenteral solution the same.

	Maximum Suggested Dextrose Load
Preemie	4-6 mg/kg/min
Term/Neonate	12-14 mg/kg/min
Older Infant/Child	5-12 mg/kg/min

	Suggested PN Advancing Guidelines for Dextrose	
Preemie	Initial	4-6 mg/kg/min
	Advance	1-2 mg/kg/min
Term/Neonate	Initial	5%
	Advance	2-5%
Older Infant/Child	Initial	5-10%
	Advance	5%
Adolescent & Older	Initial	10%
	Advance	5-10%

The recommended maximum dextrose load for adults is 5 mg/kg/min. For pediatric patients, 25% dextrose concentration is the suggested maximum concentration with central TPN. Peripheral TPN dextrose concentrations must be kept much lower to avoid thrombophlebitis. Each gram of dextrose provides 3.4 kcal per gram.

Complications such as hyperglycemia which can lead to osmotic diuresis, loss of electrolytes and hyperosmolar coma can be avoided by glucose tests until goal rate and concentration are reached.

Protein

Protein Goals - General Guidelines

Premature/Neonate	2.5-3.0 g/kg/day
Infants	2.0-2.5
Children 2-13 yr	1.5-2.0
Adolescents	1.0-1.5

Estimated protein requirements during catch-up growth can be calculated using a similar equation to assess catch-up growth for calories:

a. Plot child's height and weight on the NCHS growth chart
b. Determine at what age the present weight would fall at the 50th percentile (= child's weight age).
c. Determine recommended protein for weight age using the RDA's.
d. Determine the ideal weight at the 50th percentile for the child's present age (= child's ideal weight for chronological age)
e. Multiply the recommended protein for weight age by the ideal weight
f. Divide this value by the child's actual weight

$$\frac{\text{Protein requirement}}{(\text{g/kg})} = \frac{\text{Protein required for Weight Age (g/kg)} \quad x \quad \text{Ideal Weight for age (kg)}}{\text{Actual Weight (kg)}}$$

Protein requirements for infants and children range from 0.5 to 3.0 gms/kg/day. Protein requirements are based per kg of weight. For optimal utilization of protein for anabolism, energy requirements must be met by a simultaneous infusion of non-protein energy sources. An optimal calorie to nitrogen ratio for pediatric patients is 100-200:1.

Suggested Nonprotein Calorie to Nitrogen Ratio

<10 kg	150:1 during acute stress, sepsis
	175-200:1 for maintenance, repletion
10-20 kg	120:1 during acute stress, sepsis
	150-175:1 for maintenance, repletion
>20 kg	100:1 during acute stress, sepsis
	150:1 for maintenance, repletion

Suggested PN Advancing Guidelines for Amino Acids
(AA gm/kg/day)

Preemie	Initial	0.25-0.5
	Advance in 1-2 days	0.5
Term/Neonate	Initial	0.5-1.0
	Advance/day	0.5-1.0
Older Infant/Child	Initial	1.0
	Advance/day	0.5-1.0
Adolescent/	Initial	1.0
Older	Advance/day	1.0

In addition to the amino acid formulations currently marketed for use in adults and older pediatric patients (over 6-8 years of age), there are two formulations marketed for use in preterm infants on long term TPN, or high risk infants <12 months: Aminosyn PF and TrophAmine. TrophAmine is considered the industry standard protein source for premature/stressed, neonates, and stressed smaller children. These solutions contain amino acids that may be conditionally essential for the premature infant.

Modifications of these pediatric amino acid solutions include:

> Increased branch chain and essential amino acids
> Decreased glycine, methionine and phenyalanine content
> Added taurine, tyrosine, aspartate, glutamate and cysteine*
> *Cysteine must be added separately at the time of compounding.

Complications such as hyperammonemia, acidosis, and azotemia can occur with protein intakes greater than 3-3.5 gm/kg/day for neonates and >4 gm/kg/day for pediatrics. Monitor serum BUN and Creatinine until goal is reached, then monitor weekly.

Fatty Acids

The use of parenteral lipid emulsions is indicated in the prevention or treatment of essential fatty acid deficiency (EFA), and as a calorie source. When used to prevent EFA deficiency, at least 2-4% of the total daily calorie goal should be supplied as EFA or linoleic acid. In infants and children, 0.5-1.0 grams/kg/day of fat emulsion is sufficient to prevent EFA deficiency. In general, only the 20% fat emulsions are used with the pediatric population. The dose should not exceed 4.0 grams/kg/day. The daily dose of parenteral fat emulsion should be administered over as much of the 24 hour period as possible. When used as a calorie source, fat should not exceed 60% of the nonprotein calorie intake. Intravenous fat infusion should be limited to 0.5-1.0 grams/kg/day in neonates who weigh less than 1000 grams with hyperbilirubinemia (>8mg%). The lipids can be advanced after actual bilirubin levels start to decline. For preterm infants weight less than 1000 grams maximum dose is 1.5-2.5 grams/kg/day or 100 mg/kg per hour. For preterm infants greater than 1000 grams, the maximum dose is 3.0-3.5 grams/kg/day or 150 mg/kg per hour. Infant maximum dose is 4 gms/kg/day; children and teens maximum dose is 2.5-3.0 gms/kg/day. Children and teenagers maximum dose is 2.5-3.0 gms/kg/day.

Lipid Clearance

Less than or equal to 32 week gestation and less than 1500 grams - the rate of lipid clearance is ≈ 0.16 gm/kg/hr

> Greater than 33 week gestation - the rate of clearance is ≈ 0.3 gm/kg/hr
> A term newborn's clearance is similar to an adults.

Suggested Guidelines for Advancing PN Lipids

		(Fat gm/kg/day)
Preemie	Initial	0.5
	Advance	0.5
Term/Neonate	Initial	0.5-1.0
	Advance	0.5
Older Infant/	Initial	1.0
Child	Advance	0.5-1.0
Adolescent/	Initial	1.0
Older	Advance	1.0

Potential Complications
- Altered pulmonary function
- Impaired immune function
- Increased kernicterus in newborns due to displacement of bilirubin by free fatty acids
- Hyperphospholipidemia
- Hypercholesterolemia
- Abnormal platelet function
- Allergic reaction

Fluid Requirements
1. 100 ml/kg for each kg up to 10 kg, plus
   50 ml/kg for each kg from 10-20 kg, plus
   20 ml/kg for each added kg greater than 20 kg.
2. Older children estimated 1 ml/kcal
3. Cardiac and renal patients must be individualized

Electrolytes
Electrolyte requirements are increased with severe diarrhea, vomiting, nasogastric losses and fistula losses. Decreased requirements are indicated with congestive heart failure and renal failure. The average daily requirements for electrolytes:

Electrolyte	Preterm Amount (per kg/day)	Term-3 yrs Young Children Amount (per kg/day)	Older Children >4 years Amount (per kg/day)
Sodium	2-4 mEq	2-5 mEq	2-4 mEq
Potassium	2-4 mEq	2-4 mEq	2-4 mEq
Magnesium	0.25-0.5 mEq	0.25-1.0 mEq	0.25-1 mEq
Phosphorus	1.3-1.5 mEq	0.5-2.0 mEq	0.5-2.0 mEq
Calcium*	1.0-3.0 mEq	0.5-1.0 mEq	0.2-0.5 mEq
Acetate	varies with acid/base status		
Chloride	"	"	"

*Preterm infants have significantly higher calcium and phosphorus needs. A general guideline for maximum concentrations for TPN solutions are:
   2.5 mEq per 100 ml Calcium concentration
   1.0 mM per 100 ml Phosphorus concentration
A maximal combined dose of 45 mMol of calcium and phosphorus is usually recommended.

NOTE: The maximum levels of calcium and phosphorus that can be added to TPN without precipitation vary based on the pH of the solution, amino acid concentration, dextrose concentration, and the type of parenteral components used for compounding. Consult with the pharmacy staff at your institution for guidelines regarding maximizing calcium and phosphorus in TPN.

Vitamins
For infants and children 2.5 kg to <40 kg or 11 years of age, 5 ml (1 vial) of reconstituted MVI-Pediatric product supplies the following per day (approximates requirements):

Vitamin A	2300 IU (or 0.7 mg Vit. A - retinol)
Vitamin D	400 IU/Kg (or 10 mcg)
Vitamin E	7 IU
Thiamine	1.2 mg
Riboflavin	1.4 mg
Pyridoxine (B6)	1.0 mg
Niacin	17.0 mg
Pantothenate	5.0 mg
Biotin	20.0 mcg
Folic Acid	140.0 mcg
Cyanocobalamin (B12)	1.0 mcg
Vitamin K	200.0 mcg
Ascorbic Acid	80.0 mg

Preterm Infants

Suggested to dose based on weight. 1.5 ml/kg/d of reconstituted MVI-Pediatric up to 2.5 kg. If infant weighs ≥ 2.5 kg, then give full 5 ml dose as described above.

Recommended Daily Dosage for Preterm Infants:

Vitamin A	1400 IU
Vitamin D	400 IU
Vitamin E	5 IU
Thiamine	0.6 mg
Riboflavin	0.8 mg
Pyridoxine	0.6 mg
Niacin	10 mg
Pantothenate	2.0 mg
Biotin	3.0 mcg
Folic Acid	65 mcg
Cyanocobalamin (B12)	0.4 mcg
Vitamin K	5 mcg/kg
Ascorbic Acid	50.0 mg

For Children >11 years of age or >40 kg

The 10 ml dose of MVI-12 used for adult TPN solutions is appropriate to meet requirements. Each 10 ml dose of the MVI-12 product supplies the following per day:

Vitamin A	3300 IU - or 10 mg Vitamin A - retinol
Vitamin D	200 IU - or 5 mcg)
Vitamin E	10 IU
Thiamine	3.0 mg
Riboflavin	3.6 mg
Pyridoxine (B6)	4.0 mg
Niacin	40.0 mg
Pantothenate	15.0 mg
Biotin	60.0 mcg
Folic Acid	400.0 mcg
Cyanocobalamin (B12)	5.0 mcg
Vitamin K	none
Ascorbic Acid	100.0 mg

Trace Elements

Guidelines for the use of parenteral trace elements in preterm/pediatrics are as follows:

Nutrient	Dose/Day
Zinc	
Premature infants <3 kg	400 mcg/kg
Term infants <3 months	250 mcg/kg
3 months-5 years	100 mcg/kg
Children	2.5-4.0 mg/day
Copper*	20 mcg/kg
Chromium*	0.2 mcg/kg
Manganese*	2-10 mcg/kg
Selenium**	2 mcg/kg
Molybdenum**	0.25 mcg/kg
Iodide	1.0 mcg/kg
Iron	
Premature infants <3 kg	None
Term infants <3 mos	1-1.5 mg/day
Children >1 yr	1.0 mg/day

*Omit in patients with obstructive jaundice.
**Limit in patients with impaired renal function.

When parenteral nutrition is limited to 1-2 weeks or is supplemental, only zinc need be added to the parenteral nutrition solution. If parenteral nutrition continues for longer than one month, selenium, iodide, and chromium can be added, and in the absence of cholestasis, copper and manganese can also be added. . Several pediatric multiple trace element products are available. For children >11 years of age or > 40 kg, one of the adult trace element mixtures may be used.

Iron

Iron, given as iron dextran, is usually only given as a treatment for iron deficiency anemia. Anaphylaxis has been reported in some patients given iron dextran. Guidelines for dosage and administration of iron dextran can be found in the manufacturer's package insert

Carnitine

Carnitine may be used with preterm infants or infants on long term TPN (>2 weeks). Suggested dose is 3-10 mg/kg. The goal for use is to improve fat oxidation and nitrogen balance.

Patient Monitoring

Growth

Weight	Daily
Height	Weekly - infants Monthly - over 1 year of age
Head circumference	Weekly - infants Monthly - under 2 years of age
Triceps skinfold, mid-arm muscle circumference, muscle circumference	Monthly if trained professional available

Parameter	Initiation	When Stable
Blood Glucose	4x/day	Daily
Urine, glucose, protein, ketones, specific gravity, pH	4x/day (if glucose > 130 mg)	3x/day
Vital Signs	Hourly x 4, then every 4 hours	3x/day
Intake and Output	Hourly	3x/day
Administration System	Hourly	3x/day
Infusion Site/ Dressing	Hourly	3x/day

Suggested Laboratory Monitoring

Pre-parenteral nutrition	Initiation phase	Maintenance phase
CBC Platelet count BUN Creatinine Glucose Calcium Phosphorus Cholesterol Uric acid Total protein Albumin ALT AST Alkaline phosphatase LDH Total bilirubin Conjugated bilirubin GGTP Triglycerides Magnesium Electrolytes Prealbumin Trace elements Ammonia	*Daily measurement of labs listed below until glucose and amino acid goal reached:* Electrolytes Glucose BUN Creatinine Calcium Phosphorus Magnesium Triglycerides CBC 2x/wk Ammonia 2x/wk	Electrolytes weekly CBC weekly BUN weekly Creatinine, glucose, calcium, , magnesium, Phosphorus, cholesterol, uric acid, total Protein, albumin, ALT, AST, alkaline Phosphatase, LDH, total bilirubin, conjugated Bilirubin, GGTP, triglycerides, magnesium and prealbumin weekly Vitamin A & E (for neonates > 1.5 kg) Zinc, copper, B_{12}, serum folate levels monthly Hematology studies iron, TIBC, ferritin) when imbalance Suspected Ammonia weekly
Acid-base status Serum-turbidity	Daily acid-base status Daily serum turbidity	Weekly acid-base status Weekly serum turbidity

TPN Cycling/Discontinuation

Cycling
- This administration provides for planned interruption of nutrient infusion.
- May stimulate normal patterns of food ingestion during day if TPN runs at night.
- Can allow child to use a normal daytime routine when run at night.
- Older children may be able to better tolerate a more concentrated solution in a shortened time period.

Discontinuation
- Wean down the infusion rate over a period of time to lesson the possibility of hypoglycemia; ex. TPN rate @ 140 cc/hr, decrease to 70 cc/hr x 1 hr, then 25 cc/hr x 1 hr.
- * If TPN discontinued abruptly, a 5% dextrose solution should be infused to prevent hypoglycemia.

Composition of Common Parenteral Nutrition Solutions

Calorie value of dextrose solutions

% Dextrose	Calories per ml
5	0.170
7.5	0.2553
10	0.340
12.5	0.425.
15	0.510
17.5	0.595
20	0.680
22.5	0.765
25	0.850

Fat emulsions

Product	Oil Source	% Linoleic Acid	% Linolenic Acid	Total kcal/ml	Osmolarity (mOsm/L)
Liposyn II 10% (Abbott)	Safflower Soybean	65.8	4.2	1.1	276
Liposyn II 20% (Abbott)	Safflower Soybean	65.8	4.2	2.0	258
Liposyn III 10% (Abbott)	Soybean	54.5	8.3	1.1	284
Liposyn III 20%	Soybean	54.5	8.3	2.0	292
Intralipid 10% (Clinitec)	Soybean	50	9	1.1	260
Intralipid 20% (Clinitec)	Soybean	50	9	2.0	260

Intravenous Nutritional Therapy

Protein Substrates

	CRYSTALLINE	AMINO	ACID	INFUSIONS	
	Aminosyn 3.5% (Abbott)	Aminosyn II 3.5% (Abbott)	Aminosyn 5% (Abbott)	Aminosyn II 5% (Abbott)	Travasol 5.5% (Clinitec)	TrophAmine 6% (McGaw)
Amino Acid Concentration	3.5%	3.5%	5%	5%	5.5%	6%
Nitrogen (g/100 ml)	0.55	0.54	0.79	0.77	0.925	0.93
Amino Acids (Essential) (mg/100 ml)						
Isoleucine	252	231	360	330	263	490
Leucine	329	350	470	500	340	840
Lysine	252	368	360	525	318	490
Methionine	140	50	200	86	318	200
Phenylalanine	154	104	220	149	340	290
Threonine	182	140	260	200	230	250
Tryptophan	56	70	80	100	99	120
Valine	280	175	400	250	252	470
Amino Acids (Nonessential) (mg/100 ml)						
Alanine	448	348	640	497	1140	320
Arginine	343	356	490	509	570	730
Histidine	105	105	150	150	241	290
Proline	300	253	430	361	230	410
Serine	147	186	210	265		230
Taurine						15
Tyrosine	31	95	44	135	22	140
Aminoacetic Acid (Glycine)	448	175	640	250	1140	220
Glumatic Acid		258		369		300
Asparatic Acid		245		350		190
Cysteine						< 14

Electrolytes (mEg/L)						
Sodium	7	16.3		19.3		5
Potassium			5.4			
Chloride					22	<3
Acetate	46	25.2	86	35.9	48	56
Phosphate (mM.L)						
Osomolarity (mOsm/L)	357	308	500	438	575	525
Supplied in (ml)	1000[2]	1000[3]	500[4] 1000[4]	500[3] 1000[3]	500[6] 1000[6] 2000[6]	500[6]
Labeled Indications						
Peripheral Parenteral Nutrition	Yes	Yes	Yes	Yes	Yes	Yes
Central TPN	No	No	Yes	Yes	Yes	Yes
Protein Sparing	Yes	Yes	Yes	Yes	Yes	No

1. Histidine is considered an essential amino acid in infants and in renal failure.
2. With 7 mEg/L sodium from the antioxidant sodium hydrosulfite.
3. Includes 20 mg/dl sodium hydrosulfite.
4. Includes 5.4 mEg/L potassium from the antioxidant potassium metabisulfite.
5. With =3 mEg/L sodium bisulfite.
6. With < 50 mg sodium metabisulfite per 100 ml.

Protein Substrates (cont.)

Crystalline Amino Acid Infusions

	Aminosyn 7% (Abbott)	Aminosyn PF 7% (Abbott)	Aminosyn II 7% (Abbott)	Aminosyn 8.5% (Abbott)
Amino Acid Concentration	7%	7%	7%	8.5%
Nitrogen (g/100ml)	1.1	1.07	1.07	1.34
Amino Acids (Essential) (mg/100ml)				
Isoleucine	510	534	462	620
Leucine	660	831	700	810
Lysine	510	475	735	624
Methionine	280	125	120	340
Phenylalanine	310	300	209	380
Threonine	370	360	280	460
Tryptophan	120	125	140	150
Valine	560	452	350	680
Amino Acids (Nonessential) (mg/100ml)				
Alanine	900	490	695	1100
Arginine	690	861	713	850
Histidine[1]	210	220	210	260
Proline	610	570	505	750

	Aminosyn 7% (Abbott)	Aminosyn PF 7% (Abbott)	Aminosyn II 7% (Abbott)	Aminosyn 8.5% (Abbott)
Serine	300	347	371	370
Taurine		50		
Tyrosine	44	44	189	44
Aminoecetic Acid (Glycine)	900	270	350	1100
Glutamic Acid		576	517	
Asptartic Acid		370	490	
Cysteine				
Electrolytes (mEg/L)				
Sodium		3.4	31.3	
Potassium	5.4			5.4
Chloride				35
Acetate	105	32.5	50.3	90
Phosphate (mM/L)				
Osmolarity (mOsm/L)	700	586	612	850
Supplied in (ml)	500[2]	250[3] 500[3]	500[4]	500[2] 1000[2]
Labeled Indications				
Peripheral Parenteral Nutrition	Yes	Yes	Yes	Yes
Central TPN	Yes	Yes	Yes	Yes
Protein Sparing	Yes	No	Yes	Yes

Copyright © October 1992 by Facts and Comparisons

1. Histidine is considered an essential amino acid in infants and in renal failure.
2. Includes 5.4 mE/g/L potassium from the antioxidant potassium metabisulfite.
3. From the antioxidant sodium hydrosulfite.
4. Includes 20 mg/dl sodium hydrosulfite.

Protein Substrates (Cont.)

CRYSTALLINE AMINO ACID INFUSIONS

	TrophAmino 10% (McGaw)	Aminosyn 10% (Abbott)	Aminosyn PF 10% (Abbott)	Aminosyn II 10% (Abbott)	Aminosyn (pH8) 10% (Abbott)
Amino Acid Concentration	10%	10%	10%	10%	10%
Nitrogen (g/100 ml)	1.55	1.57	1.52	1.53	1.57
Amino Acids (Essential) (mg/100ml)					
Isoleucine	820	720	760	660	720
Leucine	1400	940	1200	1000	940
Lysine	820	720	677	1050	720
Methionine	340	400	180	172	400
Phenylalanine	480	440	427	298	440
Threonine	420	520	512	400	520
Tryptophan	200	160	180	200	160
Valine	780	800	673	500	800
Amino Acids (Nonessential) (mg/100ml)					
Alanine	540	1280	698	993	1280
Arginine	1200	980	1227	1018	980
Histidine[1]	480	300	312	300	300
Proline	680	860	812	722	860
Serine	380	420	495	530	420
Taurine	25		70		
Tyrosine	240	44	40	270	44
Aminoacetic Acid (Glycine)	360	1280	385	500	1280
Glumatic Acid	500		620	738	
Asparatic Acid	320		527	700	
Cysteine	<16				
Electrolytes (mEg/L)					
Sodium	5		3.4	45.3	
Potassium		5.4			2.7
Chloride	<3				
Acetate	97	148	46.3	71.8	111
Phosphate (mM/L)10					
Osmolarity (mOsm/L)	875	1000	829	873	993
Supplied in (ml)	500[2]	500[3] 1000[3]	1000[4]	500[5] 1000[5]	500[6] 1000[6]
Labeled Indications					
Peripheral Parenteral	Yes	Yes	Yes	Yes	Yes
Central TPN	Yes	Yes	Yes	Yes	Yes
Protein Sparing	No	Yes	No	Yes	Yes

Copyright © October 1992 by Facts and Comparisons

1. Histidine is considered an essential amino acid in infants and in renal failure.
2. With <50 mg sodium metabisulfite per ml.
3. Includes 5.4 mEg/L potassium from the antioxidant potassium metabisulfite.
4. With 230 mg sodium hydrosulfite per 100 ml.
5. With 20 mg sodium hydrosulfite per 100 ml.
6. Potassium derived from the antioxidant potassium metabisulfite.

Professional references

1. Cochran EB, Phelps SJ, Helms RA. Parenteral Nutrition in the Pediatric Patient. <u>Clin Pharm</u> 7:351, 1988.
2. Committee on Nutrition, American Academy of Pediatrics. Pediatric Nutrition Handbook. 3rd Edition. Elk Grove Village: American Academy of Pediatrics, 1993.
3. Fisher AA, Poole RL, Machie R, Tsang C, Baugh N, Utley K, Kerner J. Clinical Pathway for Pediatric Parenteral Nutrition. <u>Nutr Clin Pract</u> 12:76-80, 1997.
4. Fomon SJ, et al. Body composition of Reference Children from Birth to Age Ten Years. <u>Am J Clin</u> Nutr35:1174, 1982.
5. Greene HL, Hambridge KM, Schandler et al. Guidelines for the Use of Vitamins, Trace Elements, Calcium, Magnesium and Phosphorus in Infants and Children Receiving Total Parenteral Nutrition. <u>Am J Clin Nutr</u> 48:1324, 1988.
6. Greene HL, Moore C, Phillips B, et al. Evaluation of a Pediatric Multiple Vitamin Preparation for Total Parenteral Nutrition. II. Blood levels of Vitamins A, D, E. <u>Pediatrics</u> 77:539, 1986.
7. Guidelines for the Use of Parenteral & Enteral Nutrition in Adult and Pediatric Patients. <u>JPEN</u> 17 Suppl: 31SA, 1993.
8. Hanning RM, Zlotkin SH. Amino Acid and Protein Needs of the Neonate: Effects of Excess and Deficiency. <u>Sem in Perinatol</u> 13: 131, 1989.
9. Heird WC, Dell RB, Helms RA, et al. Evaluation of an Amino Acid Mixture Designed to Maintain Normal Plasma Amino Acid Patterns in Infants and Children Receiving Parenteral Nutrition. <u>Pediatrics</u> 80: 401, 1987.
10. Heird WC, Parenteral Support of the Hospitalized Child IN Textbook of Pediatric Nutrition, 2nd Ed., Suskind (ed.), Raven Press, New York, 1993. pp. 225-238.
11. Hendricks KM. Estimation of Energy Needs IN Manual of Pediatric Nutrition, 2nd Ed, Hendricks & Walker (eds.), B.C. Decker, Inc., Philadelphia, PA, 1990. pp. 59-71.
12. Hill ID, Madrazo-de la Garza JA, Lebenthal E. Parenteral Nutrition in Pediatric Patients IN Parenteral Nutrition, 2nd Ed., Rombeau and Caldwell (Eds.), W.B. Saunders Co., Philadelphia, PA, 1993. pp. 770-790.
13. Johnson GC, Anderson JD. Compounding Considerations for Parenteral Nutrition. IN Nutrition Support Handbook, Teasley-Strausburg (eds.), Harvey Whitney Books Co., Cincinnati, OH,1992. pp. 133-146.
14. Kerner JA. Parenteral Nutrition IN Pediatric Gastrointestinal Disease, Vol. 2, Walker (ed.), B.C. Decker, Philadelphia, PA, 1991. pp. 1645-1675.
15. Payne-James JJ, Khawaja HT. First Choice for Total Parenteral Nutrition: The Peripheral Route. <u>JPEN</u> 17:468, 1993.
16. Pollack MM. Nutritional Support of Children in the Intensive Care Unit. IN Textbook of Pediatric Nutrition, 2nd Ed., Suskind (ed.), Raven Press, New York, 1993. pp. 207-216.
17. Gottschlich, MM, Matarese, LE, Shronts, EP, Nutrition Support Dietetics: Core Curriculum, Second Edition, A.S.P.E.N. Publications, 1993.
18. Fisher, AA, et. al., Clinical Pathway for Pediatric Parenteral Nutrition, Nutr in Clinical Practice, Apr 97, Vol. 12, No. 2, pp. 76-80.
19. Ford, Edward G., Nutrition Support in Pediatric Patients, Nutr in Clinical Practice, Oct 96, Vol. 11, pp. 183-191.
20. Conference Pediatric Parenteral Nutr, MCAspen, Lori Gross. MSRD, Nov. 1991.
21. Conference on Pediatric Nutr. Support, MCAapen, Lori Gross, MSRD., Sept. 1994.
22. Queen (Etc) Handbook of Pediatric Nutr. pp. 279-308.
23. Facts on Comparison Handbook, March 1997

FOOD AND NUTRITION BOARD, NATIONAL ACADEMY OF SCIENCES – NATIONAL RESEARCH COUNCIL
RECOMMENDED DIETARY ALLOWANCES,[a] Revised 1989[b]

Designed for the maintenance of good nutrition of practically all healthy people in the United States

Category	Age (years) or Condition	Weight (kg)	Weight (lb)	Height (cm)	Height (in)	Protein (g)	Fat-Soluble Vitamins				Water-Soluble Vitamins							Minerals						
							Vitamin A (µg R.E.)[c]	Vitamin D (µg)[d]	Vitamin E (mg α-TE)[e]	Vitamin K (µg)	Vitamin C (mg)	Thiamin (mg)	Riboflavin (mg)	Niacin (mg N.E.)[f]	Vitamin B6 (mg)	Folate (µg)	Vitamin B12 (µg)	Calcium (mg)	Phosphorus (mg)	Magnesium (mg)	Iron (mg)	Zinc (mg)	Iodine (µg)	Selenium (µg)
Infants	0.0-0.5	6	13	60	24	13	375	7.5	3	5	30	0.3	0.4	5	0.3	25	0.3	400	300	40	6	5	40	10
	0.5-1.0	9	20	71	28	14	375	10	4	10	35	0.4	0.5	6	0.6	35	0.5	600	500	60	10	5	50	15
Children	1-3	13	29	90	35	16	400	10	6	15	40	0.7	0.8	9	1.0	50	0.7	800	800	80	10	10	70	20
	4-6	20	44	112	44	24	500	10	7	20	45	0.9	1.1	12	1.1	75	1.0	800	800	120	10	10	90	20
	7-10	28	62	132	52	28	700	10	7	30	45	1.0	1.2	13	1.4	100	1.4	800	800	170	10	10	120	30
Males	11-14	45	99	157	62	45	1,000	10	10	45	50	1.3	1.5	17	1.7	150	2.0	1,200	1,200	270	12	15	150	40
	15-18	66	145	176	69	59	1,000	10	10	65	60	1.5	1.8	20	2.0	200	2.0	1,200	1,200	400	12	15	150	50
	19-24	72	160	177	70	58	1,000	10	10	70	60	1.5	1.7	19	2.0	200	2.0	1,200	1,200	350	10	15	150	70
	25-50	79	174	176	70	63	1,000	5	10	80	60	1.5	1.7	19	2.0	200	2.0	800	800	350	10	15	150	70
	51+	77	170	173	68	63	1,000	5	10	80	60	1.2	1.4	15	2.0	200	2.0	800	800	350	10	15	150	70
Females	11-14	46	101	157	62	46	800	10	8	45	50	1.1	1.3	15	1.4	150	2.0	1,200	1,200	280	15	12	150	45
	15-18	55	120	163	64	44	800	10	8	55	60	1.1	1.3	15	1.5	180	2.0	1,200	1,200	300	15	12	150	50
	19-24	58	128	164	65	46	800	10	8	60	60	1.1	1.3	15	1.6	180	2.0	1,200	1,200	280	15	12	150	55
	25-50	63	138	163	64	50	800	5	8	65	60	1.1	1.3	15	1.6	180	2.0	800	800	280	15	12	150	55
	51+	65	143	160	63	50	800	5	8	65	60	1.0	1.2	13	1.6	180	2.0	800	800	280	10	12	150	55
Pregnant						60	800	10	10	65	70	1.5	1.6	17	2.2	400	2.2	1,200	1,200	320	30	15	175	65
Lactating	1st 6 months					65	1,300	10	12	65	95	1.6	1.8	20	2.1	280	2.6	1,200	1,200	355	15	19	200	75
	2nd 6 months					62	1,200	10	11	65	90	1.6	1.7	20	2.1	260	2.6	1,200	1,200	340	15	16	200	75

551

[a] The allowances, expressed as average daily intakes over time, are intended to provide for individual variations among most normal persons as they live in the United States under usual environmental stresses. Diets should be based on a variety of common foods in order to provide other nutrients for which human requirements have been less well defined. See text for detailed discussion of allowances and of nutrients not tabulated.

[b] Weights and heights of Reference Adults are actual medians for the U.S. population of the designated age, as reported by NHANES II. The median weights and heights of those under 19 years of age were taken from Hamill et al. (1979) (see pages 16-17 of reference 1). The use of these figures does not imply that the height-to-weight ratios are ideal.

[c] Retinol equivalents. 1 retinol equivalent = 1 µg retinol or 6 µg β-carotene. See text for calculation of vitamin A activity of diets as retinol equivalents.

[d] As cholecalciferol. 10 µg cholecalciferol = 400 I.U. of vitamin D.

[e] α-Tocopherol equivalents. 1 mg d-α tocopherol = 1 α-T.E. See text for variation in allowances and calculation of vitamin E activity of the diet as α-tocopherol equivalents.

[f] 1 N.E. (niacin equivalent) is equal to 1 mg of niacin or 60 mg of dietary tryptophan.

*Reprinted with permission from the National Academy of Sciences, Washington, D.C.

The 10th edition of Recommended Dietary Allowances can be purchased for $19.95 plus $2.00 shipping from the National Academy Press, 2101 Constitution Ave., NW, Washington, DC 20418. To order by telephone, call toll free: 1-800-624-6242.

Median Heights and Weights and Recommended Energy Intake[a]

Category	Age (years) or Condition	Weight (kg)	Weight (lb)	Height (cm)	Height (in)	REE (kcal/day)	Multiples of REE	Average Energy Allowance (kcal)[b] Per kg	Per day[c]
Infants	0.0-0.5	6	13	60	24	320		108	650
	0.5-1.0	9	20	71	28	500		98	650
Children	1-3	13	29	90	35	740		102	1,300
	4-6	20	44	112	44	950		90	1,800
	7-10	28	62	132	52	1,130		70	2,000
Males	11-14	45	99	157	62	1,440	1.70	55	2,500
	15-18	66	145	176	69	1,760	1.67	45	3,000
	19-24	72	160	177	70	1,780	1.67	40	2,900
	25-50	79	174	176	70	1,800	1.60	37	2,900
	51+	77	170	173	68	1,530	1.50	30	2,300
Females	11-14	46	101	157	62	1,310	1.67	47	2,200
	15-18	55	120	163	64	1,370	1.60	40	2,200
	19-24	58	128	164	65	1,350	1.60	38	2,200
	25-50	63	138	163	64	1,380	1.55	36	2,200
	51+	65	143	160	63	1,280	1.50	30	1,900
Pregnant	1st trimester								+0
	2nd trimester								+300
	3rd trimester								+300
Lactating	1st 6 months								+500
	2nd 6 months								+500

a Calculation of REE (Resting Energy Expenditure) based on FAO equations, then rounded.
b In the range of light to moderate activity the coefficient of variation is ±20%.
c Figure is rounded.

Estimated Safe and Adequate Daily Dietary Intakes of Selected Vitamins and Minerals[a]

		Vitamins		Trace Elements[b]				
Category	Age (years)	Biotin (µg)	Pantothenic Acid (mg)	Copper (mg)	Manganese (mg)	Fluoride (mg)	Chromium (µg)	Molybdenum (µg)
Infants	0-0.5	10	2	0.4-0.6	0.3-0.6	0.1-0.5	10-40	15-30
	0.5-1	15	3	0.6-0.7	0.6-1.0	0.2-1.0	20-60	20-40
Children and adolescents	1-3	20	3	0.7-1.0	1.0-1.5	0.5-1.5	20-80	25-50
	4-6	25	3-4	1.0-1.5	1.5-2.0	1.0-2.5	30-120	30-75
	7-10	30	4-5	1.0-2.0	2.0-3.0	1.5-2.5	50-200	50-150
	11+	30-100	4-7	1.5-2.5	2.0-5.0	1.5-2.5	50-200	75-250
Adults		30-100	4-7	1.5-3.0	2.0-5.0	1.5-4.0	50-200	75-250

a Because there is less information on which to base allowances, these figures are not given in the main table of RDA and are provided here in the form of ranges of recommended intakes.
b Since the toxic levels for many trace elements may be only several times usual intakes, the upper levels for the trace elements given in this table should not be habitually exceeded.

Estimated Sodium, Chloride, and Potassium Minimum Requirements of Healthy Persons[a]

Age	Weight (kg)[a]	Sodium (mg)[a,b]	Chloride (mg)[a,b]	Potassium (mg)[c]
Months				
0-5	4.5	120	180	500
6-11	8.9	200	300	700
Years				
1	11.0	225	350	1,000
2-5	16.0	300	500	1,400
6-9	25.0	400	600	1,600
10-18	50.0	500	750	2,000
>18[d]	70.0	500	750	2,000

a No allowance has been included for large, prolonged losses from the skin through sweat.
b There is no evidence that higher intakes confer any health benefit.
c Desirable intakes of potassium may considerably exceed these values (~3,500 mg for adults).
d No allowance included for growth. Values for those below 18 years assume a growth rate at the 50th percentile reported by the National Center for Health Statistics (Hamill et al., 1979 in reference 1) and averaged for males and females.

552

GIRLS: BIRTH TO 36 MONTHS
HEAD CIRCUMFERENCE FOR AGE &
WEIGHT FOR LENGTH

NAME_____ RECORD #_____

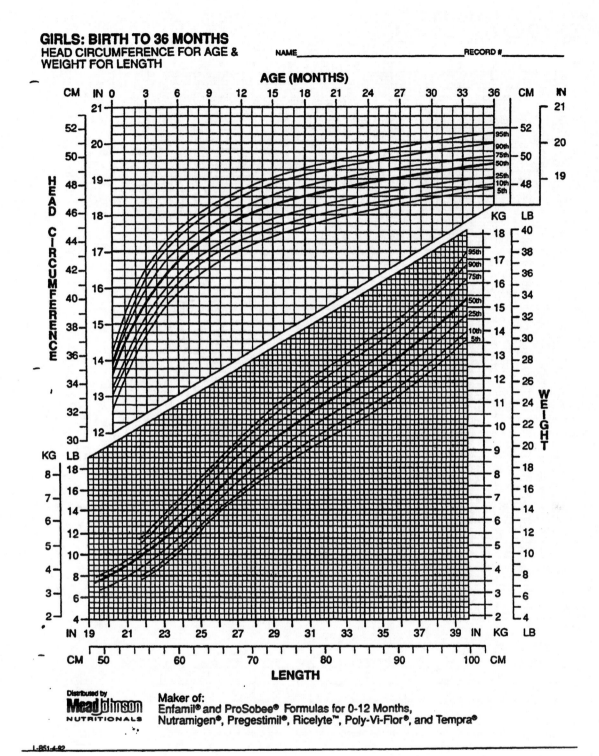

AGE (MONTHS)

HEAD CIRCUMFERENCE

LENGTH

WEIGHT

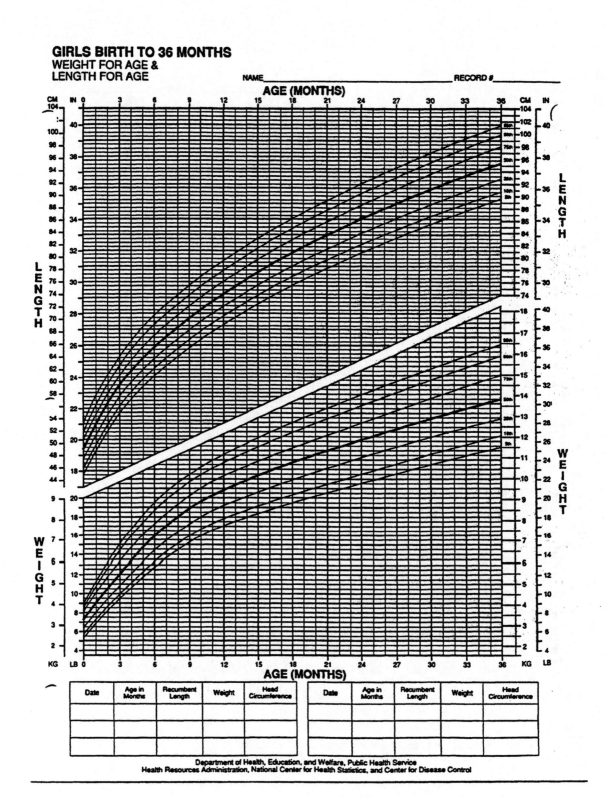

GIRLS BIRTH TO 36 MONTHS
WEIGHT FOR AGE &
LENGTH FOR AGE

NAME_____ RECORD #_____

AGE (MONTHS)

Date	Age in Months	Recumbent Length	Weight	Head Circumference		Date	Age in Months	Recumbent Length	Weight	Head Circumference

Department of Health, Education, and Welfare, Public Health Service
Health Resources Administration, National Center for Health Statistics, and Center for Disease Control

GIRLS: PREPUBESCENT
PHYSICAL GROWTH
NCHS PERCENTILES*

NAME_____ RECORD #_____

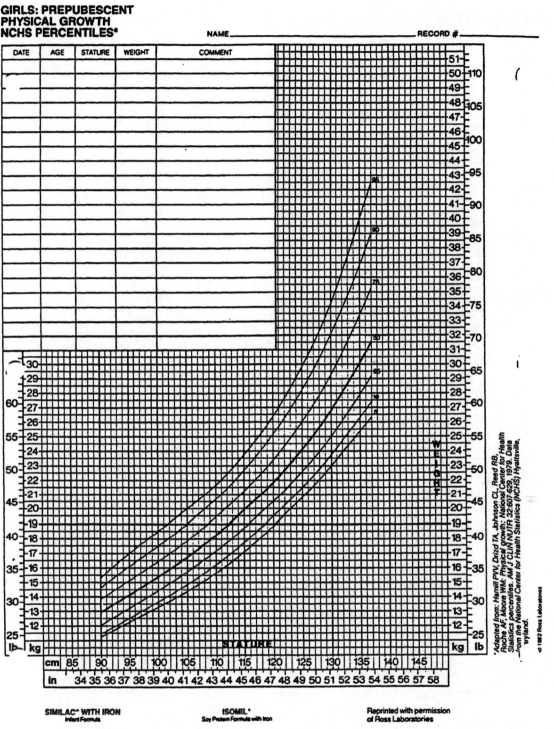

*Adapted from: Hamill PVV, Drizd TA, Johnson CL, Reed RB, Roche AF, Moore WM: Physical growth: National Center for Health Statistics percentiles. AM J CLIN NUTR 32:607-629, 1979. Data from the National Center for Health Statistics (NCHS) Hyattsville, Maryland.

© 1982 Ross Laboratories

SIMILAC® WITH IRON
Infant Formula

ISOMIL®
Soy Protein Formula with Iron

Reprinted with permission
of Ross Laboratories

GIRLS: 2 TO 18 YEARS
PHYSICAL GROWTH
NCHS PERCENTILES*

NAME_____ RECORD #_____

Used with permission of Ross Products Division,
Abbott Laboratories, Columbus, OH 43216 from NCHS Growth Charts,
© 1982 Ross Products Division, Abbott Laboratories.

*Adapted from: Hamill PVV, Drizd TA, Johnson CL, Reed RB,
Roche AF, Moore WM: Physical growth: National Center for Health
Statistics percentiles. AM J CLIN NUTR 32:607-629, 1979. Data
from the National Center for Health Statistics (NCHS), Hyattsville,
Maryland.

© 1982 Ross Laboratories

NAME_____ RECORD #_____

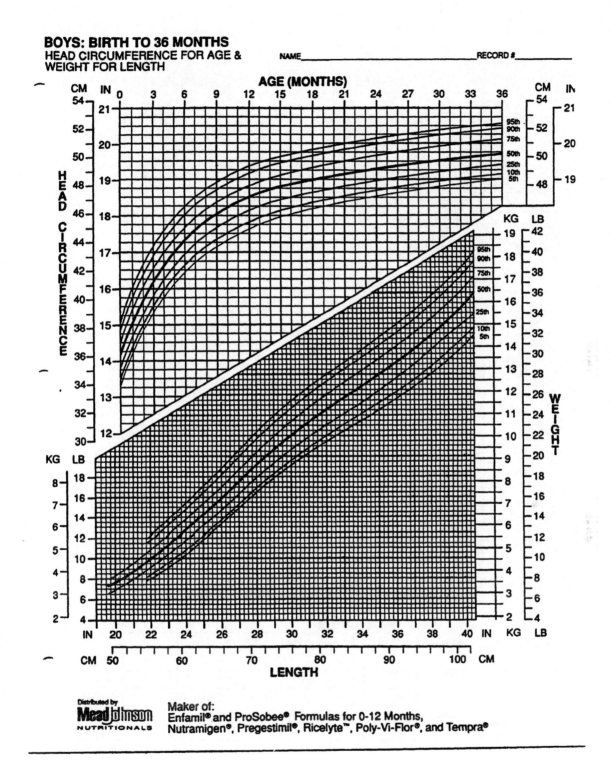

BOYS BIRTH TO 36 MONTHS
WEIGHT FOR AGE &
LENGTH FOR AGE

NAME_____ RECORD #_____

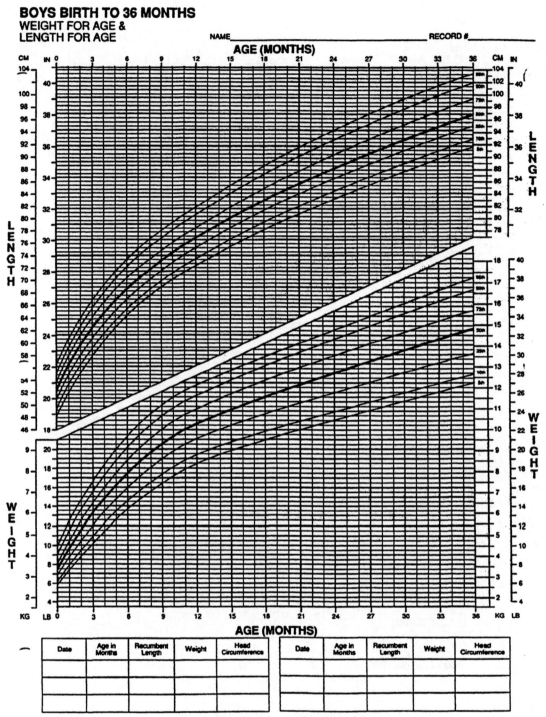

	Date	Age in Months	Recumbent Length	Weight	Head Circumference		Date	Age in Months	Recumbent Length	Weight	Head Circumference

Department of Health, Education, and Welfare, Public Health Service
Health Resources Administration, National Center for Health Statistics, and Center for Disease Control

BOYS: 2 TO 18 YEARS
PHYSICAL GROWTH
NCHS PERCENTILES*

NAME _____ RECORD # _____

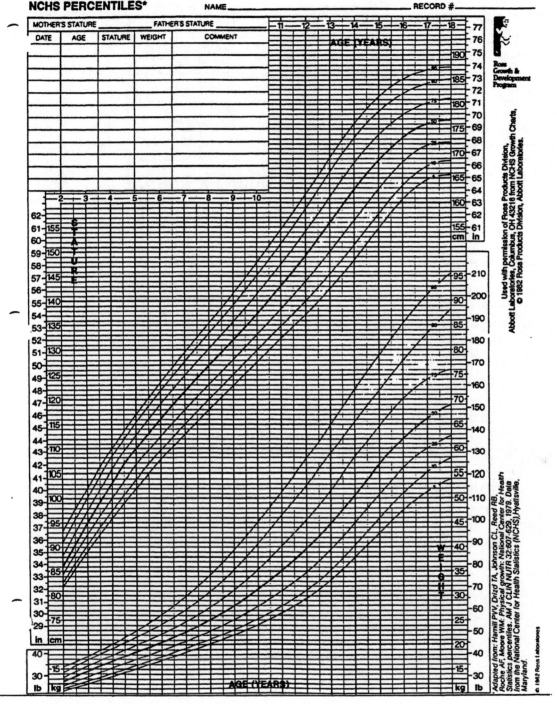

Ross
Growth &
Development
Program

523

BOYS: PREPUBESCENT
PHYSICAL GROWTH
NCHS PERCENTILES*

NAME_____ RECORD #_____

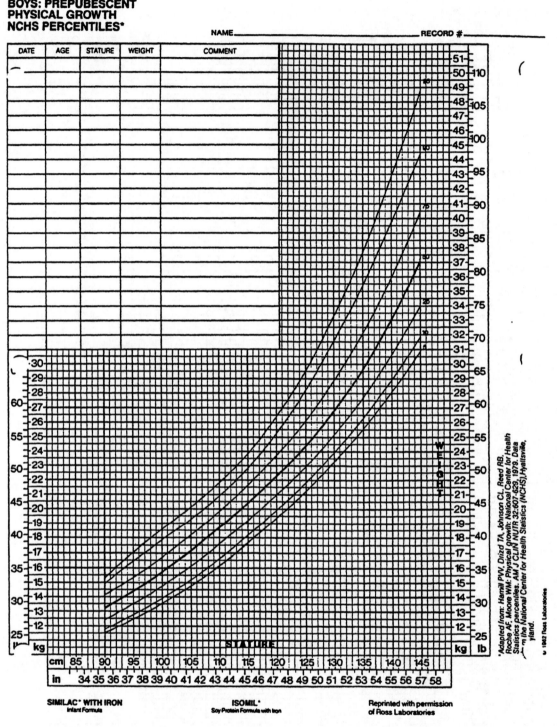

SIMILAC* WITH IRON
Infant Formula

ISOMIL*
Soy Protein Formula with Iron

Reprinted with permission
of Ross Laboratories

*Adapted from: Hamill PVV, Drizd TA, Johnson CL, Reed RB, Roche AF, Moore WM: Physical growth: National Center for Health Statistics percentiles. AM J CLIN NUTR 32:607-629, 1979. Data from the National Center for Health Statistics (NCHS), Hyattsville, Maryland.

© 1982 Ross Laboratories

LAB VALUES
Deviations in Disease

(B=Blood; P=Plasma; S=Serum; U=Urine)

CONSTITUENT	DECREASED IN	INCREASED IN
Chemistry		
Acetone (S)		Starvation Uncontrolled diabetes
Alkaline phosphatase (S)	Hypothyroidism Protein-calorie malnutrition Gross anemia Vitamin C deficiency: scurvy Cretinism Hypervitaminosis—vitamin D Celiac disease Milk-alkali syndrome (excess calcium and antacids)	Hyperparathyroidism Metastatic liver disease Hepatic disease Obstructive jaundice Cushing's syndrome Growth periods Pregnancy Carcinoma with bone metastasis Vitamin D deficiency: rickets, osteomalacia Paget's disease of bone Osteogenic sarcoma
Ammonia (B)		Liver cirrhosis Hepatic encephalopathy
Amylase (U)	Liver disease Renal disease	Carcinoma—pancreas Acute pancreatitis Common bile duct stones
Amylase (S)	Necrotic pancreatitis Hepatitis Severe burns Congestive heart failure Adrenocortical stress Toxemia of pregnancy	Gross alcohol intake Renal disease Cholecystitis Diabetic coma Acute pancreatitis Obstruction of pancreatic ducts Post-gastrectomy
Bilirubin (S) (total)		Massive hemolysis Hepatitis Carcinoma of liver or pancreas Biliary tract obstruction Obstructive liver disease Hemolytic disease Hepatotoxic drugs

CONSTITUENT	DECREASED IN	INCREASED IN

Calcium (S)	Hypoparathyroidism
	Renal insufficiency
	Hypoproteinemia
	Acute pancreatitis
	Malnutrition
	Malabsorption syndrome
	  (steatorrhea)
	Pregnancy
	
	Respiratory alkalosis
	Magnesium deficiency
	Vitamin D deficiency: rickets,
	  osteomalacia
		Hyperparathyroidism
		Osteolytic disease
		Metastatic cancer to bones
		Multiple myeloma
		Hypervitaminosis - vitamin D
		Malignant tumors
		Milk-alkali syndrome
		
		Paget's disease of the bones
		Sarcoidosis
		Thyrotoxicosis
		Bone fractures
		Immobilization

Chloride (S)	Gastrointestinal disease with
	  fluid loss: diarrhea, vomiting
	Emphysema
	Congestive heart failure
	Chronic obstructive pulmonary
	  disease (COPD)
	Addison's disease
	Iatrogenic: hypokalemic-
	  chloremic alkalosis (diuretics)
	Potassium-saving diuretics
	  (no chloride replacement)
		Dehydration
		Primary hyperparathyroidism
		Renal tubular acidosis
		Iatrogenic: inappropriate
		  IV fluids

Cholesterol (S)	Hyperthyroidism
	Malnutrition
	Severe sepsis
	Idiopathic steatorrhea
	Extensive liver disease
	Anemia (megaloblastic,
	  hypochromic)
		Hypothyroidism
		Liver disease with
		  biliary obstruction
		Nephrotic stage of
		  glomerulonephritis
		Diabetes mellitus
		Chronic pancreatitis
		Familial hypercholesterolemia
		High dietary intake

Cholesterol (HDL) (S)	Liver failure Heredity	Exercise
Copper (S)	Anemia Wilson's disease Skeletal lesions	
Creatinine (S or P)	Hyperparathyroidism Acromegaly	Renal disease Uremia Severe congestive heart failure Muscle-wasting diseases

CONSTITUENT	DECREASED IN	INCREASED IN
Creatinine phospho- kinase (S)		Myocardial Infarction Necrosis: heart, skeleton, muscle, bone Alcohol withdrawal Shock, convulsions Exercise Muscle trauma
Glucose (B)	Pancreatic islet cell tumor Hyperinsulinism Addison's disease Extensive liver disease Reactive hypoglycemia	Diabetes mellitus Hyperthyroidism Pancreatic insufficiency Cushing's syndrome Acute stress Pheochromocytoma
Iodine - PBI (S)	Hypothyroidism Dietary deficiency	Hyperthyroidism Thyroiditis
Iron (S)	Iron-deficiency anemia Nephrosis Chronic renal insufficiency Infections	Hemochromatosis Hemolytic disease Liver disease Transfusions Hemosiderosis Thalassemia Untreated macrocytic anemia
Iron-binding capacity	Transfusions Hemochromatosis Malnutrition Infection Liver cirrhosis Nephrosis Rheumatoid arthritis Protein-losing enteropathies Uremia	Hepatitis Hemorrhage Iron-deficiency anemia Pregnancy Hypoxia

CONSTITUENT	DECREASED IN	INCREASED IN
Lactic dehydrogenase (S)		Tissue necrosis (particularly with heart, red cells, kidney, skeleton, muscle, liver, and skin) Hemolytic disorders Pernicious anemia Myocardial infarction Infectious hepatitis Liver disease Acute pancreatitis Pulmonary infarction Tumors Shock Surgical trauma Cerebral vascular accident
Lipase (S)		Acute pancreatitis Intestinal obstruction Duodenal ulcer Pancreatic duct obstruction (gallstones)

Magnesium (S)	Chronic alcoholism
	Primary aldosteronism
	Inadequate dietary intake
	Vomiting, diarrhea
	Increased urinary losses:
	  diabetic ketoacidosis,
	  hyperthyroidism
		Renal failure

Nonprotein nitrogen - (B, P, and S)		Dehydration Renal disease Intestinal obstruction Metallic poisoning
Phospholipids	Malnutrition	Obstructive jaundice Nephrosis Diabetic acidosis

Phosphorus	Hyperparathyroidism
	Vitamin D deficiency:
	  rickets, osteomalacia
	Malabsorption: celiac
	  disease, sprue
	Malnutrition
	Renal tubular acidosis
		Sarcoidosis
		Renal insufficiency
		Chronic glomerular disease
		Hypoparathyroidism
		Hypervitaminosis—D
		Milk-alkali syndrome

CONSTITUENT	DECREASED IN	INCREASED IN
Potassium (S)	Starvation Malabsorption syndromes Cushing's syndrome Chronic fever Malignant hypertension Poor dietary intake Anti-inflammatory drugs Renal tubular acidosis	Adrenal insufficiency - (Addison's disease) Renal failure Acute infection

Potassium (S)—continued	Liver disease with ascites
	Unusual losses: vomiting,
	  chronic diarrhea, chronic
	  use of non-potassium sparing
	  diuretics	

AST (formerly SGOT)		Myocardial infarction
		Infections (post-trauma and
		  generalized
		Skeletal muscle diseases:
		  muscular dystrophy
		Myocarditis
		Cardiomyopathies
		Pericarditis
		Pulmonary infarction
		Shock, burns, crushing injuries
		Liver necrosis or disease:
		  cirrhosis, hepatitis,
		  metastatic liver disease

Sodium (S)	Adrenal insufficiency
	Renal insufficiency
	Renal tubular acidosis
	Diabetic acidosis
	Starvation with acidosis
	Dilutional hyponatremia:
	  excessive water administration,
	  congestive heart failure,
	  diuretics with sodium
	  restriction, hepatic failure with
	  ascites, oliguria
		Dehydration
		Hyperadrenocorticalism
		Iatrogenic

Triglycerides		Hyperlipoproteinemia

CONSTITUENT	DECREASED IN	INCREASED IN
Urea Nitrogen (BUN)	Cirrhosis Hepatic failure Starvation Nephrosis not complicated with renal insufficiency Overhydration	Acute or chronic renal failure Congestive heart failure Tumor: urinary obstruction Bleeding gastric ulcer Dehydration Mercury poisoning High protein catabolism
Uric Acid	Acute hepatitis	Gout Increased cell breakdown: leukemia, chemotherapy Polycythemia Renal insufficiency Arthritis Eclampsia
Vitamin A	Cirrhosis Infectious hepatitis Pancreatic insufficiency Chronic obstructive pulmonary disease Congestive heart failure Thyrotoxicosis Malnutrition	
Vitamin C	Infection Leukemia Dietary deficiency	
Protein (S)	Malnutrition Malabsorption syndrome Glomerulonephritis Nephrosis Leukemia Chronic liver disease	Dehydration Multiple myeloma Hepatic disease Systemic lupus erythematosis

Albumin (S)	Liver disease
	Malnutrition
	Chronic loss: nephrotic
	  syndrome, burns
	Congestive heart failure
	Cirrhosis
	Pancreatic insufficiency
	Malabsorption syndrome:
	  protein-losing enteropathies
	Eclampsia
	Overhydration
		Dehydration

CONSTITUENT	DECREASED IN	INCREASED IN
Globulin (S)		Liver disease: cirrhosis, hepatitis Infection Multiple myeloma Hodgkin's disease Leukemia Collagen disease Advanced carcinoma Sarcoidosis Lymphomas Hyperlipidemia Tuberculosis

Hematology

CONSTITUENT	DECREASED IN	INCREASED IN
Hemoglobin	Protein-calorie malnutrition Hemorrhage Anemia Hypochromic, microcytic anemia: iron deficiency, sickle cell anemia, thalassemia, hemoglobin C disease Normochromic, normocytic anemia: hemorrhage, hemolysis, aplastic anemia Macrocytic anemia (with increased MCV & increased MCHC): folic acid deficiency, vitamin B_{12} deficiency (pernicious anemia)	Polycythemia Dehydration
Hematocrit	Anemias Hemorrhage Fluid overload	Polycythemia Dehydration
Platelet	Absolute absence: aplastic bone marrow Thrombocytopenia	Polycythemia Essential thrombocytosis Splenectomy
Red blood count	Hemorrhage Anemias Chronic infections	Polycythemia Dehydration
White blood count	Susceptibility to infection Malnutrition	Acute infection Leukemia

CONSTITUENT	DECREASED IN	Dehydration INCREASED IN
Chemistry— Urine		
Albumin		Toxic dehydration Chronic uncontrolled diabetes Nephrotic syndrome
Bile		Presence indicates hepatic obstruction
Glucose		High blood sugar Low renal threshold
Ketones		Decreased CHO metabolism
Nitrates		Urinary tract infection
pH—Urine	Acidosis	Alkalosis
Protein		Renal failure Circulatory changes
Urobilinogen	Obstructive jaundice Hepatic jaundice	Tumor Congestive heart failure Hepatocellular failure
Vanillylmandelic acid		Pheochromocytoma
Other		
CO_2	Metabolic acidosis Hyperventilation	Metabolic alkalosis Hypoventilation Excessive diarrhea
Creatinine clearance (S and U)		Renal insufficiency
Fat, quantitative		Cystic fibrosis Celiac disease
pH—blood	Acidosis	Alkalosis
Sweat chloride		Cystic fibrosis

PROFESSIONAL REFERENCES

1. Fischback F. A manual of laboratory diagnostic tests. 2nd ed. St. Louis: J.B. Lippincott, 1984.

2. Monsen, ER. The journal adopts SI units for clinical laboratory values. J Am Dietetic Assoc 1987; 87(3):356-8.

3. Tilkian, SM, Conover MB, Tilkian AG. Clinical implications of laboratory tests. 4th ed. St. Louis: C.V. Mosby, 1987.

4. Young DS. Implications of SI units for clinical laboratory data style specifications and conversion tables Ann Intern Med 1987; 106:114.

POTENTIAL RENAL SOLUTE LOAD (PRSL)

DESCRIPTION

Potential Renal Solute Load (PRSL) should be considered in circumstances when water balance is a primary concern.

Indications for Use

1. Relatively low fluid intake
2. Greater than normal extra-renal losses of fluid
3. Low renal concentrating ability
4. Consumption of a diet that yields a large renal solute load

Major Constituents

	Premature Infant (not growing)*	Full-term Infant (growing)
Protein	5.7 mOsm/gm.	4 mOsm/gm.
Sodium	1 mOsm/gm.	1 mOsm/mEq
Potassium	1 mOsm/mEq	1 mOsm/mEq
Chloride	1 mOsm/mEq	1 mOsm/mEq
Phosphorus	0.032 mOsm/mg.	--**

*   The growing premature infant retain 1 mOsm/gm. protein for growth.

**   Phosphorus contributes the same amount of solute to the PRSL as is retained by sodium, potassium, and chloride combined. Therefore, phosphorus does not need to be considered for a full-term infant.

Other non-nitrogenous urinary solutes are ordinarily of minor importance relative to sodium, chloride, potassium, and phosphorus.

Calculation of PRSL

For Premature Infants

PRSL/100 ml. = (Protein gm./100 ml. x 5.7) + [Na (mEq/100 ml.) + K (mEq/100 ml.) + Cl (mEq/100 ml.)] + P mg./100 ml. x 0.032)

For Full-term Infants:

PRSL/100 ml. = (Protein gm./100 ml. x 4) + [Na (mEq/100 ml.) + K (mEq/100 ml.) + Cl (mEq/100 ml.)]

PROFESSIONAL REFERENCES

1. Bergman KE, Ziegler EE, Fomon SJ. Water and renal solute load. In: Fomon SJ. Infant nutrition, 2nd ed. Philadelphia: W.B. Saunders Co., 1974:245.

2. Ziegler EE, Fomon SJ. Fluid intake, renal solute load, and water balance in infancy. J Pediatr 1971; 78:561.

3. Ziegler EE, Ryu JE. Renal solute load and diet in growing premature infants. J Pediatr 1976; 89:609.

CONVERSION FACTORS

OUNCES TO GRAMS

To convert ounces to grams, multiply ounces by 30 (the exact figure is 28.35).

POUNDS TO KILOGRAMS

To convert pounds to kilograms, multiply pounds by 0.45, or divide by 2.2.

INCHES TO CENTIMETERS

To convert inches to centimeters, multiply inches by 2.54.

KILOCALORIE TO JOULE

One kilocalorie = 4.184×10^3 joules, or 4.184 kilojoules (kjoule).

MILLIGRAMS TO MILLIEQUIVALENTS

To convert milligrams to milliequivalents, multiply milligrams by the valence and divide by the atomic weight:

$$\underline{\text{Milligrams x Valence}} = \text{Milliequivalents}$$
$$\text{Atomic Weight}$$

MILLIEQUIVALENTS TO MILLIGRAMS

To convert milliequivalents to milligrams, multiply atomic weight by milliequivalents and divide by valence:

$$\underline{\text{Atomic Weight x Milliequivalents}} = \text{Milligrams}$$
$$\text{Valence}$$

	Atomic Weight	Valence
Calcium	40.07	2
Chlorine	35.5	1
Magnesium	24.3	2
Phosphorus	31.04	2
Potassium	39.0	1
Sodium	23.0	1

SODIUM CHLORIDE TO SODIUM

To convert sodium chloride to sodium, multiply by 0.393.
Example: 5 grams of sodium chloride = 5 x 0.393 = 2,000 milligrams of sodium

SODIUM TO SODIUM CHLORIDE

To convert sodium to sodium chloride, multiply by 2.54.
Example: 1,000 milligrams of sodium = 1,000 x 2.54 = 2,540 milligrams of sodium chloride.

IU (INTERNATIONAL UNITS) TO RE (RETINOL EQUIVALENTS)

To convert international units of retinol to retinol equivalents, divide IU by 3.33.

To convert international units of B-carotene to retinol equivalents, divide IU by 10.

IU (INTERNATIONAL UNITS) TO a-TE (a-TOCOPHEROL EQUIVALENT)

To convert international units of vitamin E to a-tocopherol equivalents, multiply IU by 0.70.

TABLE OF WEIGHTS AND MEASURES

Common Measurement	Milliliters (ml)	Grams (g)	Teaspoons (tsp.)	Tablespoons (tbsp.)	Cups (c.)	Ounces (oz.)	Pounds (lb.)
1 teaspoon	5	5	1	1/3	1/48	0.167	-
1 tablespoon	15	15	3	1	1/16	0.5	-
1/4 cup	60	60	12	4	1/4	2.0	1/8 (0.125)
1/3 cup	80	80	16	5-1/3	1/3	2.67	-
1/2 cup	120	120	24	8	1/2	4.0	1/4 (0.250)
3/4 cup	180	180	36	12	3/4	6.0	-
1 cup	240	240	48	16	1	8.0	1/2 (0.500)
1 pint	480	480	96	32	2	16.0	1
1 quart	960	960	192	64	4	32	2
1 liter	1,000	1,000	200	66.67	4.167	35.2	2.2
1 gallon	3,840	3,840	763	256	16	128	8

For convenience, 1 milliliter is considered equivalent to 1 gram (1 ml = 1 g). One ounce equals 28.35 grams. For easy computing purposes, however, 30 grams (or 30 ml) is considered equivalent to 1 ounce.

Prenatal Weight Gain Grid Instructions

1. Select appropriate gain grid based on the individuals' height and pregravid weight status.

Height w/o shoes	Standard Weight (in pounds)	Underweight <90% Standard	Overweight >120% Standard	Very Overweight >135% Standard
4'9"	104	94	125	140
4'10"	107	96	128	144
4'11"	110	99	132	148
5'0"	113	102	136	153
5'1"	116	103	139	157
5'2"	118	106	142	159
5'3"	123	111	148	166
5'4"	128	115	154	173
5'5"	132	119	158	178
5'6"	136	122	163	184
5'7"	140	126	168	189
5'8"	144	130	173	194
5'9"	148	133	178	200
5'10"	152	137	182	205
5'11"	156	140	187	211
6'0"	160	144	192	216

2. Plot weight gain

If pregravid weight is known:
a. Calculate the amount of weight gained or lost.
b. Find the vertical line on the grid that corresponds with the number of weeks gestation for the visit.
c. Place a mark where the weeks gestation intersect the number of pounds of weight gained or lost.
d. At each prenatal visit, the weight gain or loss is plotted at the appropriate weeks gestation.

If pregravid weight in unknown, or if reported pregravid weight seems unreasonable:
a. Use the weight measured at the first clinic visit to select the correct grid.
b. Place a mark on the grid at the point where the weeks gestation intersect with the curve in the first trimester or middle of the established range during the second and third trimester.

If gestational age is changed due to ultrasound testing during the course of the pregnancy, begin plotting for the new gestational age on the same grid and note the reason for the change.

3. Inform woman of recommended total weight gain ranges for her pregravid weight.

Pregravid Status	Pounds
Underweight (<90%)	28-40
Standard weight (90-120%)	25-35
Overweight (>120%)	15-25
Very Overweight (>135%)	15-20

4. Monitor rate of weight gain.

The rate of weight gain is just as important as total weight gain. Women with excessive or inadequate weight gains will need personalized counseling in order to determine the cause and to help them normalize their gain. These women should be referred to their health care provider for assistance.

1st trimester		2-5 pounds
2nd and 3rd trimester	Underweight:	Slightly more than 1 lb/week
	Standard Weight:	Approximately 1 lb/week
	Overweight	Slightly more than 1/2 lb/week
	Very overweight:	Plot on overweight grid, however, individual weight gain rate (curve) should be set by her caregiver.

Used with permission of: The California Department of Health Services, Maternal and Child Health Branch

B

baby bottle tooth decay, 30
    cerebral palsy and, 440
beriberi, thiamin and, 37
bile acid sequestrants, 231–232
binge eating syndrome (BED), 431–432
binge eating, bulimia nervosa and, 429–431
biotin, 37
bland diet, 105–108
blindness, night, vitamin A and, 38
blood glucose goals, diabetes and, 147
body mass index (BMI), 412, 415
bone deformation, calcium and, 39
bone demineralization, phosphorus and, 39
bone development problems, vitamin A and, 38
bottle feeding, cleft lip and/or palate, 444
bottle mouth, nursing, 30
breastfeeding, 11–13, 16–21
bruising, vitamin C and, 37
bulbar dysphagia diet, 96–98
bulimia nervosa, 429–431

C

cachexia, 403
caffeine
    adolescent exercise and, 420
    lactation and, 12
    pregnancy and, 9
calciferol, 38
calcium, 39
    needs, adolescents and, 409–410, 416, 516
    pregnancy and, 7
    vegetarianism and, 43–44
calcium-controlled diets, 253–261
calcium-rich foods, 260–261
calorie intakes
    diabetes and, 148–150
    estimating, 77–78
    recommended, 409–410, 416, 516
calorie-controlled meal plans, 203–216
calorie-rich, protein-rich diets, 327–329
Cambodian food practices, 59–68
cancer, 403–408
carbohydrate, 1
    counting, diabetes and, 174–175, 177–178